Therapeutic Gastrointestinal Endoscopy

Therapeutic Gastrointestinal Endoscopy

Edited by

Stephen E. Silvis, M.D.

Chief, Special Diagnostic Treatment Unit
Veterans Administration Medical Center

Professor of Medicine
University of Minnesota
Minneapolis, Minnesota

IGAKU-SHOIN　　　　　New York • Tokyo

Text and Cover Design by Wanda Lubelska Design
Typesetting by Achorn Graphic Services, Inc. in Palatino
Printing and Binding by Mandarin Offset Inc.

Published and distributed by

IGAKU-SHOIN Ltd.,
5-24-3 Hongo, Bunkyo-ku, Tokyo

IGAKU-SHOIN Medical Publishers, Inc.,
1140 Avenue of the Americas, New York, N.Y. 10036

First edition 1985 by IGAKU-SHOIN Ltd., Tokyo.

Library of Congress Cataloging in Publication Data
Main entry under title:

Therapeutic gastrointestinal endoscopy.
  Includes index.
  1. Endoscope and endoscopy.   2. Gastrointestinal
system—Diseases—Treatment.   I. Silvis, Stephen E.
[DNLM: 1. Endoscopy.   2. Gastrointestinal Diseases—
therapy. WI 100 T3975]
RC804.E6T44   1984   616.3'306'028   84-12843

ISBN: 0-89640-105-7 (New York)
      4-260-14105-8 (Tokyo)

Printed and bound in Hong Kong

10 9 8 7 6 5 4 3 2 1

Contributors

John H. Bowers, M.D.
Associate Clinical Professor of
  Medicine
Adjunct Associate Professor of
  Surgery
University of Utah School of
  Medicine
Salt Lake City, Utah 84132

Patrick G. Brady, M.D., F.A.C.P.
Associate Professor of Medicine
University of South Florida College
  of Medicine
Chief, Section of Digestive Diseases
  and Nutrition
James A. Haley Veteran's Hospital
Tampa, Florida 33612

Richard I. Breuer, M.D.
Associate Professor of Medicine
Northwestern University Medical
  School
Senior Attending Gastroenterology
Evanston Hospital
Evanston, Illinois 60201

Frank Chateau, P.A.
Senior Physician's Assistant
Department of Medicine
Beth Israel Medical Center
Mt. Sinai School of Medicine of the
  City University of New York
New York, New York 10028

Robert M. Craig, M.D.
Associate Professor of Medicine
Northwestern University Medical
  School
Senior Attending, Gastroenterology
Northwestern Memorial Hospital
Chicago, Illinois 60611

David Y. Graham, M.D.
Professor of Medicine
Baylor College of Medicine
Chief, Digestive Diseases Section
Veterans Administration Medical
  Center
Houston, Texas 77211

Dov Z. Grant, M.D.
Assistant Attending in Medicine
Department of Medicine
Beth Israel Medical Center
Mt. Sinai School of Medicine of the
  City University of New York
New York, NY 10028

Rollin W. Hughes, Jr., M.D.
Consultant in Gastroenterology
Mayo Clinic
Rochester, Minnesota 55901

**Bergein P. Overholt, M.D.,
  F.A.C.P.**
Weisgarber Medical Center
Knoxville, Tennessee 37919

John P. Papp, M.D., F.A.C.P., F.A.C.G.
Associate Clinical Professor of Medicine
Michigan State University School of Human Medicine
Director, Endoscopy Unit
Blodgett Memorial Medical Center
Grand Rapids, Michigan 49506

Jeffrey L. Ponsky, M.D.
Director, Department of Surgery
Mt. Sinai Medical Center
Associate Professor of Surgery
Case Western Reserve University School of Medicine
Cleveland, Ohio 44106

Jerome H. Siegel, M.D., F.A.C.P.
Assistant Clinical Professor of Medicine
Mt. Sinai School of Medicine of the City University of New York
New York, New York 10028

Stephen E. Silvis, M.D.
Chief, Special Diagnostic Treatment Unit
Veterans Administration Medical Center
Professor of Medicine
University of Minnesota
Minneapolis, Minnesota 55417

Michael V. Sivak, Jr., M.D.
Head, Section of Gastrointestinal Endoscopy
Department of Gastroenterology
The Cleveland Clinic Foundation
Cleveland, Ohio 44106

Francis J. Tedesco, M.D.
Professor of Medicine
Chief, Gastroenterology
Medical College of Georgia
Augusta, Georgia 30912

Jack A. Vennes, M.D.
Professor of Medicine
University of Minnesota
Staff Physician in Gastroenterology
Veterans Administration Medical Center
Minneapolis, Minnesota 55417

Albert M. Waitman, M.D.
Chief, Medical Endoscopy
Attending in Medicine
Department of Medicine
Beth Israel Medical Center
Assistant Clinical Professor of Medicine
Mt. Sinai School of Medicine of the City University of New York
New York, New York 10028

Preface

This book has been prepared for the use of endoscopists who already have expertise in diagnostic endoscopy and for the use of trainees who are in the latter years of their education. The authors have assumed that readers have an excellent understanding of the techniques used to perform the various diagnostic procedures, the basic principles of endoscopy, patient preparation, indications and contraindications. To perform therapeutic gastrointestinal endoscopy, the physician or surgeon should have an in-depth knowledge of gastrointestinal disease.

Therapeutic Endoscopy has been under discussion for three years. Initially, it was the editor's opinion that the field was moving so rapidly that it would be preferable to wait for further developments before compiling a textbook on this exciting field.

A major portion of the book is devoted to techniques that have been developed in the past decade or that at least came into widespread use during that period. Some of them have been introduced only in the past few years. Two such techniques are newer methods for biliary drainage and endoscopic gastrostomy. A more intermediate group of techniques includes gastric polypectomy and colonic polypectomy, which have revolutionized the management of these problems and have made abdominal surgery unnecessary in the vast majority of patients. Endoscopic sphincterotomy has now been used for a decade. With this therapy, there have been dramatic reductions of morbidity and mortality due to recurrent common duct stones. The field of electrocoagulation for gastrointestinal bleeding and laser therapy for hemorrhage from tumors remains in a developmental stage, but it is progressing rapidly. It is the editor's opinion that this area of endoscopy is the wave of the future, in which accurate diagnosis by endoscopic methods can be followed immediately with a therapeutic maneuver that shortens the time of hospitalization, reduces morbidity and mortality and decreases costs.

Some of the techniques that are described in this book, such as esophageal dilatation for strictures and removal of foreign bodies, are very old; however, over the past decade, even these techniques have been modified radically. Easy endoscopic access to the esophagus has allowed most foreign bodies to be removed by use of flexible endoscopes without anesthesia and with marked reduction of the risk to patients. A much more critical analysis of the instrumentation, techniques, goals and results of esophageal dilatation has been performed during the past few years.

It was the aim of the editor to produce a textbook that would give the personal experience of experts in particular areas, to review the available literature and to compare the various treatment modalities and techniques. It is the editor's opinion that the authors have accomplished these goals to an admirable degree. They have presented their material in a clear, concise manner with enthusiasm tempered by critical evaluation. Obviously, almost all the techniques require further study, both in regard to the details of their performance and in regard to the patient groups in which the techniques are appropriately applied. The editor anticipates that the therapeutic use of endoscopy will evolve with the development of numerous, ingenious techniques for the management of the various gastrointestinal diseases.

I wish to thank all the contributors and Mr. John Gardner of Igaku-Shoin Medical Publishers, Inc., who has guided this project from its inception. Mrs. Judith Sundae, Mrs. Angela Curran, Ms. Valarie Wesley, and Mrs. Sheila Haroldson, my secretaries, have made the entire project possible through all their telephone and stenographic assistance and have my lasting appreciation.

In addition, I wish to thank my wife, Marilyn, to whom I dedicate this book, for her many hours of excellent proofreading, critical advice and support throughout this project.

Stephen E. Silvis, M.D.
Editor

Contents

Therapeutic
Gastrointestinal
Endoscopy

1

Dilatation for the Management of Benign and Malignant Strictures of the Esophagus

David Y. Graham

The function of the esophagus is to transport food from the mouth to the stomach. When the ability to perform this function is disturbed, an affected person complains of dysphagia. Dysphagia, by definition, relates to difficulty associated with the act of swallowing. It is easily distinguished from globus hystericus, an overdiagnosed condition usually present in neurotic, tense persons. A person with globus hystericus complains of a lump in the hypopharynx or behind the sternum and, importantly, finds that swallowing often relieves the symptom.

Dysphagia is a reliable symptom that usually indicates an esophageal disorder. Therefore, elicitation of the symptom of dysphagia should always stimulate a thorough diagnostic evaluation. The complete workup of a patient with dysphagia is beyond the scope of this chapter, but several points deserve emphasis. The history and physical examination yield the correct diagnosis at least 80% of the time. For example, in dysphagia stemming from incoordination of the oropharynx, ingestion of fluids usually is poorly tolerated. If this condition is suspected, the examiner should watch the patient attempt to drink water; it may even reflux from the patient's nose. Most structural lesions in the body of the esophagus compromise the esophageal lumen, and solids are less well tolerated than are liquids. Achalasia is suggested by a long history of dysphagia for liquids and solids. Intermittent dysphagia suggests an esophageal ring, a web or spasm. Unremitting or progressive dysphagia suggests organic narrowing.

The choice of diagnostic procedures for evaluating a patient with dysphagia is quite broad. Spiro has noted that "When it comes to diagnostic studies, however, the physician should have a clear order of priority so that he will not fire the entire blunderbuss down the throat of the unfortunate patient" (1). The evaluation of most patients with dysphagia should include a barium esophagogram and fiberoptic endoscopy. Radiologic examination usually is the first diagnostic procedure to be employed because it illustrates the anatomic structures and in most cases demonstrates organic lesions. A barium swallow is incomplete and should not be regarded as normal unless the examiner has administered a solid bolus (i.e., a 12 mm diameter barium pill or a barium-coated marshmallow). Fluoroscopic examination of the esophagus provides additional benefits: movement of the bolus can be viewed directly, and motility of the esophagus can be evaluated in the supine and upright positions.

If the x-ray studies and an endoscopic examination (including a retroflexed view of the esophagogastric junction) are normal, this author recommends passage of a large (50 French), mercury-filled bougie. This maneuver often results in elimination or reduction of the complaints of dysphagia.

A variety of esophageal lesions have been successfully managed with bougienage. The most common cause of benign stricture is peptic stenosis stemming from gastroesophageal reflux; this cause is followed in frequency by surgical intervention for reflux esophagitis and by corrosive injury. In addition, there are a number of uncommon causes, such as stricture-associated moniliasis and indwelling tubes. Dilatation is potential therapy for esophageal narrowing of any origin, including benign stricture of almost any cause, rings, webs, or cancer. Achalasia and diffuse esophageal spasm may respond to vigorous dilatation with pneumatic dilators (2,3).

The goal of dilatation is to restore the ability to eat and drink normally. Patients vary remarkably in their tolerance to dysphagia, but in most cases dysphagia will not be completely relieved until a minimal luminal diameter equivalent to 38 or 40 French is achieved. The author's goal is to achieve a minimal esophageal diameter of at least 40 French; in most instances, I continue dilatation until a 50 French bougie can be passed.

The sizes of esophageal dilators are expressed in metric units (millimeters) or French units, the latter being based on the circumference of the instrument (diameter in millimeters multiplied by pi). For convenience in converting from millimeters to French units, a factor of 3 (rather than 3.14) times the diameter is often used. This distinction is of no consequence except with large dilators, for which there may be a considerable discrepancy. In this chapter, I will indicate the sizes of French dilators according to both systems (e.g., 15 mm or 45 to 47 French).

TECHNIQUE

When one considers that an esophageal stricture develops over many months or years, it seems prudent not to rush too fast to achieve a normal luminal diameter. At the time of endoscopic examination, the diameter of the stricture can be estimated and compared to the diameter of the endoscope. The diameter of a standard endoscope can be easily ascertained by measuring it or by reading the accompanying literature. Pentax endoscopes are named according to their size; for example, an F34A fiberscope is 34 French diameter. An Olympus Q fiberscope has an external diameter of 11 mm (33 to 35 French).

It is best to start dilatation with a dilator that is one or two sizes smaller than the diameter of the stricture. The first dilator that meets resistance determines the actual diameter of the stricture. With mercury-filled bougies, it is easier to "feel" the dilator actually engaging a stricture (when dilatation is done with the patient in the seated position). I pass no more than one or two sizes larger than the first dilator that meets resistance per dilatation episode.

Esophageal dilatation can be repeated daily, every other day or several times per week, depending on the patient, the severity of the stricture and the sense of resistance that is felt. If a mecury-filled dilator cannot be pushed through a stricture with the thumb and forefinger, it is probably best to change to Eder-Puestow metal olives or balloon dilators. On the second or subsequent dilatation episodes, it is best to begin with a dilator that is one or two sizes smaller than the largest dilator passed at the previous session.

A wide variety of esophageal dilatation devices are available, and new instruments are continually being introduced (4–7), although most fail to gain widespread acceptance. Mercury-filled bougies are the most commonly used dilators. Mercury-filled dilators include those with a rounded (Hurst) or tapered (Maloney) end (Fig. 1), and dilators with an olive tip may be obtained by special order in England (7). Dilators are filled with mercury to achieve the correct balance between flexibility and rigidity, not because the weight is an aid in dilatation. Recently manufactured mercury-filled bougies may be different from older models because the company that made the rubber tube apparently no longer does so. Many newer dilators are too flexible and are not useful. When purchasing new or replacement dilators, it is important to inspect each dilator on receipt. In the author's experience, many have been rejected immediately.

A Maloney dilator, with its tapered end, seems to be easier for patients to swallow than a Hurst dilator. It also may be easier to dilate a small-diameter stricture with a Maloney dilator than with a Hurst device. Although no studies have demonstrated that one type of mercury-filled dilator is safer than another, a Maloney dilator is theoretically safer in that its tapered tip is more likely to enter a stricture. Conversely, however, the tip also is more likely to bend and cause the dilator to be misdirected.

A reasonably well equipped unit should have a set of Maloney or Hurst dilators (preferably both) ranging in size from 34 to 60 French. Smaller sizes usually are too flexible, and small-diameter strictures require directed dilatation. The unit also should have a set of Eder-Puestow metal olives (including the newly available, largest sizes) and a set of balloon dilators ranging in size from 4 to 20 mm.

MERCURY-FILLED BOUGIES

To reduce the risk for aspiration if vomiting occurs, esophageal dilatation should be done in a fasting patient. Esophageal dilatation with mercury-filled

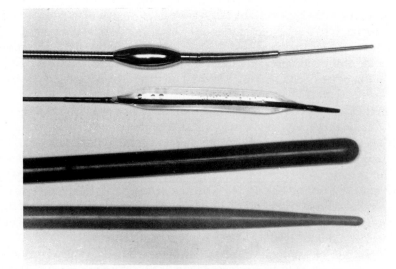

Fig. 1a. A variety of bougies, including an Eder-Puestow dilator, a polyethylene balloon dilator, a Hurst and a Maloney mercury-filled bougie.

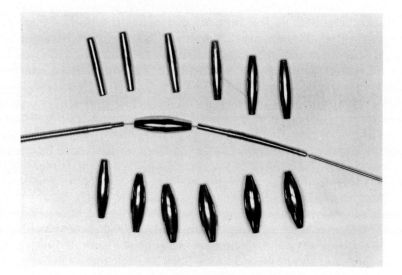

Fig. 1b. A set of Eder-Puestow dilators.

bougies frequently is done in a sitting position. This position is convenient for the patient and the physician; in addition, the weight of the dilator is helpful in traversing the esophagus to the level of the stricture. The risk for aspiration may be further reduced by performing dilatation in the lateral decubitus position. When endoscopic examination immediately precedes esophageal dilatation, the dilatation procedure should be performed in the left lateral decubitus position because there is no reason to have a patient be recumbent for endoscopy and then upright for dilatation, particularly if the patient has been sedated.

Before use, the distal end of the mercury-filled dilator is well lubricated. The bougie is introduced into the mouth and directed into the pharynx with the forefinger. It usually is easily swallowed and is gently passed down the esophagus. Hurst and Maloney dilators can be used safely only by experienced operators. An experienced physician can "feel" when the dilator engages a stricture, and slight withdrawal of the dilator confirms whether engagement has occurred. The dilator is held lightly between the thumb and fingers (which prevents application of excessive force), and the stricture is dilated. Grasping the dilator with the whole hand, as though it were a ski pole, may promote the use of excessive force and has resulted in at least one unusual complication (i.e., a broken nose) (8). In that case, the upper shaft of the dilator had been lubricated, and when the operator's hand slipped, it struck the patient's nose. Unlike a rubber, mercury-filled bougie, the shaft of an Eder-Puestow dilator may be grasped with the hand because more force can be safely applied as the dilator is advanced over a guide wire (Fig. 1b). It is preferable to be hesitant with the dilator rather than to inadvertently perforate the esophagus. Only experienced operators should attempt to continue advancing a dilator when substantial resistance is met.

In adults, the esophagus averages 40 cm in length, measured from the teeth to the stomach. A mark should be placed on the shaft of each dilator (approximately 40 cm from the tip of a Hurst dilator or 45 to 50 cm from the tip of a tapered Maloney dilator) to allow the operator to ascertain the relative positions of the tip of the dilator, the lower esophageal sphincter and the stomach.

METAL OLIVES

Mercury-filled bougies having diameters less than 32 French are too limber to be useful in the dilatation of small-diameter strictures. Such strictures are best dilated with metal olives or balloon dilators. The Eder-Puestow dilator apparatus is designed to be used over a guide wire that can be easily passed through the biopsy channel of an endoscope into the stomach under direct vision. Strictures are best evaluated with small-diameter endoscopes because such endoscopes often can pass through the narrowing and permit examination of the distal extent of the stricture and the stomach beyond. Although the biopsy channel of pediatric instruments is of sufficient diameter to allow passage of a guide wire, the diameter of the proximal orifice of the biopsy channel may be less than that of the guide wire. This problem can be overcome by replacing the valve piece with one that has a larger internal diameter (e.g.,

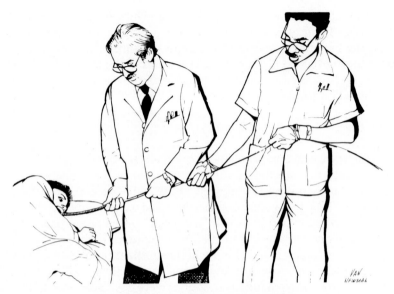

Fig. 2. The technique of esophageal dilatation performed with an Eder-Puestow
dilator passed over a guide wire, em-
phasizing the role of the assistant in
managing the guide wire.

exchange the valve of an Olympus P endoscope with one from an Olympus D,
Q or K instrument).

Although the guide wire often is placed under direct vision through the
fiberscope, fluoroscopy can be used to observe the wire and confirm that it has
passed through the strictures. In this way, endoscopy becomes unnecessary
and the expense that it would have entailed can be used instead for follow-up
dilatations. Several investigators (9) have employed electrosurgery to increase
the luminal diameter so that a spring-tipped guide wire can be introduced. This
technique makes use of a diathermy snare or a sphincterotome, and three or
four small cuts are made around the circumference of the stricture. This approach has been associated with a high complication rate and probably is
outmoded now that small balloon dilators are available.

Esophageal dilatation with metal olives is a two-person procedure (Fig. 2).
One person has responsibility for the wire. He or she must keep it taut so that
the dilator can be safely advanced over the wire to ensure that the dilator and
wire do not move forward as a unit; if the two components move forward
together, the purpose of the guide wire is defeated (it must stay in a relatively
constant position). That person also is responsible for the distal (outside) tip of
the wire, which is sharp and which may flail about, causing injury to the
endoscopist, the assistant or the patient. The operator has the simpler job of
pushing the dilator.

Because they can now be obtained with shafts of the same length as those of
the Eder-Puestow dilators, balloon dilators may some day replace metal olives.

I predict that balloon dilators will ultimately largely replace Eder-Puestow metal olives as well as mercury-filled bougies.

BALLOONS

The use of small balloons to dilate esophageal strictures is a relatively new technique, and its true place in our armamentarium is not yet known (see section on achalasia for forceful dilatation in that disorder). The older technique of esophageal dilatation with mercury-filled dilators or Eder-Puestow olives is well established and known to be effective. It is always difficult for a new technique to gain widespread acceptance if the old technique is effective. Initially, balloons designed for dilatation of blood vessels (10) were used to dilate very narrow strictures so that an Eder-Puestow guide wire could be passed and traditional dilatation begun. Balloon dilators with wider diameters (4 to 20 mm) have only recently become commercially available, and their ultimate usefulness is not yet established (11–13). Balloon dilators have several theoretical advantages, the most important being that applied force is directed only radially. In addition, balloons are effective for the management of complex strictures and those with luminal diameters less than that of a spring-tipped guide wire.

Balloon dilatation can be accomplished under direct vision if a balloon dilator is passed through the biopsy channel of an endoscope. A 6- or 8-mm balloon catheter passes through the 2.8-mm channel of an Olympus endoscope; a 12-mm balloon catheter (36 to 37 French) passes through the 3.5-mm channel of a Pentax fiberscope. Alternatively, the balloon catheter can be passed over a highly torquable guide wire (1.5 mm diameter) that has been directed through the stricture under endoscopic or fluoroscopic guidance. The spring-tipped guide wire that is sold with a balloon catheter usually can be inserted through even the most complex strictures. It is particularly useful for dilating obstructing esophageal carcinoma (see below). An Eder-Puestow guide wire is too short to accommodate some balloon catheters, but, if needed, a balloon catheter can be loaded onto an Eder-Puestow guide wire before passage and its insertion monitored by fluoroscopic guidance. It is best to have a number of balloon catheters of various lengths (i.e., those long enough to go through an endoscope and those short enough to be passed over a guide wire).

A syringe is used to inflate a balloon dilator. The balloon can be inflated with air, water or contrast material, and the pressure that is generated can be monitored with a manometer or pressure gauge (Fig. 3). I prefer using water-soluble contrast material, diluted 1:3 with saline, coupled with a pressure gauge to ensure that the pressure is maintained below the level that would rupture the low-compliance balloon. A sudden fall in pressure signifies that the stricture has dilated. If fluoroscopic guidance is used, the stricture and its response can be observed directly. With this technique, the stricture is apparent as a narrowing or waist in the balloon (Fig. 4a). The balloon is partially filled with contrast material and moved back and forth within the stricture to position the waist in approximately the middle of the balloon. Additional pressure is then applied; this pressure is associated with effacement of the waist, indicating dilatation of

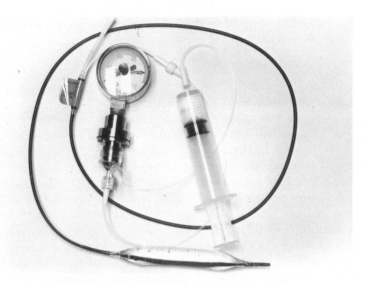

Fig. 3. A balloon dilator and pressure gauge.

the stricture (Fig. 4b). A series of progressively larger balloons can be used to achieve complete dilatation; the largest balloon currently available is 20 mm (60 to 61 French). Alternative techniques permit direct visualization of the procedure; the balloon may be passed through the biopsy channel of an endoscope or over a guide wire beside the endoscope. Whichever route is chosen, passage of the balloon is facilitated by use of the guide wire. When fluoroscopic guidance is not used, the operator can judge the effect of treatment by observing a fall in pressure on the pressure gauge (which may be difficult to see) and, more importantly, by being able to slide the distended catheter easily back and forth within the previously strictured area.

Balloon dilatation of benign strictures also can be performed without fluoroscopic or endoscopic guidance. The guide wire may be placed by means of the endoscope; the endoscope is then withdrawn, leaving the guide wire in place. The balloon is inserted, inflated in the proximal segment of the esophagus and advanced until the stricture is encountered. The balloon is then deflated, advanced 2 to 4 cm, reinflated and deflated again. Advancements in 2- to 4-cm increments are repeated until the inflated balloon can be drawn back and forth within the area of the stricture without difficulty.

The author prefers the method he calls Blind Retrograde Balloon Dilatation. For this approach, (i) an Eder-Puestow spring-tipped guide wire is placed into the stomach with the use of the endoscope; (ii) the distance from the incisor teeth to the stricture is measured, (iii) the shaft of the dilator is marked to identify the distance from the incisors to the point where the middle of the balloon is positioned in the stricture; (iv) a deflated balloon is advanced into the stomach over the guide wire; (v) the balloon is inflated and withdrawn to the obstruction; (vi) the balloon is then partially deflated and withdrawn 2-4 cm

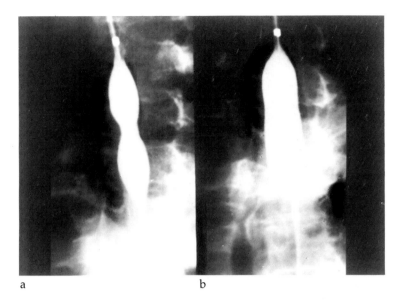

Fig. 4. A contrast-filled balloon dilator is seen in an esophageal stricture, with the stricture appearing (a) as a waist in the balloon and (b) after successful dilatation (courtesy of Microvasive, Inc.).

so as to be positioned in the stricture; (vii) the balloon is alternately inflated, deflated, withdrawn an additional 2-4 cm and reinflated, (viii) finally, the balloon is deflated, pushed back into the stomach, reinflated and used to calibrate the stricture by pulling the inflated balloon through the previously strictured area without difficulty. Patient discomfort is used as a guide as to the final diameter of dilatation for a dilatation episode. Currently, I attempt to achieve an esophageal diameter of 15 mm (45 French) at the initial dilatation episode (see below).

There usually is little or no blood on the balloon after removal, and endoscopic evaluation of the esophagus immediately after dilatation usually reveals minimal changes in the appearance of the mucosa compared to before dilatation. Dilatation with a balloon is well tolerated by patients and can be done with only local pharyngeal anesthesia. This approach permits patient discomfort to guide the number of dilatations attempted during a session. If a patient feels discomfort, the procedure is stopped and rescheduled for another day. Until we have data to the contrary, it is prudent to dilate only two or three French sizes per session.

OTHER TYPES OF DILATORS

An endoscope can be used as a dilator under certain circumstances. If the diameter of a stricture is only slightly less than that of the endoscope, an attempt can be made to push the endoscope through to dilate the stricture. This approach is particularly appropriate for mucosal webs and rings. It should be emphasized that endoscopes are not designed to be used as dilators and that severe damage to fiber bundles may occur if excessive force is applied. This method is not recommended, and, at best, gentle force exerted with the thumb and forefinger is all that should be applied, taking care to maintain the esophageal lumen within the center of the field. If this approach fails to permit passage, another type of dilator must be used.

Dilators whose diameters increase in stepwise fashion have been introduced (5,6). Examples are separate dilators, the Celestin stepped dilator (6) and a dilator used as an overtube on an endoscope. The major postulated advantage of these devices is to allow progressive dilatations during a single session. It is unlikely that they will prove safer or superior to traditional dilators, and I doubt that they will be widely used.

DEFINITION OF SUCCESSFUL TREATMENT

One of the main problems encountered in attempting to define success of dilatation is the lack of a consensus on what constitutes relief of dysphagia. The best results usually are reported with small series of patients with short and incomplete follow-up. The author and his colleagues (14) define a good response to dilatation as either freedom from dysphagia or infrequent dysphagia that does not warrant further dilatation. An unsatisfactory response is defined as inability to relieve dysphagia with periodic dilatation. British surgeons (7) have recently agreed to use the following grading system: 0, normal; 1, occasional difficulty swallowing solids; 2, unable to swallow solid food; 3, unable to swallow minced food; 4, unable to swallow pureed or liquid food; 5, unable to swallow liquids or saliva. Luna (9) has suggested use of the following three-level grading scale: (i) good, able to eat a normal diet without dysphagia—no further dilatation needed; (ii) moderate, rare or slight dysphagia with solid foods—occasional dilatations needed; (iii) bad, inability to achieve a caliber of 50 French and persistent dysphagia even with semisolid food—frequent dilatations needed. Several other grading systems have been proposed. A standard system is needed, but it seems that symptoms, not luminal size, should be the primary consideration.

COMPLICATIONS

Physicians seldom encounter problems with the equipment used for esophageal dilatation, but the equipment should be inspected carefully before each

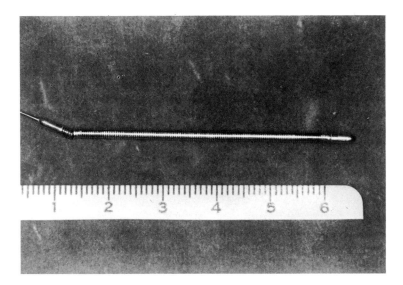

Fig. 5. The tip of an Eder-Puestow wire has been broken, and the wire must be replaced.

use, nevertheless. For example, cracks may appear in the rubber of mercury-filled bougies, or the spring-tip of a guide wire may become bent, necessitating replacement (Fig. 5) (15).

Esophageal dilatation is safest when performed under fluoroscopic guidance. This general rule holds for dilatation with balloons, Eder-Puestow olives and mercury bougies. Fluoroscopic guidance often is not possible, or practical, because many endoscopy units do not have fluoroscopy capabilities. The author uses fluoroscopic guidance routinely only in the management of complicated strictures and in instances when placement of the guide wire is uncertain. Examples of esophageal abnormalities that necessitate fluoroscopic intervention are carcinoma and long strictures.

It is important to attempt to identify all factors that might increase the risk for dilatation before starting the procedure (16). The first, and most obvious, risk factor is an anatomic abnormality that precludes safe, unguided dilatation (i.e., epiphrenic diverticulum). Figure 6 illustrates a number of abnormalities that might occur in the lower portion of the esophagus, each of which would increase the risk for perforation if a dilator is introduced without endoscopic or fluoroscopic guidance.

The most common site of esophageal perforation is the area immediately proximal to a stricture. It is unknown whether perforation is caused by the tip of the instrument or by the side of the instrument when the shaft is bowed because of undue pressure. The risk for perforation (per procedure) is low, being on the order of four to six perforations per 1000 dilatations (8,16,17). In 764 dilatations performed by the author and his colleagues, there have been five perforations (14); one resulted from use of excessive force to pass a flexible

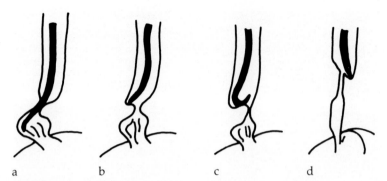

a   b   c   d

Fig. 6. Complications that may occur with a mercury-filled dilator, including (a) impaction of the tip of the dilator in a hiatal hernia sac distal to the stricture, preventing insertion of a Maloney dilator to its full diameter, (b) impaction of the tip of the dilator in an eccentric ulcer or a diverticulum proximal to a stricture, (c) retroflexion of the tip of the dilator without passage through a stricture and (d) impaction of the tip of the dilator on a shelf proximal to a malignant stricture. Adapted from Tulman and Boyce (16), with permission.

endoscope through a stricture, while four were caused by Hurst dilators. Interestingly enough the dilators involved in the perforation incidents had diameters greater than 38 French; in three cases, wider-diameter dilators had been passed safely on earlier occasions. Esophageal perforation with wide-diameter dilators may relate to their increased stiffness or to the fact that with such dilators, there is an increased radial (tearing) force for a given insertion force (18). The rate of perforations reported in various series may reflect the accuracy and completeness of the records that are maintained, as well as whether the experience is that of trainees or practicing gastroenterologists or surgeons.

Esophageal perforation has occurred when dilatation immediately followed a suction biopsy of the esophagus, a procedure that provides a relatively deep specimen (19). Barkin and associates (20) have reported that there was no increase in morbidity when dilatation followed forceps biopsy. Unfortunately, that conclusion may not be valid because of the small number of patients examined; a change in perforation rate from four per 1000 to 12 per 1000 (300% increase) would not have been detected. Newer endoscopes have large biopsy channels, and it is now possible for endoscopists to use a large (jumbo) biopsy forceps, yielding a biopsy more closely resembling that obtained by the suction technique. We have no logical denominator to use to assess the actual risk associated with dilatation after deep biopsy. Because there is no compelling reason to perform biopsy and dilatation during the same session, the author believes that it is prudent to delay one or the other procedure unless the biopsy is of a large exophytic lesion.

Because perforation is the main complication of dilatation, it is critically important that perforation be identified as soon as is possible; delayed diagnosis is associated with increases in morbidity and mortality. Cervical perforation usually is obvious and is associated with fever, chest pain, leukocytosis, pain on swallowing, change in quality of voice and air in the subcutaneous tissues of the neck. Radiographic examination usually reveals air in the retroesophageal space. The most common symptom of esophageal perforation is persistent pain after dilatation, even mild pain. When perforation is suspected, it is important to obtain upright and lateral x-ray films of the chest to serve as a baseline and to search for free air under the diaphragm, pneumothorax or pleural effusion. Pleural fluid often has an elevated amylase concentration because of leakage of salivary amylase from the esophagus. A contrast esophagogram is then performed. The author uses barium because it provides the best definition of the mucosa and tears that may have occurred (21,22). Radiologists may prefer a "first look" with water-soluble contrast material, but if the results are negative, the test should be repeated with barium.

Many times, suspected or actual esophageal perforation can be managed conservatively (nonsurgically) with antibiotics and nasogastric suction or suction placed at the site of perforation. In the author's opinion, this approach usually is inappropriate and is based, in part, on the concept that to employ surgical therapy is to admit defeat. I believe that dilatation and surgical management of benign esophageal strictures (or achalasia) are alternative forms of therapy that achieve the same end. A suspected or proven perforation prompts me to switch immediately to the alternative therapy. It has been shown that surgical therapy can be performed immediately after perforation with minimal or no increase in morbidity or mortality. If surgical intervention is delayed until it is obviously necessary, morbidity and mortality are greatly increased. With benign esophageal stricture, surgeons often extend the defect and repair the stricture with a Thal procedure. In the case of achalasia, surgeons may close the defect caused by the dilator and perform a Heller myotomy (23,24). There also may be an incomplete perforation, in the form of an intraesophageal hematoma (25), that may rupture after some time.

When the position of the guide wire can be controlled with fluoroscopic guidance, the tip should extend 4 to 6 inches beyond the lower sphincter. A greater length of guide wire usually is inserted when endoscopic guidance is used to monitor its placement, to provide a margin of safety to ensure that the guide wire remains in the stomach throughout the dilatation procedure. If a considerable length of the guide wire is in the stomach, the dilator may strike it at an angle and cause it to become kinked (Fig. 7). Withdrawal of the wire then results in the formation of a loop that might cause esophageal perforation (Fig. 8) (15,26). Formation of a loop can be prevented by withdrawing the guide wire flush with the end of the dilator and removing the dilator and the guide wire together. Kinks in the guide wire can be straightened easily; if not, the guide wire must be replaced.

Bleeding rarely complicates esophageal dilatation for the management of benign lesions. When bleeding occurs, it usually is minor and transfusions are rarely needed. Bacteremia has developed after esophageal dilatation, but it is a serious problem only in immunocompromised patients (27,28). The bacteria in the blood may originate from the dilator or the oropharynx. It is important to clean the dilator adequately after each use to prevent the instruments from being a potential source of infection. The author recommends vigorous scrub-

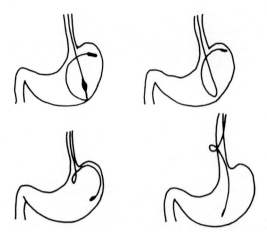

Fig. 7. The sequence of events that leads to esophageal perforation when a guide wire forms a loop. This complication can be prevented by withdrawing the guide wire into the shaft and removing the two instruments as a unit. Adapted from Sanderson and Trotter (15), with permission.

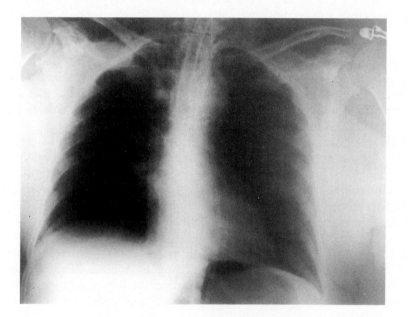

Fig. 8. X-ray film of the chest demonstrates a loop in the guide wire perforating the esophagus. Reprinted from *British Journal of Surgery* 67:300–301, 1980 (15), with permission.

bing with a germicidal solution, followed by air drying; more rigorous sterilization is probably unnecessary.

DISEASES REQUIRING ESOPHAGEAL DILATATION

DIVERTICULA, RINGS AND WEBS

Esophageal diverticula may be associated with motor abnormalities of the esophagus and represent a hazard to patients only when inexperienced endoscopists encounter them or when esophageal dilatation is performed blindly. Esophageal stenosis may be caused by mucosal abnormalities, such as rings or webs. Rings and webs usually cause intermittent dysphagia, with the difficulty occurring only when an affected person swallows a piece of food that has a diameter equal to or greater than the diameter of the opening. The etiologic basis of webs is unknown. Two areas of ringlike mucosal abnormalities have received sufficient attention to deserve names. The proximal mucosal web, a feature of Plummer-Vinson syndrome (also called Patterson-Kelly syndrome), is associated with iron deficiency anemia (sideropenic dysphagia). The upper esophageal web usually is a thin, filmy mucosal web located below the upper sphincter. Treatment consists of administration of iron (for the anemia) and esophageal dilatation. Usually, passage of an endoscope breaks such webs; to ensure that the web is seen, the endoscope must be introduced carefully into the upper portion of the esophagus. Patients with a history of an upper esophageal web have an increased risk for esophageal carcinoma.

The most common ring in the distal portion of the esophagus is Schatzki's ring, which is a thin (less than 4 mm thick) mucosal ring in the lower segment of the esophagus that usually proves to be the squamocolumnar (esophagogastric) junction (Fig. 9) (29). The diagnosis can be made on the basis of radiographic or endoscopic examination, and the treatment of choice, if the ring causes symptoms, is dilatation. As with the proximal web, Schatzki's ring usually can be ruptured with an endoscope without difficulty. Alternatively, a single pass with a 50 to 60 French, mercury-filled dilator usually suffices. To confirm or make the diagnosis on the basis of endoscopic findings, it is necessary to examine the distal esophagus with care when the lumen is well distended with air.

In some instances, particularly with Schatzki's ring, the diameter of the opening is narrow (2 to 4 mm) and the ring is quite firm (Figs. 10 and 11). It is difficult to believe that such a small-diameter opening is a congenital abnormality; many patients have long histories of symptomatic gastroesophageal reflux (29,30). Some endoscopists consider such rings to be short peptic strictures. Whatever the pathogenesis, rings with very narrow intraluminal diameters should be managed by an approach similar to that used for benign esophageal strictures (i.e., bougienage over a wire or balloon dilator, followed by progres-

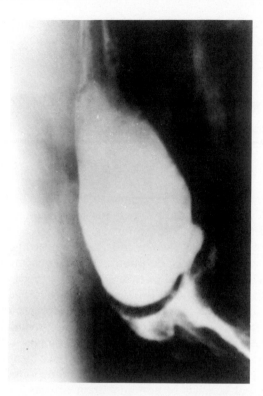

Fig. 9. A radiograph shows a Schatzki's ring with a luminal diameter of approximately 3 mm.

sively larger mercury-filled dilators). It has been reported that pneumatic dilatation, with dilators designed for the management of achalasia, has been needed for relief in some patients (29); the author has not encountered such a patient.

CORROSIVE INJURY

Lye or strong alkaline agents contained in dishwasher detergents, household cleaners and ammonia are the most common causes of chemical injury to the esophagus. Such agents usually are ingested accidentally by children or during suicide attempts by adults. Strong acids are components of drain cleaners. Acids are much less damaging to the esophagus than are alkaline agents because alkali dissolves squamous epithelium and fat.

After ingestion of a corrosive agent, the usual presenting complaints are severe pain in the mouth and chest, followed by pain on swallowing or inability to swallow. Depending on the degree of damage, signs of esophageal perforation may appear. It should be noted that the degree of damage to the mouth does not correlate with the degree of damage to the esophagus. Although the absence of pharyngeal burns makes a diagnosis of ingestion unlikely, ingestion

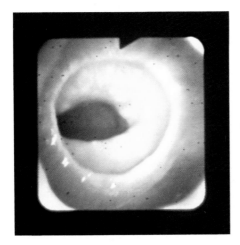

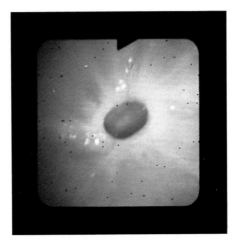

Fig. 10. A Schatzki's ring as normally seen through an endoscope.

Fig. 11. A very narrowed Schatzki's ring with a luminal diameter of approximately 3 to 4 mm.

should be considered as a possibility until it has been ruled out, and an attempt should be made to determine the extent of injury.

The form of treatment that is administered depends on the hospital service that accepts responsibility for the patient (ear, nose and throat, thoracic surgery, general surgery, medicine). Esophagoscopy usually is performed within the first 24 hours to delineate the extent of esophageal injury. If there is a deep burn or circumferential injury, esophagoscopy is immediately terminated. With serious injury, broad-spectrum antibiotics are administered parenterally (often in combination with methylprednisolone) immediately after the diagnosis of esophageal burn has been confirmed. Many centers require patients to swallow a weighted string to act as a guide for subsequent bougienage. After 3 or 4 days, a patient's symptoms usually regress and liquids and solids can be taken by mouth. After about 1 week, corticosteroid therapy is discontinued and a barium esophagogram is performed. Esophagoscopic examination also can be repeated at this time. If a stricture is discovered, bougienage is begun. Long, firm caustic strictures often are the hardest to dilate, and because of that fact, they may have the highest complication rate. Psychiatric care should be obtained for patients who have attempted suicide. Patients suffering lye damage to the esophagus have an increased risk for esophageal cancer.

DIFFERENTIATION BETWEEN BENIGN AND MALIGNANT STRICTURES

The history, the barium contrast radiographic study and the endoscopic view help distinguish benign from malignant strictures of the esophagus. The most common presentation of a patient with benign or malignant esophageal stenosis is dysphagia. Patients with benign peptic strictures usually have a history of a slowly progressive dysphagia, often superimposed on a long history of symptoms of gastroesophageal reflux. Radiographic studies demonstrate short, smoothly tapered strictures in most such patients. By contrast, patients with malignant strictures usually relate a recent onset of symptoms. Radiographic examination in such patients reveals mucosal destruction and evidence of intraluminal tumor mass. Endoscopic studies readily identify a mass in most such patients, and the endoscopist's opinion is that of "cancer."

In every instance, it behooves gastroenteroscopists to ensure that a seemingly benign esophageal stricture is truly benign; confirmation of the benign nature of a stricture can be accomplished only by taking a biopsy sample, collecting specimens by means of aspiration or brush for cytologic examination or by both measures. The remaining esophageal lumen may be so narrow that it is difficult to obtain adequate biopsy specimens. In such instances, the biopsy should be repeated after the stricture has been dilated successfully. Other techniques that can be used to obtain adequate specimens include aspiration with a biopsy needle and removal of material from within the stricture for cytologic examination.

BENIGN STRICTURE

The natural course of peptic esophageal stricture appears to be variable; there have even been reports of resolution of such strictures (31). The author and his colleagues have studied the natural course of esophageal stricture in 154 patients in whom bougienage was used as primary therapy. Dilatation was considered successful with respect to major or total relief of dysphagia in 84.5% of 103 patients who had been followed up for 6 months or longer (median follow-up period was 26 months) (Table 1) (14). Life table analysis showed that approximately one-third of the patients required no dilatation during a projected 4-year follow-up period (Fig. 12). The patients seemed to fall into two groups: in one group, the natural course was to improve or become asymptomatic after the initial series of dilatations; a few patients in this group eventually had recurrent symptoms. In the second group (which contained slightly fewer than

TABLE 1. Results of Treatment of 103 Patients Followed for 6 Months or Longer After Successful Dilatation

Dysphagia	Number	Percentage
None	52	50.5
Very mild or intermittent, not requiring dilatation	12	11.5
Requiring continued dilatation with benefit	23	22.5
Present, but refused further treatment	3	3.0
Surgical intervention not requiring further dilatation	9	8.5
Surgical intervention, requiring continued dilatation	4	4.0

Reprinted from *Gastroenterology* 85:346–350, 1983 (14), with permission.

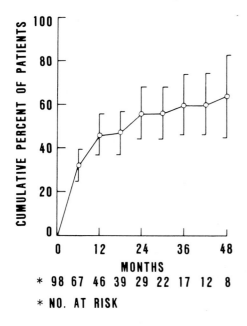

Fig. 12. Life table plot of the interval until redilatation for 98 patients with initial dilatation to 40 French or greater. Reprinted from *Gastroenterology* 85:346–350, 1983 (14), with permission.

one-half of the patients), further dilatations were required for the management of dysphagia during the first year of the follow-up period. Although two-thirds of these patients needed regular dilatation in subsequent years, the median frequency of dilatation for the total group was less than once per year. Our experience is consistent with our previous report of a different group of 92 patients (32) and with the collective results of 10 series (14). Overall, one can expect between an 80% and a 90% success rate. Repeat dilatation is rarely a problem and can be handled simply. An important observation is that we were unable to identify any factor, such as initial severity of the stricture, cause of the stricture, presence or absence of active esophagitis or initial caliber of dilatation, that could serve to predict the need for subsequent dilatation. Surgical intervention may be necessary for recalcitrant stricture or for the management of other severe symptoms of reflux.

Esophageal stricture may be associated with peptic ulcer. In our experience, 23% of the patients with peptic stricture have had documented peptic ulcer disease in the stomach or duodenum.

TUMORS

The primary therapy for benign esophageal stricture is esophageal dilatation. (5,14,32–36). With malignant stricture, however, the primary therapy is management of the malignant disease (radiation therapy or surgical intervention); esophageal dilatation or surgical or endoscopic bypass of the obstruction (prosthetic device insertion) is used strictly as a palliative measure.

The etiologic basis of carcinoma of the esophagus remains unknown; in clinical practice, the development of esophageal cancer is related to the use of alcohol and cigarettes and to chronic esophageal irritation. Carcinoma of the esophagus usually occurs in persons over the age of 50, with men being affected more often than women. Dysphagia, usually progressive, is the most common symptom. Other signs and symptoms associated with spread of the primary tumor include pain, bronchopulmonary symptoms (tracheoesophageal fistula) and hoarseness. Weight loss is a common occurrence, whereas serious bleeding is a rare manifestation. Many patients delay seeking medical attention; of those who do present early, a delay in diagnosis often occurs as a result of the physician's failure to order appropriate studies. A question concerning dysphagia should always be included in the review of systems. Squamous cell carcinoma predominates; adenocarcinoma usually represents either spread of carcinoma from the fundus of the stomach or the spontaneous development of a tumor from Barrett's epithelium.

The form of management that is used depends on the location of the tumor and its size and on the extent of spread. Surgical intervention is used to manage tumors located in the distal or middle one-third of the esophagus, whereas radiation therapy is most often reserved for tumors in the proximal one-third of the esophagus. In general, the results of the two treatment modalities are similar, with 5-year survival rates of less than 5%. Chemotherapy is currently ineffective. Most patients present with advanced and inoperable disease. Therapy for palliation of esophageal obstruction consists of bougienage or the placement of stents to maintain the patency of the esophageal lumen.

In most cases, the primary therapy for squamous cell carcinoma is high-voltage radiation therapy. This treatment modality is effective and in most instances eradicates the primary tumor. Unfortunately, because of the advanced state of most squamous cell carcinomas at the time of diagnosis, this therapy is palliative, and few patients survive 5 years. The goal of palliative therapy for esophageal carcinoma is to allow the patient to eat and drink normally; radiation therapy is effective in achieving this goal, even when the esophagus is completely obstructed. From 25% to 50% of patients who undergo radiation therapy subsequently have esophageal strictures, usually within 6 months of therapy. Fortunately, however, the strictures are easily managed with dilatation and usually do not recur. In developed and Western countries, the primary therapy should be radiation therapy or surgical intervention (other forms of therapy should be reserved for specific problems in management).

A variety of endoscopically applied palliative therapies are available; examples are thermal techniques accomplished with electrocautery or laser energy to remove a tumor mass (37). Cryotherapy also has been used in a similar manner. The two most widely accepted palliative therapies for carcinoma of the esophagus are dilatation and placement of an esophageal prosthesis (37–41). Esophageal dilatation with mercury-filled bougies, metal olives or balloon dilators can be performed before, during or after radiation therapy. At the time of presentation, most patients can swallow liquids and, if they are unable to eat solid food, a nutritious liquid diet can be prescribed until the carcinoma has responded to radiation therapy. The author's policy has been to reserve dilatation for patients with difficulty swallowing secretions or liquid meals. Recently,

Hunt and associates (42), in a preliminary communication, suggested that early dilatation (during radiation therapy) may help prevent weight loss, promote weight gain or have both effects. Whether early dilatation has an effect on patient well-being or survival is unknown and requires additional study.

Esophageal dilatation may be performed safely throughout the period of radiation therapy. In some areas of the world, insertion of an esophageal prosthesis is considered the primary therapy for carcinoma of the esophagus. By contrast, the author believes that the primary indications for insertion of a prosthesis are (i) esophagorespiratory fistula, (ii) dysphagia that necessitates frequent dilatation despite radiation therapy, especially if the tumor recurs after successful radiation therapy, as occurs in approximately 15% of patients with cancer (43), or (iii) adenocarcinoma of the esophagus. It is the author's working hypothesis that if the esophagus can be dilated, a prosthesis is not required; if it cannot be dilated, insertion of a prosthesis is impossible.

The technique of endoscopy-assisted insertion of an esophageal prosthesis is relatively straightforward. First, the lumen encroached upon by the tumor must be dilated so that the prosthesis will fit through the tumor. The luminal diameter required depends on the prosthesis; the requirement is greatest for the Atkinson prosthesis, with its rather firm distal flange.

A variety of prostheses are available (Fig. 13). The most commonly used are the Celestin tube (latex rubber), the Atkinson prosthesis (silicone rubber), the Procter-Livingstone tube (latex rubber) and polyvinyl chloride tubes (formed, as needed, from laboratory tubing) (39,41). The proximal end of the prosthesis is widened into a funnel, whereas the distal end may be cut off flush (e.g., commercial tubes) or at an angle (e.g., "homemade" polyvinyl chloride tubes).

Some investigators perform esophageal dilatation and insert a prosthesis during one session. The author prefers a more conservative approach and recommends that esophageal dilatation be performed slowly over several days to a week; this conservative approach may help reduce the frequency of esophageal perforation.

At the time of insertion of a prosthesis, a dilator is passed that has a diameter equal to or greater than the diameter of the prosthesis. Esophagoscopy is then performed, and the distance from the teeth to the proximal and distal margins of the tumor is measured so that a prosthesis of the correct length can be chosen. It is best to use a prosthesis that extends 3 to 5 cm below the inferior margin of the tumor. There are a variety of techniques for inserting a prosthesis into a tumor. Each technique possesses the following three characteristics: ability to direct a prosthesis accurately into the channel, use of a device (pusher) to push the prosthesis into place and some means to remove or reposition the prosthesis.

A common approach is to insert a prosthesis over a Maloney or Hurst bougie and to rely on a string or umbilical tape to recover the prosthesis (41). A gum rubber introducer with an inflatable end frequently is used with a Celestin tube, and a Nottingham introducer often is used with an Atkinson prosthesis (Fig. 14). The Nottingham introducer, designed specifically for insertion of prostheses (44), is basically a flexible metal rod that is introduced over a spring-tipped guide wire. The distal end contains a segment that expands to grip the

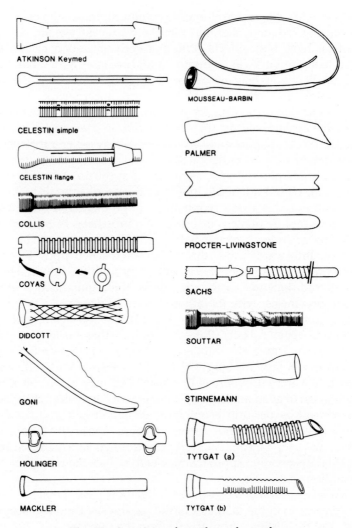

Fig. 13. A variety of esophageal prostheses. Reprinted from *British Journal of Surgery* 69:61–68, 1982 (39), with permission.

prosthesis firmly and thus allows it to be positioned, repositioned or removed without difficulty.

The author prefers to insert a prosthesis by using a small-diameter (pediatric) endoscope as a guide (Fig. 15). After measurements are taken, the prosthesis and the pusher, a piece of inside-braided Tygon tubing (Fisher catalog no. 14-169-20c), are mounted on a well-lubricated endoscope. The distance from the distal end of the prosthesis to the proximal margin of the tumor is marked on the pusher, as is the distance from the funnel of the prosthesis to the proximal margin of the tumor. The prosthesis, pusher and endoscope are well lu-

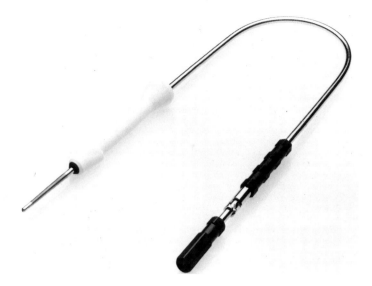

Fig. 14. A silicone-rubber Atkinson esophageal prosthesis mounted on a Nottingham introducer (courtesy of KeyMed).

bricated, and the endoscope is inserted normally. The prosthesis is advanced into position over the endoscope; the endoscope is withdrawn through the prosthesis to check the position and any necessary adjustments are then made (Fig. 16). The prosthesis can be removed after being grasped with a rat-toothed forceps (Olympus catalog no. FG9U). In this procedure, the Pentax 34F is fitted with a pusher overtube, the edge of the prosthesis is grasped with the forceps and pulled onto the overtube and the overtube, endoscope and prosthesis are then removed as a unit.

The true mortality associated with insertion of prostheses is unknown. Although Atkinson and colleagues (45) have reported a 10% procedure-related mortality, prostheses can be inserted safely in selected patients, as evidenced by the fact that Palmer (46) inserted 75 consecutive prostheses without a fatality. By contrast, recent reports have noted higher mortalities (e.g., 9%, 16% and 30% as 7-, 14- and 30-day mortalities, respectively) (47). Insertion of a prosthesis clearly is neither an antitumor therapy nor a substitute for radiation therapy. Whether insertion of a prosthesis is safer or more effective than dilatation is unknown, but most patients do not require either form of treatment. Clinical trials with well-defined subgroups are needed to address this question. The routine use of esophageal dilatation or insertion of prostheses in patients with carcinoma of the esophagus is not recommended.

If the prosthesis must remain in place for many months, one made of silicone rubber is preferred. Silicone rubber is nearly inert, whereas latex rubber may dissolve and expose the nylon coil used to strengthen Celestin prostheses (48,49). By contrast, the plasticizer contained in polyvinyl chloride tube prostheses is slowly leached out, and such tubes gradually lose their normal pliabil-

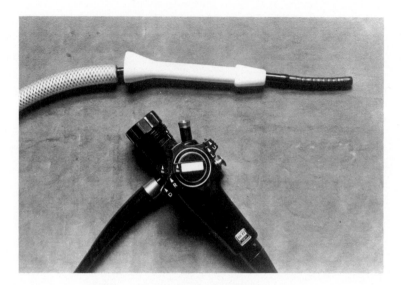

Fig. 15. An Atkinson esophageal prosthesis and a pusher tube are seen mounted on a pediatric endoscope before insertion.

ity and become quite firm. It is prudent, therefore, to inspect latex rubber or polyvinyl chloride tube prostheses at least bimonthly and to replace them after 4 to 6 months. Considering the natural course of the underlying tumor, this precaution is not needed frequently.

Proximal displacement of a prosthesis is not a serious problem. Atkinson and Celestin tubes are manufactured with distal collars; Uhlich and Gietzen (50) recently recommended adding a collar to "homemade" polyvinyl chloride tube prostheses. Proximal displacement is more of a problem, however, if the prosthesis crosses the esophagogastric junction. In that instance, longer prostheses with collars are recommended.

Prostheses have a relatively narrow internal diameter and, because of this aspect, the most common complication is blockage with food. Patients should be cautioned to chew food well before swallowing. If blockage occurs, a nasogastric tube may be used to push the material through. Alternatively, one might attempt administering proteolytic enzymes or carbonated beverages or using a small-diameter endoscope to clean out the lumen.

ACHALASIA

Gastroenterologists are often called upon to differentiate achalasia from other causes of dysphagia. Achalasia is a disorder of esophageal motility characterized by failure of lower esophageal sphincter relaxation and of the normally progressive peristalsis of the smooth muscle in the body of the esophagus. This double failure impedes the flow of liquids and solids from the esophagus into

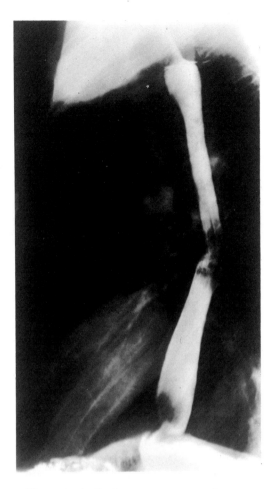

Fig. 16. A barium-contrast esophago-gram shows a Celestin esophageal prosthesis bridging a tracheoesophageal fistula.

the stomach. The pressure of the lower sphincter usually is quite elevated, and the esophagus may dilate greatly, even to the point of becoming a fluid-filled, sigmoid-shaped mass easily seen on a routine x-ray film of the chest. The etiologic basis of achalasia is unknown; in South America, Chagas' disease may cause similar findings.

Achalasia usually is easily diagnosed in patients with a long history of dysphagia associated with characteristic radiographic and manometric appearances (3). Manometry confirms that the upper esophageal sphincter is normal. The body of the esophagus frequently shows an elevated baseline pressure (which returns to normal when the esophagus is emptied) with no apparent peristaltic contraction waves; simultaneous, low-amplitude contractions usually are recorded. The lower sphincter shows an elevated resting pressure

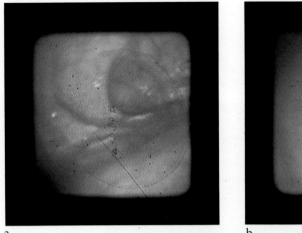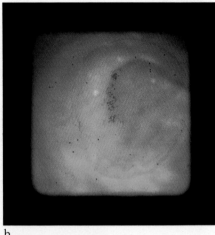

a   b

Fig. 17. Achalasia where the body of the esophagus is widely dilated and partially filled with fluid (a). The esophagogastric junction is seen at a sharp angle to the left (b).

(usually above 40 mm Hg), with incomplete relaxation after a swallow. Although endoscopic examination is rarely needed to establish the diagnosis, it is particularly helpful for ruling out coexisting carcinoma of the esophagus or gastric fundus, which may simulate achalasia.

Dysphagia with liquids and solids is the most common presenting complaint. It is possible to elicit a history of regurgitation of food that is unchanged (not "soured" by gastric juice) as well as pulmonary symptoms secondary to overflow of esophageal contents and chronic aspiration. An x-ray film of the chest may suggest the diagnosis by demonstrating a dilated esophagus with an air/fluid level in the midthorax or the absence of a gastric air bubble. Barium studies reveal esophageal dilatation of a variable degree with a distal segment tapered in the shape of a cone (beak deformity). In addition, barium remains in the esophagus for an extended time, even in the upright posture; the height of the barium column is a rough measure of the hydrostatic pressure needed to overcome the lower esophageal sphincter.

Endoscopic studies usually demonstrate esophageal dilatation and residual food particles and fluid (Fig. 17a). The emptied esophagus is seen to narrow to a cone-shaped structure, ending in a rosette that in its sigmoid segment may be displaced laterally (Fig. 17b). When an esophagoscope enters the sphincter, the sphincter relaxes and allows the endoscope to pass through without resistance. Resistance to passage of an endoscope (or of a large-diameter dilator) should raise a strong suspicion of cancer.

Pneumatic dilatation carries a greater risk for perforation than does standard dilatation (3,16). Many different balloon dilators are available; most systems use a balloon whose diameter is determined and fixed by a silk or nylon cover.

Vantrappen and Hellemans (3) have had much experience with dilatation for the management of achalasia; they use a Sippy dilator manufactured from a nylon bag and two condoms. The low-compliance polyethylene balloons previously discussed in reference to dilatation for the management of benign and malignant esophageal strictures are just now becoming available in sizes useful for patients with achalasia and in the author's experience are very easy to use.

The aim of therapy is to weaken the lower esophageal sphincter. Medical therapy consists of forceful (pneumatic) dilatation and yields "cures" in 80% to 85% of cases. Surgical therapy consists of cutting the lower sphincter (Heller myotomy). There is still considerable debate as to whether medical or surgical therapy is the treatment of choice. Most gastroenterologists believe that forceful dilatation of the esophagus should be the primary therapy for achalasia, with surgical intervention being reserved for patients in whom achalasia persists after several unsuccessful attempts at pneumatic dilatation, for patients in whom carcinoma cannot be excluded and for children and psychotic patients who are uncooperative for the dilatation procedure. Some investigators consider a widely dilated sigmoid esophagus to be a relative contraindication to pneumatic dilatation; the author disagrees. I believe that medical therapy should be tried at least twice before surgical intervention is contemplated because medical therapy is effective in most cases, because lower-sphincter pressure remains 10 to 15 mm Hg above intragastric pressure, which reduces the frequency of post-treatment gastroesophageal reflux and resultant stricture formation, and because if dilatation fails or a complication is experienced, surgical therapy is still available. Heller myotomy yields an 80% to 85% "cure" rate and about a 30% incidence of esophageal reflux. To prevent reflux, the Heller procedure is sometimes modified to include an antireflux procedure.

Almost all patients describe some relief from dysphagia after therapy, even after ineffective therapy, such as passage of a Maloney dilator. Thus, symptoms are not a reliable indicator of the effectiveness of therapy, and the results of medical and surgical therapy should be evaluated on the basis of manometric measurements, relief of symptoms and studies of esophageal emptying (barium swallow or radioisotope scintigraphy). Ineffective therapy may allow the disease to continue with additional dilatation of the esophagus.

Use of Pneumatic Dilators

Many types of balloon dilators have been used for pneumatic dilatation in the management of achalasia, and balloons are available that have diameters on inflation that range from 3 to 5 cm. It is best to start with the 3 cm diameter balloon and to increase in 0.25-cm increments as needed. The 5-cm (150 to 157 French) balloon should rarely be needed. The actual dilatation procedure is simple. The patient should be fasting to ensure that an operation can be performed immediately if esophageal perforation occurs. The procedure is done under local anesthesia with atropine and meperidine given preoperatively; diazepam may be administered at the time of the procedure, if desired. The esophagus is first emptied of liquids. A large-diameter dilator is passed (i.e., a 50 to 60 French, mercury-filled bougie) and, if any resistance is met, the diagnosis is questioned and dilatation is stopped. A pneumatic dilator should always be introduced over a guide wire, and the procedure should be performed under fluoroscopic guidance. The first goal is to ensure that the balloon is placed in the correct position across the lower sphincter. The balloon is inflated under fluoroscopic guidance, and inflation is maintained for 1 minute. There often is blood on the surface of the balloon on removal, but this blood is of no consequence. Some investigators (51,52) immediately follow dilatation with a radiographic contrast study to assess the adequacy of dilatation and for early recognition of perforation, which occurs in 1% to 5% of cases. If perforation occurs or is strongly suspected, Heller myotomy can be performed with little or no increase in risk (24).

In summary, malignant and benign esophageal obstructions usually are responsive to dilatation. Thus, medical therapy is the initial therapy of choice (not all surgeons have yet acquiesced). The introduction of the balloon dilating systems may ultimately alter our standard practice of using Eder-Puestow metal olives and mercury-filled bougies.

REFERENCES

1. Spiro HM: *Clinical Gastroenterology,* ed 2. New York, Macmillan, 1977, pp 17–18.
2. Ebert EC, Ouyang A, Wright SH, et al: Pneumatic dilatation in patients with symptomatic diffuse esophageal spasm and lower esophageal sphincter dysfunction. *Dig Dis Sci* 28:481–485, 1983.
3. Vantrappen G, Hellemans J: Treatment of achalasia and related disorders. *Gastroenterology* 79:144–154, 1980.
4. Ciaglia P, Entwhistle J: Esophageal dilator: Improved screw type. *N Y State J Med* 79:25–26, 1979.
5. Buess G, Thon J, Hutterer F: A multiple-diameter bougie fitted over a small-caliber fiberscope. *Endoscopy* 15:53–54, 1983.
6. Cotton PB, Williams CB: Therapeutic upper gastrointestinal endoscopy, in Cotton PB, Williams CB (eds): *Practical Gastrointestinal Endoscopy,* ed 2. Oxford, Blackwell, 1982, p 51.
7. Earlam R, Cunha-Melo JR: Benign oesophageal strictures: Historical and technical aspects of dilation. *Br J Surg* 68:829–836, 1981.
8. Palmer ED: Broken nose in the endoscopy clinic. *Gastrointest Endosc* 17:69, 1970.
9. Luna LL: Endoscopic therapy of benign esophageal stricture. *Endoscopy* 15:203–206, 1983.
10. London RL, Trotman BW, DiMarino AF Jr, et al: Dilatation of severe esophageal strictures by an inflatable balloon catheter. *Gastroenterology* 80:173–175, 1981.
11. Owman T, Lunderquist A: Balloon catheter dilation of esophageal strictures—A preliminary report. *Gastrointest Radiol* 7:301–305, 1982.
12. Merrell N, McCray RS: Balloon catheter dilation of a severe esophageal stricture. *Gastrointest Endosc* 28:254–255, 1982.

13. Cohen R, Gray S, Hersh T: Balloon dilation of benign and malignant esophageal strictures—A new technique. *Gastrointest Endosc* 29:181, 1983.

14. Patterson DJ, Graham DY, Smith JL, et al: Natural history of benign esophageal stricture treated by dilatation. *Gastroenterology* 85:346–350, 1983.

15. Sanderson CJ, Trotter GA: Eder-Puestow oesophageal dilatation: A new hazard. *Br J Surg* 67:300–301, 1980.

16. Tulman AB, Boyce HW Jr: Complications of esophageal dilation and guidelines for their prevention. *Gastrointest Endosc* 27:229–234, 1981.

17. Silvis SE, Nebel O, Rogers G, et al: Endoscopic complications. Results of the 1974 American Society for Gastrointestinal Endoscopy survey. *J Am Med Ass* 235:928–930, 1976.

18. Kozarek RA, Phelps JE, Partyka EK, et al: Intraluminal pressures generated during esophageal bougienage. *Gastroenterology* 81:833–837, 1981.

19. Jones JD, Bozymski EM: Instrumental esophageal perforation. *Dig Dis Sci* 24:319–320, 1979.

20. Barkin JS, Taub S, Rogers AI: The safety of combined endoscopy, biopsy, and dilation in esophageal strictures. *Am J Gastroenterol* 76:23–26, 1981.

21. Seltzer SE, Jones B, McLaughlin GC: Proper choice of contrast agents in emergency gastrointestinal radiology. *CRC Crit Rev Diagn Imaging* 12:79–99, 1979.

22. Vassal K, Montali RJ, Larson SM, et al: Evaluation of barium and Gastrografin as contrast media for the diagnosis of esophageal ruptures or perforations. *Am J Roentgenol Radium Ther Nucl Med* 123:307–319, 1975.

23. Slater G, Sicular AA: Esophageal perforations after forceful dilatation in achalasia. *Ann Surg* 195:186–188, 1982.

24. McKinnon WMP, Ochsner JL: Immediate closure and Heller procedure after Mosher bag rupture of the esophagus. *Am J Surg* 127:115–117, 1974.

25. Bradley JL, Haw SY: Intramural hematoma (incomplete perforation) of the esophagus associated with esophageal dilatation. *Radiology* 130:59–62, 1979.

26. Bancewicz J: A hazard of the Eder-Puestow system of oesophageal dilation. *Br J Surg* 66:66, 1979.

27. Raines DR, Bronche WC, Anderson DL, et al: The occurrence of bacteremia after esophageal dilation. *Gastrointest Endosc* 22:86–87, 1975.

28. Golladay ES, Tepas JJ, Pichard LR, et al: Bacteremia after esophageal dilation: A clinical and experimental study. *Ann Thorac Surg* 30:19–23, 1980.

29. Arvanitakis C: Lower esophageal ring: Endoscopic and therapeutic aspects. *Gastrointest Endosc* 24:17–18, 1977.

30. Postlethwait RW, Sealy WC: Experiences with the treatment of patients with lower esophageal webs. *Ann Surg* 165:786–796, 1976.

31. Palmer ED: The hiatal hernia-esophagitis stricture complex; twenty year prospective study. *Am J Med* 44:566–579, 1968.

32. Lanza FL, Graham DY: Bougienage is effective therapy for most benign esophageal strictures. *J Am Med Ass* 240:844–847, 1978.

33. Benedict EB: Peptic stenosis of the esophagus; a study of 233 patients treated with bougienage, surgery, or both. *Am J Dig Dis* 11:761–770, 1966.

34. Olsen HW, Lawrence WA, Bottarini G, et al: The fiberoptic approach to dilation of stenotic lesions of the esophagus. *Gastrointest Endosc* 23:201–202, 1977.

35. Cadranel S, Rodesch P, Peeters JP, et al: Fiber-endoscopic monitored dilation of oesophageal strictures in children. *Endoscopy* 9:127–130, 1977.

36. Huchzemeyer H, Freise J, Becker H: Dilation of benign esophageal strictures by peroral fiberendoscopic bougienage. *Endoscopy* 9:207–210, 1977.

37. Fleisher D, Kessler F: Endoscopic Nd:YAG laser therapy for carcinoma of the esophagus: A new form of palliative treatment. *Gastroenterology* 85:600–605, 1983.

38. Graham DY, Dobbs SM, Zulber M: What is the role of prosthesis insertion in esophageal carcinoma? *Gastrointest Endosc* 29:1–5, 1983.

39. Earlam R, Cunha-Melo JR: Malignant oesophageal strictures: A review of techniques for palliative intubation. *Br J Surg* 69:61–68, 1982.

40. Boyce WH: Peroral prosthesis for palliating malignant esophageal and gastric obstruction. *Gastroenterology* 77:1141–1153, 1979.

41. Peura DA, Heit HA, Johnson LF, et al: Esophageal prosthesis in cancer. *Am J Dig Dis* 23:796–800, 1978.

42. Hunt LB, Shirazi SS, Tewfik, et al: The role of esophageal dilation in treatment of esophageal carcinoma. *Gastrointest Endosc* 29:167, 1983.

43. Cassidy DE, Nord HJ, Boyce WH Jr: Management of malignant esophageal strictures. *Am J Gastroenterol* 76:173, 1981.

44. Atkinson M, Ferguson R, Parker GC: Tube introducer and modified Celestin tube for use in palliative intubation of oesophagogastric neoplasms at fibreoptic endoscopy. *Gut* 19:669–671, 1978.

45. Atkinson M, Ferguson R, Ogilvie AL: Management of malignant dysphagia by intubation at endoscopy. *J R Soc Med* 72:894–897, 1979.

46. Palmer ED: Peroral prosthesis for the management of incurable esophageal carcinoma. *Am J Gastroenterol* 59:487–498, 1973.

47. den Hartog Jager FCA, Bartelsman JFWM, Tytgat GNJ: Palliative treatment of obstructing esophagogastric malignancy by endoscopic positioning of a plastic prosthesis. *Gastroenterology* 77:1008–1014, 1979.

48. Mackenzie I, Whyte AS, Tankel HI: Structural deterioration in Celestin tubes. *Br J Surg* 63:851–852, 1976.

49. Branicki FJ, Ogilvie AL, Willis MR, et al: Structural deterioration of prosthetic oesophageal tubes: An in vitro comparison of latex rubber and silicone rubber tubes. *Br J Surg* 68:861–864, 1981.

50. Uhlich GA, Gietzen TH: The prevention of esophageal tube migration. *Gastrointest Endosc* 29:227–229, 1983.

51. Stewart ET, Miller WN, Hogan WJ, et al: Desirability of roentgen esophageal examination immediately after pneumatic dilation for achalasia. *Radiology* 130:589–591, 1979.

52. Cohen NN: An end point for pneumatic dilation of achalasia. *Gastrointest Endosc* 22:29, 1975.

2

Sclerotherapy for Esophageal Varices

Michael V. Sivak, Jr.

VARICEAL HEMORRHAGE: A PERSPECTIVE

Variceal hemorrhage presents a difficult problem. Although much is known about the causes of portal hypertension and the development of esophageal collateral channels, virtually nothing is known of the precise factors that initiate hemorrhage.

Many patients never bleed from varices. Although Graham and Smith (1) found that the serum level of albumin tended to predict death from liver failure and that death due to hemorrhage tended to be associated with massive ascites, there are in general no reliable clinical indications of forthcoming hemorrhage. Attempts have been made to relate variceal hemorrhage to portal pressure. Wedged hepatic vein studies have not been helpful in defining patients at high risk for bleeding, although elevation of pressure undoubtedly must occur before portal hypertension and a potential for hemorrhage can be said to exist (2–4). Reports indicate that there is a relationship between the length and diameter of varices and the likelihood of bleeding (5–7). Other investigators (8) suggest that certain features in the endoscopic appearance of varices can be used to predict hemorrhage.

These observations have not been used as selection criteria for a trial of any form of therapy. Thus, prophylactic therapy against variceal hemorrhage is inherently indiscriminate, and where such therapy has been attempted (e.g., the prophylactic portosystemic shunt), the results have been unsatisfactory (9–11).

Thus, therapy for variceal hemorrhage is obliged to be after the fact, imposing the foremost difficulty in evaluating any existing or proposed trial of therapy, namely, the timing of intervention in relation to the natural course of variceal bleeding. Mortality resulting from this event in patients with advanced cirrhosis is 42% at 6 weeks from onset (1). Approximately three-fourths of the deaths occur in the first week, and almost two-thirds are due to hemorrhage. After 6 weeks, death is due equally to bleeding, hepatic failure and other causes. Further, the survival curve after 6 weeks approximates that for patients with similar liver disease who have not had any bleeding. Smith and Graham (12) demonstrated that varying the time of entry of patients into a study will in itself change the survival curve. If therapy is delayed, survival from the point of treatment appears to improve, irrespective of other variables, because an appreciable number of patients, presumably the poor-risk patients, have died. Thus, many studies of various methods of treatment pertain to selected patient populations, a fact that is sometimes not obvious.

Because, in most instances, therapy is initiated in response to, and not in anticipation of, bleeding and because mortality and cause of death vary considerably before and after 6 weeks from the onset, management must be divided into immediate and long-term measures. The immediate concern is to stop the bleeding. Ideally, acute therapy would also prevent recurrent bleeding and would have a low complication rate. The three goals of long-term therapy are to prevent further hemorrhage, to influence survival favorably and to do both with a minimum of complications and side effects. It has been impossible thus far to attain all these goals by a single approach. For example, a favorable reduction of hemorrhage may entail an unacceptable decrease in survival or an increase in frequency and severity of side effects.

The interrelationships of survival, reduction of hemorrhage, complications and side effects also are influenced by the severity of the underlying liver disease. Most patients with variceal hemorrhage have an underlying, chronic, fatal disease. Liver disease, which further compounds the difficulty of evaluating the efficacy of any form of management, is the single most important determinant of overall survival. Severity of liver disease does not, however, predict the manner of death.

Finally, the difficulties in assessing the results of therapy are compounded as new approaches and methods are introduced. New approaches must not only be considered in relation to the natural course of variceal hemorrhage but must also be compared one to another.

MANAGEMENT OF ESOPHAGEAL VARICEAL HEMORRHAGE

Endoscopy is the only practical way to establish that hemorrhage is variceal in origin. An appreciable number of patients with upper gastrointestinal hemorrhage who are known to have varices are actually bleeding from another source. Certainty exists only if hemorrhage from a varix is actually observed. But, by nature, this type of bleeding is intermittent. More often, varices are found to be the only potential source of established blood loss when bleeding has stopped. This finding usually is acceptable evidence.

Methods for immediate control of hemorrhage include balloon tamponade, intravenous vasopressin, emergency portosystemic shunt surgery and sclerotherapy. There are other potentially useful methods, including laser photocoagulation and electrocoagulation, but these techniques have not been studied extensively and will not be considered here. Percutaneous transhepatic obliteration of varices has been used in some centers, and although there was initial enthusiasm, it appears that this technique will be abandoned. Portal vein thrombosis developed in about one-third of the patients, more than one-half resumed bleeding, and it is not possible to repeat the procedure (13,14).

Intravenous vasopressin controls bleeding at least initially in 50% to 75% of instances. It decreases flow in the superior mesenteric artery and portal vein by approximately 40% and reduces portal pressure by about 25%. It also lowers cardiac output and raises blood pressure and must be used with care when cardiac ischemia may not be well tolerated. Newer agents may enhance effectiveness and decrease the frequency and severity of some of the side effects of this class of drugs (15).

Balloon tamponade with the Sengstaken-Blakemore tube and its variations has been available for many years. Because of the variety of potential complications and because it is more difficult to use than intravenous vasopressin, it is generally performed after or in addition to administration of vasopressin, often as a lifesaving measure to stop severe bleeding. Early retrospective studies emphasized that the complication rate and mortality were excessive (16,17). However, more recent trials have demonstrated that tamponade is not only effective in about 90% of cases but that it also is reasonably free of serious complications (18,19). However, it requires monitoring by personnel who are familiar with the device and who have knowledge of its limitations, particularly that it can be considered only a temporary measure. The major problem, then, becomes resumption of hemorrhage with its removal. Almost two-thirds of patients in one series resumed bleeding after tamponade was discontinued, this sequence of events being associated with high mortality (20).

Emergency portacaval shunt surgery is considered by Orloff and colleagues (21) to be an option in the management of acute variceal bleeding. Of 180 unselected patients operated on between 1963 and 1978, the operative survival was 58%, 1-year survival was 45% and 5-year (actuarial) survival was 38%. Two percent of the patients resumed bleeding during the follow-up period, and about two-thirds had encephalopathy, which was said to be severe in only 7% of patients. It is difficult to evaluate these results. Although bleeding is obviously controlled, survival does not appear to be substantially greater than that for the natural course of variceal hemorrhage. Probably only a minority of patients now undergo emergency portacaval shunt procedures, indicating that this approach is generally considered to be an unattractive option.

Until the resurgence of sclerotherapy, the only method for long-term control of hemorrhage had been surgery (22,23). Conn (24), in a review of these early studies, encountered serious problems with interpretation of the data. A study by Reuff and associates (25) revealed a decrease in bleeding coupled with an increase in the frequency of encephalopathy, as well as a slight decrease in survival that was not statistically significant. The most recent report of a trial by

Reynolds and coworkers (26) demonstrated complete control of hemorrhage in patients with shunts, although moderate to severe encephalopathy developed in 37% of such patients. A small increase in survival was demonstrated. In summary, such procedures appear to control bleeding at some cost in terms of side effects, with at best a small survival advantage. Patients were to some degree selected in each of these trials.

Various modifications of the portosystemic shunt have been developed to circumvent the problem of encephalopathy. Warren and colleagues (27) have reported their experience with the distal splenorenal shunt. Operative mortality was about 4%, with good long-term patency of the shunt and excellent prevention of hemorrhage. Encephalopathy occurred in only 12% of patients. This procedure is not suitable for all patients, and large experiences have not been reported by other groups. There are no reports of controlled trials.

Other operations, chiefly devascularization and/or transection procedures, are available (28). Devascularization of the proximal one-half of the stomach and/or mobilization of the distal portion of the esophagus may be technically more difficult after than before sclerotherapy. Some devascularization procedures are extremely complicated and prolonged; the Sugiura operation involves transabdominal devascularization of the proximal one-half of the stomach, splenectomy, transthoracic devascularization of the distal portion of the esophagus, vagotomy, esophageal transection and pyloromyotomy (29). Excellent results are reported, although confirmatory series have not been published. The stapling gun has been used to transect and reanastomose the esophagus to interrupt variceal flow. When this approach is used alone, it is associated with high complication and rebleeding rates (30). It can be combined with devascularization, although this procedure is more complicated. Johnston (31) reported late follow-up bleeding in only 6% of patients undergoing this combined procedure. Sixty-nine percent of the patients were still alive at 3-year follow-up, and esophageal strictures developed in 16% of the patients. He advised the operation for less than ideal shunt candidates, who might be suitable for a lesser procedure. Experience with these new procedures is limited, and many questions remain regarding them. It is therefore difficult at present to fit them into a general scheme of management of variceal bleeding. These questions also are not germane to the treatment of patients who are not eligible for any operative procedure.

Drug therapy may attain a place in the long-term prevention of recurrent variceal hemorrhage. Lebrec and associates (32) reported a trial with propranolol and found that repeat hemorrhage occurred in 50% of a placebo group as compared to only 4% of a treated group of good-risk patients. These findings have not yet been confirmed in other trials. Potential problems with this approach include diminished cardiovascular response should hemorrhage recur and enhancement of salt retention and ascites (33). The drug cannot be used for the management of acute hemorrhage. Because propranolol has not received approval for this purpose from the U.S. Food and Drug Administration and because the data are not yet corroborated by other trials, this drug cannot be recommended for prophylaxis of esophageal hemorrhage at the present time, except in controlled trials. There also are no data as yet to support its use in conjunction with sclerotherapy.

INDICATIONS FOR SCLEROTHERAPY

Several factors should be considered in assigning sclerotherapy a role in the management of variceal hemorrhage: the timing of the procedure, whether it should be done in response to acute hemorrhage, even perhaps as an initial measure, whether it should be reserved for long-term prophylaxis after hemorrhage ceases or has been stopped by other means, whether it is suitable for all patients across the spectrum of poor to good liver function and whether it would achieve the best results if it were combined with other procedures in either short-term or long-term management.

Sclerotherapy for control of acute variceal bleeding has been reported by a number of investigators (34–38). Several investigators used the rigid endoscope, and all of them employed balloon tamponade initially to control bleeding, with the exception of Lewis and coworkers (37). Although the latter authors did not discuss tamponade in advance of the procedure, they fixed a balloon in the cardia during sclerotherapy to stem or decrease loss of blood so that injections could be undertaken.

Sclerotherapy is extremely difficult when there is ongoing hemorrhage, chiefly because the field must be cleared of blood. The presence of blood is a serious problem when a fiberscope is used because most instruments do not have adequate suction capability. Although one may seek to avoid this situation, variceal bleeding may resume at any time, especially during the early period after onset. Often, a clot is found protruding from a varix. The clot often gives way during the first sclerotherapy procedure. Hemorrhage also may be precipitated by the needle puncture. Therefore, difficulty of performing sclerotherapy in such circumstances cannot always be avoided. Fleig and associates (39) reported on 25 patients in whom massive hemorrhage persisted despite tamponade. None of the patients received vasopressin. Immediate control of bleeding by sclerotherapy was achieved by employing a rigid endoscope and general anesthesia in 92% of the patients. Bleeding resumed in 17.4% of them, and the complication rate was 12%. Sixty percent of the patients survived, an impressive figure considering their poor condition. It is clearly possible to stop severe spurting-type bleeding from an esophageal varix with a twin suction channel fiberscope, but this method is difficult. It requires some modification of technique and may entail an increase in the complication rate.

All things considered, sclerotherapy should not be used as the first procedure for acute hemorrhage, if possible. Intravenous vasopressin and balloon tamponade are adequate and relatively safe measures, provided their limitations as temporary expedients are recognized. Because recurrent bleeding carries a high mortality, sclerotherapy is first indicated in the emergent period after bleeding has been stopped or slowed with vasopressin and/or tamponade. In general, this period lasts 4 to 6 hours, during which time the patient can be hemodynamically stabilized, and proper preparations for the procedure can be made. It should be noted that a somewhat opposite view is supported by data from Barsoum and colleagues (40), who found that emergency sclerotherapy was more effective for short-term control of bleeding than was tamponade.

Most authors recommend that endoscopic sclerotherapy be continued during the follow-up period in an effort to prevent recurrent hemorrhage. Although the outcome for repeat sclerotherapy procedures in relation to the natural course of variceal hemorrhage has been studied, there are no reports that compare sclerotherapy to portosystemic shunt procedures. However, surgical intervention is not an option for many patients. Sclerotherapy can be considered for such patients, especially in view of the fact that there are data to support a favorable response with respect to transfusion requirements.

In summary, sclerotherapy is indicated in the emergent, but not necessarily in the acute management of the majority of patients. It has been shown to be of benefit in long-term management after hemorrhage. For selected, good-risk patients, surgical therapy also may be an option, especially a selective shunt procedure. Sclerotherapy has not been compared to such procedures. In cases in which surgical intervention cannot be considered because of poor liver function, prior operation or technical reasons, long-term sclerotherapy is indicated. Even though there is a report of prophylactic sclerotherapy that has demonstrated a good result in patients without prior hemorrhage, not enough data are available to recommend this technique for general usage (41).

TECHNIQUE OF SCLEROTHERAPY

The difficulties entailed in evaluating this rediscovered procedure are exacerbated by extreme variability in methodology. It is not known whether better results and fewer complications are achieved with one method as compared to another. The variables include choice of endoscope, sclerosing agent or agents, schedule of procedures, placement of injections intravariceally as opposed to paravariceally, pattern of injections in the esophagus, injection volume and the use of various methods of compression. Unfortunately, nearly every aspect of the various described techniques is empiric.

Sugawa and coworkers (42) demonstrated that thrombosis, perivenous fibrosis and thickening of the intima of the veins could be produced in an animal model by injection of 5% sodium morrhuate. Repeated intravariceal injections were made an average of three times per animal, and endoscopic follow-up was performed at weekly intervals. They noted that ulcers developed frequently at injection sites but that the ulcers healed in about 3 weeks.

The development of an ulcer appeared to depend, at least to some degree, on the volume of sclerosant injected.

Another investigation in animals by Jensen and associates (43) compared the efficacy of sclerotherapy, ferromagnetic tamponade, argon and Nd:YAG laser treatment, monopolar electrocoagulation and a heater probe for control of variceal hemorrhage. The Nd:YAG laser treatment and sclerotherapy were more reliable to a significant degree in controlling bleeding, whereas all other methods were effective 50% or less of the time. Injections were made intravariceally. The investigators tried to reinduce bleeding by balloon inflation proximal to the bleeding point (induced before treatment by puncture with a 19-gauge needle). Hemorrhage resumed after every method of treatment, except sclerotherapy and Nd:YAG laser photocoagulation. The laser treatment was easier to apply than was sclerotherapy, but ulceration occurred more frequently and the varices were not obliterated.

The advantages of a rigid endoscope for sclerotherapy have been stressed by some authors, many of whom have reported on large series of patients (34, 44–46). A rigid instrument provides excellent suction capability, and larger-caliber endoscopes can be used for variceal compression. These endoscopes are sometimes modified by placing a slot at their distal end. The varix to be injected protrudes into the slot to facilitate injection. The injection site also is compressed as the instrument is rotated to the next injection site and, theoretically, this compression retards the disappearance of the sclerosing agent from the area. General anesthesia often is used with rigid endoscopy. The danger of aspiration, especially during acute hemorrhage, is eliminated by endotracheal anesthesia. General anesthesia also lessens some of the technical difficulties of sclerotherapy and frees the endoscopist to concentrate on the injection procedure. However, general anesthesia poses an added risk for many patients, particularly those with acute hemorrhage and poor liver function. The incidence of esophageal perforation might be expected to be higher in series in which a rigid endoscope was used. But this is not the case, as reported in several large series (34,44–46). However, expertise in rigid endoscopy is declining, except in certain specialties. It also is difficult to extrapolate the work of investigators who are highly skilled in rigid endoscopy to a general experience with the procedure. In surveys of members of the American Society for Gastrointestinal Endoscopy who perform sclerotherapy, less than 1% of those responding used a rigid endoscope (47). Where experience is lacking, the complication rate will be high. Reilly and colleagues (48) related their experience with 20 patients in whom a rigid endoscope was used initially. They later changed exclusively to a fiberoptic instrument because of problems and complications with the rigid endoscope, including difficulty with insertion, fractured teeth, pressure necrosis of the upper portion of the esophagus, inability to inject gastric varices and problems relating to general anesthesia. It is therefore likely that most sclerotherapists will use some type of fiberoptic instrument. There is no established disadvantage to doing so, although sclerotherapy for active acute hemorrhage is technically more difficult. There are no controlled trials to indicate that use of one type of instrument produces better results or is safer than another.

Before considering the question of variceal compression during sclerotherapy, it will be helpful to outline the general features of variceal anatomy. The esophageal venous system has three components: intrinsic veins, associated veins and extrinsic veins (49). A subepithelial plexus in the lamina propria and a submucosal plexus deep to the muscularis comprise the intrinsic component. These structures are interconnected, and they anastomose with the pharyngeal-laryngeal venous plexus proximally and with the subglandular plexus of the stomach distally. The connection between the intrinsic venous plexus of the esophagus and the subglandular plexus of the stomach appears to be rudimentary or may not exist in many or even most persons. This observation may explain why extensive gastric varices are not frequently associated with esophageal varices and why gastric varices may be large under certain circumstances in the absence of correspondingly large esophageal varices. The plexuses of the intrinsic component anastomose at frequent intervals along the length of the esophagus with the extrinsic veins via perforating veins. The latter usually have valves that direct flow away from the lumen. The associated veins are made up of two longitudinal vessels on the external aspect of the esophagus that anastomose with the bronchial veins proximally and with the left gastric vein distally. These veins need not be considered for practical purposes. The extrinsic veins are interconnected proximally to the thyroidal and peritracheal venous plexuses, the anterior deep cervical veins and a variety of other veins. In the midsection of the esophagus, the extrinsic veins empty into the azygous system. Distally, the extrinsic system connects with the left gastric vein. On the basis of this anatomic structure, with its many interconnections with other systems, any substance injected into the intrinsic esophageal veins may, theoretically, reach many vital sites in the body, including the heart, lungs, brain and spinal cord. Therefore, the action of any sclerosant must be considered from local and systemic points of view. The former has been studied to a much greater extent than has the latter.

A theoretical advantage with a rigid endoscope is the ability to use the instrument to compress the veins. A number of instruments and maneuvers have been designed for use in conjunction with fiberscopes in an effort to retain this presumed advantage. Examples are a balloon attached to the endoscope, an overtube sheath, a balloon fixed to the cardia during injections and a Sengstaken-Blakemore tube placed at completion of the injections.

Water-soluble radiographic contrast agents have been combined with a sclerosant in a few studies to assess movement of the material during and after injections. The validity of these studies rests on the assumption that such agents do not appreciably alter the behavior of the sclerosant. In a small number of patients studied with this methodology, Grobe and associates (50) demonstrated local accumulation at the injection site in about one-third of punctures, rapid clearance in a cephalad direction via the azygous system in about one-half of patients and passage into the gastric subglandular variceal plexus in 15% of punctures. This pattern was seen with and without proximal compression by means of a balloon attached to the endoscope. Rapid clearance to the extrinsic veins also was found in a similar study by Barsoum and coworkers (51), who believed that the local accumulation of contrast material was due to extravasation around the vessel, even though intravariceal injections were intended. They also found no caudally directed flow into gastric varices, even though a rigid endoscope was used, which would, theoretically, provide proximal compression. Silvis and colleagues (52) demonstrated in an animal model that compression resulted in retention of the active agent at the puncture site. However, the collateral venous circulation of the abdominal wall was used, which may not be analogous to the esophageal variceal circulation. The results of these studies suggest that the sclerosant is rapidly cleared from the injection site, and therefore institution of tamponade does not enhance effectiveness. This impression was confirmed when sclerotherapy without follow-up tamponade (25 patients) was compared with sclerotherapy with subsequent tamponade (25 patients) in a study by Barsoum and coworkers (40).

The use of a flexible overtube or sheath in conjunction with a fiberscope, as introduced by Clark and associates (53) and Williams and Dawson (54), is another approach for achieving compression. This device, which fits over the insertion tube of a flexible endoscope, has a window at its distal end through which successive varices can be injected as the tube is rotated. This method was compared to that of freehand injections in a study by Westaby and colleagues (55). Twenty-one patients were treated with the overtube method, and 19 patients were treated with injection alone. With the former method, there was significantly less bleeding in the first 24 hours after sclerotherapy, but this method was associated with a substantial increase in postinjection pain and esophageal stricture. The frequency of recurrence of bleeding was the same for both groups, although this was less severe with the sheath method, as evidenced by the fact that none of 11 such episodes was fatal as compared to five fatal hemorrhages among 15 such episodes in the freehand injection group. There was a trend toward earlier obliteration of varices when the sheath was used.

Various methods of achieving balloon compression during injections via a fiberscope have been developed. An inflated balloon may be fixed in the cardia during injection (56,57). This approach decreases or stops active variceal bleeding, and it also should decrease the chance for precipitation of bleeding as a result of a puncture. However, the varices will likely decrease in caliber, and it may become more difficult to identify injection sites, especially at or below the level of the esophagogastric mucosal junction. Further, all insufflated air and accumulated secretions and blood must return via the mouth, increasing the chance for aspiration. It is not known whether this method is more effective or whether its associated complication rate is any greater than those of other techniques.

Injection sclerotherapy is thought to be facilitated by proximal variceal compression during injections by making the vessels more prominent and by promoting stasis. This compression may be obtained by fixing a balloon cuff over the instrument's insertion tube just proximal to the distal tip (58–60). This technique has an added advantage in that the balloon may be positioned over a bleeding point for temporary tamponade. According to available data from animal and human studies, there is some doubt that this maneuver enhances the procedure by promoting stasis (50,51). Because these studies have shown rapid clearance of the injected material to the extrinsic veins, it is more likely that proximal compression promotes clearance rather than enhances stasis and contact of the agent with the vessel. Further, inflating the balloon before beginning injections may enhance ongoing hemorrhage or dislodge a clot from a varix.

Wang and coworkers (61) combined the sheath approach with a gastric balloon and a modified orotracheal tube. The small diameter of this device necessitates a fiberoptic brochoscope for injections. Takase and associates (62) combined a balloon cuff on the insertion tube of the endoscope with a balloon fixed in the cardia. They also performed injections under fluoroscopic guidance and used a contrast agent to be certain that the injections were intravariceal. The authors were able to use this method successfully for the management of actively bleeding varices.

Many investigators maintain that injections can be equally effective when compression is not used (63). This method is in several respects less complicated, although it requires skill and quickness in dealing with active hemorrhage from a varix.

A variety of injection devices is available commercially. Some degree of flexibility in an injector helps avoid laceration of a varix during injection as a result of motion caused by the endoscopist, the patient (especially by belching) or esophageal contractions. The best flexibility is obtained with a simple tubular system made of synthetic material, such as polyvinyl, into one end of which a needle is fixed. There is some potential for such a needle system to damage the biopsy channel of a fiberscope. Therefore, a second outer sheath is sometimes added into which the needle may be withdrawn when not in use, for example, while passing the device through the accessory channel. However, damage with a simple needle can be avoided by not inserting the needle through the channel when the tip of the fiberscope is acutely angulated. Some retractable injection devices have a spiral metal wire outer sheath. Such instruments tend to be more rigid, but they present less of a problem if some device, for example, an overtube, is used to fix the position of the varix.

Ideally, a sclerosing agent should induce rapid thrombosis, followed by intimal damage to the vein and ending in obliteration with minimal damage to the underlying esophageal musculature. The agent should be innocuous when it reaches the extraesophageal vascular system and other organs. A variety of agents and combinations of agents have been used empirically or by extrapolating data and experience from sclerotherapy for varicose veins in the legs to theories of esophageal variceal sclerosis.

Many different chemical agents are capable of causing inflammation and tissue damage, which in the case of a vein may result in thrombosis and, ultimately, fibrous obliteration. Such agents may be loosely grouped according to mechanism of action (64). Some such agents cause a direct chemical reaction with tissue components. Examples are heavy-metal salts (e.g., mercuric iodine), organic compounds (e.g., salicylate quinine hydrochloride), highly reactive halogens (e.g., Lugol's solution) and virtually any strong alkaline solution. This type of agent is not suitable for esophageal sclerotherapy. The second broad category of agents is those whose action is more physical than directly chemical in nature. Included are the more familiar fatty acids, such as sodium morrhuate and ethanolamine oleate, as well as agents that act mainly by an osmotic and dehydrating effect, for example, hypertonic glucose. This category also includes aqueous solutions, such as the high branched-chain alkyl salt sodium tetradecyl sulfate and ethanol. Other agents used empirically include such drugs as cefazolin and topical bovine thrombin.

Little scientific data are available to guide the selection of an agent or agents for esophageal sclerotherapy. Substances have been tested, more or less scientifically, to determine their effectiveness in sclerotherapy for varicosities in the legs. Cooper (64) believed that tetradecyl sulfate was superior to fatty acids because its action was more localized, an effect attributed to its neutral pH in comparison to the alkalinity of fatty acid solutions. Blenkinsopp (65) compared 1% and 3% solutions of tetradecyl sulfate with 5% ethanolamine oleate in a rat model in 1967. The 3% tetradecyl sulfate solution was most effective, followed by the 1% concentration, both of these being superior to 5% ethanolamine oleate in occluding the vein lumen. All agents tested were ineffective if injected paravariceally in this study, and no pathologic change was found in the heart or lungs of the animals. Reiner (66) found tetradecyl sulfate to be more thrombogenic than sodium morrhuate in animal experiments. The study of Jensen and colleagues (43) compared the efficacy of different sclerosants, including 5% sodium morrhuate, 5% enthanolamine oleate, 1.5% sodium tetradecyl sulfate, cefazolin, 95% and 45% ethanol and a mixture of 0.5% sodium tetradecyl sulfate and thrombin (50 units/ml) in 50% dextrose. All agents were equally effective in producing hemostasis. Another investigation (67) by this group determined the efficacy of various sclerosants and rates for ulcer and erosion formation in a canine model. Cefazolin, 47% ethanol, 5% ethanolamine oleate and a combination of 0.5% sodium tetradecyl sulfate plus thrombin plus 50% glucose were no more effective than saline injections. A combination of 1% sodium tetradecyl sulfate plus 32% ethanol, 1.5% sodium tetradecyl sulfate and 5% sodium morrhuate were more effective. There was a direct relationship between effectiveness and the frequency of esophageal damage. The ulcerogenic potential of 3% sodium tetradecyl sulfate was compared to that of 5% sodium morrhuate in one study; the latter was found to have a significantly greater potential (68).

At present, it is difficult to recommend one agent or agents in preference to others. All are capable of causing damage to tissue, and it may be true that within limits, the effects of various substances can be approximated by varying their concentration. Other factors, such as the volume, rate of injection and placement of injections, are probably of importance in determining the overall effect. Some agents, for example, fatty acid compounds, may be more suitable for paravariceal injection, whereas others might be better for intravariceal injection. Many sclerosants are not available for use worldwide, or their use is restricted.

There is considerable controversy concerning the placement of individual injections. They may be given intravariceally (34,35,38,45,48,53,56–58,60, 63,69–78), or they may be made paravariceally (39,44,79–82). A combination of both methods also is possible (36,40,83,84). Intravariceal injection is clearly the

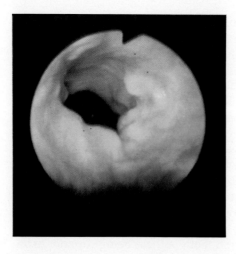

Fig. 1. Endoscopic view of the distal portion of the esophagus after six sessions of sclerotherapy.

preferred method, as evidenced by the number of reports that have described this method to date. The injection pattern can be limited to the distal few centimeters of the esophagus, or it can cover a much longer segment (36,74). The volume of sclerosant injected per puncture and the volume injected per procedure are other variables, as are the selection of a sclerosant and its concentration. Combinations of agents with theoretically different modes of action are being used (48,63,72,73).

A sequence of procedures aimed at obliterating all variceal channels, or as many as can be eliminated, appears to be beneficial. However, the safest and most effective schedule of procedures has not been established. It would be logical to perform a number of procedures at short intervals initially to prevent resumption of bleeding after initial control. However, overzealousness may result in severe ulceration and necrosis. Further, some adjustment in the schedule may be necessary, depending on the number of injections and on the type of sclerosant and its concentration.

It also may be difficult to know when to stop the series of injection procedures. A satisfactory clinical course does not necessarily indicate obliteration of varices. Further, obliteration does not occur at a fixed number of procedures. Small-caliber veins may require only a few injections, whereas many injections over the course of time are necessary with large-diameter vessels. The effect may be assessed endoscopically, and it is possible to achieve a result in which an experienced examiner cannot recognize any varices, but probably not in all cases (Fig. 1). There may be other acceptable visual end points. Variceal vessels may be visible, although puncture may not result in any bleeding. Such thrombosed vessels may be in an early stage of fibrous obliteration. Small, nodular, interrupted vessels may be seen after a series of injections. At this point, it may be difficult to ensure intravariceal injection, and further injections in the usual amounts may not greatly enhance effectiveness and might result in unacceptable esophageal damage.

The ability to determine where and when blood flow persists in a varix would be an advantage. The injection pattern could be modified to permit fewer injections without loss of effect, but perhaps with less ulceration and esophageal damage. Gertsch and associates (85) determined presclerotherapy intravariceal pressure in 18 patients by using a pressure sensor attached to the tip of the endoscope. The highest values were recorded for large-diameter varices, and a relationship was found between this variable and recurrent bleeding during or after sclerotherapy. A similar study was published by Mosimann (86) in which pressures recorded with this technique correlated with pressures obtained at operation from the superior mesenteric vein. The endoscopic use of Doppler ultrasound devices may also prove beneficial in assessing blood flow in varices (87). Variceal pressure has been determined in an animal model by inserting a needle, coupled to a pressure manometer, directly into a varix (88).

During the past five years, the author's method of sclerotherapy has been used 461 times in 120 patients. Only minor modifications have been made, chiefly in the composition of the sclerosant solution.

A patient's hemodynamic condition is first stabilized, if possible, by transfusion, intravenous vasopressin and Sengstaken-Blakemore tube tamponade, if necessary. Nevertheless, in some instances, emergency sclerotherapy for acute hemorrhage is necessary. The technique for such procedures varies somewhat from the routine method. Sclerotherapy usually is begun about 4 to 6 hours after relative hemodynamic stability has been achieved.

Two to three procedures are done in the first 10 to 15 days in an effort to gain control of a patient's course during the early high-risk period. A fourth procedure is done 6 weeks after the first one, a fifth procedure $3\frac{1}{2}$ months after the first and a sixth procedure at $6\frac{1}{2}$ months. The number and interval between procedures may be modified after the first two procedures, depending on the response to injections, as observed endoscopically. Two procedures may be enough to achieve control during the early course, depending on the size and extent of the varices. The interval between subsequent procedures may be lengthened somewhat. Total obliteration of varices may require an increase in the number of procedures. The maximal number in any one patient has been 12, and the average number is 3.7. This figure is less than the planned schedule because of early deaths from hemorrhage and hepatic failure. The maximal effect achieved with any given procedure may not be reached until several days to 1 week after injection. The effect is gradual, as evidenced by the fact that perforation almost never occurs in the first 24 to 48 hours. Rather, perforation develops after 5 to 10 days, during which time there may be little clinical evidence of impending catastrophe. Therefore, it is important not to schedule procedures too close together in the early stages lest an excessive cumulative effect lead to unnecessary esophageal damage. When the clinical course has necessitated scheduling procedures at short intervals (because bleeding has been recurrent), complications have resulted. After the varices have been obliterated and/or the clinical course has stabilized, patients are followed up endoscopically at 3- to 6-month intervals.

The equipment required for the procedure includes a twin-channel endoscope, an unsheathed, flexible injector needle (Figs. 2a and 2b) (American Endoscopy, Mentor, Ohio), a Sengstaken-Blakemore tube (for tamponade if

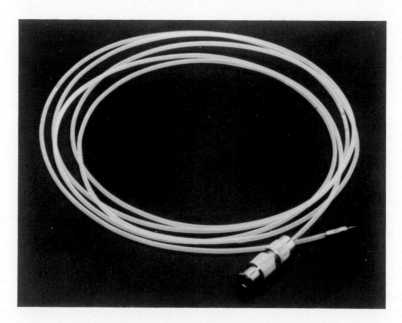

Fig. 2a. Simple injector device.

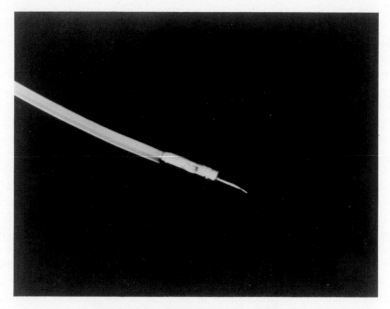

Fig. 2b. Closeup view of the distal portion of the injector shows a 5-mm, 25-gauge needle fixed in a metal collar.

hemorrhage is uncontrollable), standby vasopressin infusion and a sclerosant solution. Intravenous meperidine and diazepam are used for sedation.

The Olympus TGF-2D instrument is preferred. Its main advantage is its large (3.5 mm) second channel, which is adequate for clearing the field of blood when bleeding is active. However, its insertion tube is 16 mm in diameter, making it difficult to pass on occasion. When the Olympus TGF-2D is difficult to pass, the Olympus GIF-2T is satisfactory. The Olympus GIF-1T is also suitable for subsequent procedures when precipitation of hemorrhage during injection is less likely to occur.

The simple injector without an outer sheath has been designed by the author and his colleagues. It is flexible and responds readily to the motion that occurs during the procedure. The needle, 25 gauge and 5 mm long, is fitted into a rounded metal collar, and as a varix is punctured, the collar stops further advancement; that is, the depth of puncture is predetermined. The injector is forward loaded into the small-diameter channel, through which it will pass easily and safely as long as the distal tip of the instrument is not acutely deflected. The needle point is positioned just proximal to the tip of the instrument and is withdrawn into this position after each puncture. As the needle leaves the endoscopic field of view, it is withdrawn an additional 1 cm to ensure that it is within the endoscope.

Our sclerosant solution consists of 0.75% sotradecol (Elkins-Sinn, Cherry Hill, New Jersey) and 50% glucose. The solution must be prepared in advance, which requires some time, and must be used soon thereafter to avoid bacterial contamination. A 50-ml volume is prepared and placed in 10-ml syringes, small syringes being easier for the assistant to control during an injection. The average volume used during an initial procedure is about 30 ml.

Intravariceal injections are begun at the esophagogastric junction or within the cardia, if possible and if gastric varices are visible. When the puncture is made, it is important to keep the needle about 2 cm from the tip of the instrument to take advantage of the injector's flexibility (Fig. 3). This maneuver may be difficult near the esophagogastric junction (Fig. 4). Sudden motion during a puncture with the needle close to the more rigid tip of the endoscope is apt to cause an esophageal tear. All columns are injected at a given level, and the endoscope is then withdrawn about 2 cm for the next set of injections. Slow, steady injection pressure is maintained by the endoscopy assistant. Owing to the position of the accessory channel relative to the field of view, some vessels at a given level may be more difficult to target than others. This difference in vessel accessibility may lead to overinjection of ones that are easy to inject and underinjection of those that are difficult to inject. Varices nearest the exit point for the needle line up nicely for puncture. Therefore, it may be necessary to rotate the insertion tube to inject all vessels at a given level. A standing endoscopist can inject all such vessels easily and quickly by simply turning left and right or by raising and lowering the left shoulder. A seated endoscopist also may find more blood in his or her lap at the end of the procedure. The injection volume is determined by the diameter of the varix and by the change in its appearance during the injection. The volume ranges from 0.5 to 3.0 ml. A small varix that readily distends and blanches may require only 0.5 to 1 ml. When

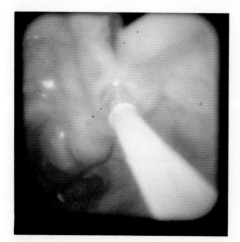

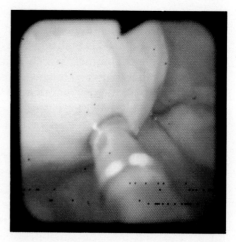

Fig. 3. Endoscopic view of injection of a varix.

Fig. 4. Endoscopic view of injection of a varix.

varices are large, there may not be much observable change as the injection is made, in which case 2 to 3 ml may be used. The author has found that a volume greater than 2 to 3 ml tends to result in increased back bleeding. If doubt arises as to whether the needle is positioned properly in a varix, a small amount of sclerosant solution should be injected.

The distal two-thirds of the esophagus is injected in this manner (Fig. 5). Although most variceal bleeding occurs in the distal few centimeters of the esophagus, injection sclerotherapy may alter this bleeding pattern. It is illogical to think that treating a limited area (e.g., a few distal centimeters) will change the pressure and flow in the more proximal varices, given the anastomosing anatomic arrangement described above.

After each injection, there frequently is some back bleeding. Oozing is permissible and stops in 1 to 2 minutes. If a stream of blood protrudes from or spurts from a puncture site, the injection pattern for active hemorrhage as described below must be considered along with intravenous vasopressin. After each set of injections at a given level has been completed, the instrument is advanced into the stomach. Air can be removed to decrease the chance of an ill-timed belch, and the volume of blood loss is best assessed by checking the amount in the gastric pool.

It is desirable to locate the bleeding point when managing active hemorrhage (Fig. 6). However, if it is impossible to locate the bleeding point, the standard injection sequence described above should be employed. If the bleeding point has been located, the first injection is made immediately above the bleeding point in the same column because it is too difficult to obtain a clear field distal to this point. Bleeding usually does not abate with one such injection, and additional ones are therefore made to the right and left of the rent. Some of these injections will be paravariceal. As flow subsides, an injection may be made distally to the bleeding point. When there is severe spurting hemor-

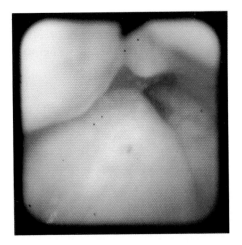

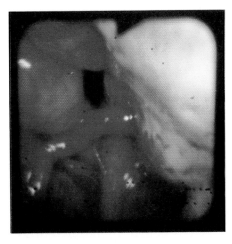

Fig. 5. Endoscopic view of the distal portion of the esophagus at the conclusion of the sclerotherapy procedure. Note the change in color of the distended varices, which nearly occlude the lumen.

Fig. 6. Endoscopic view of an actively bleeding varix.

rhage, repetition of this sequence may be required. This technique stops hemorrhage, it would seem, by causing an acute inflammatory reaction with swelling and edema. A few minutes may be required for this reaction to develop, and this delay may lead to an excessive number of injections being made by an inexperienced endoscopist anxious for a more instantaneous response. There does not appear to be any advantage in inserting the needle directly into the bleeding point because an appreciable amount of active agent may be washed away. Variceal bleeding often ceases momentarily, even when it has been severe and persistent. A clot may then be seen protruding fom a varix (Fig. 7). Injections should then be carried out as though there were active

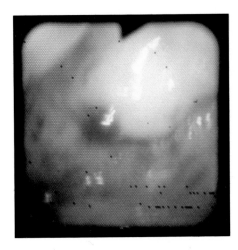

Fig. 7. Endoscopic view of a blood clot in a varix. Active hemorrhage began at this site with the first injection.

hemorrhage at the site of the clot. This situation usually is unstable, and the first or second injection may dislodge the clot. Nevertheless, the endoscopist should proceed calmly with the planned pattern of injections for active hemorrhage.

SCLEROTHERAPY: REVIEW OF THE LITERATURE BEFORE 1978

The first endoscopic sclerotherapy procedure was performed by Crafoord and Frenckner (89) in 1939. Their 16-year-old patient underwent a series of injections of quinine by means of a rigid endoscope. The injections prevented further bleeding over a 3-year follow-up period. Moersch (90) reported on sclerotherapy in 11 patients in 1941, and a series of 24 patients was reported by Patterson and Rouse (91) in 1947. In both series, repeated injections of sodium morrhuate were made with the use of a rigid endoscope. Bleeding was controlled in a large percentage of patients, with complication rates of 1.8% and 1.3%, respectively. Samson and Foree (92) reported a relatively long follow-up period in one patient in 1942. The procedure was never adopted widely, and only a few reports appeared during the 1950s (93,94). Sclerotherapy in children was described by Fearon and Sass-Kortsak (95) in 1959. The first large series of patients to be reported was that of Johnston and Rodgers (34) in 1973. Their experience comprised 217 procedures in 117 patients over a 15-year period. Ethanolamine oleate was used in conjunction with rigid endoscopy. Bleeding was controlled in 93% of the patients, whereas the complication rate was only 0.9%. The next large series in which rigid endoscopy was used consisted of 640 patients reported by Paquet and Oberhammer (44).

The number of reports and abstracts concerned with sclerotherapy has increased rapidly in the past five years, starting with two publications by Terblanche and colleagues (35,96). A rigid endoscope and general anesthesia were used for sclerotherapy in both series. However, this reawakened interest is in great measure due to the successful use of fiberoptic endoscopes for sclerotherapy, which began in the late 1970s (54,59,63).

RESULTS OF SCLEROTHERAPY

Endoscopic sclerotherapy has been reported to control variceal bleeding in the early period after the onset in about 75% of episodes (35,44,53,63,91,95,96).

In one report, sclerotherapy controlled acute hemorrhage in 16 of 19 patients for a 1-month period (twin-channel endoscope, intravariceal injections, 5% sodium morrhuate, balloon fixed in the cardia) (37). Patients received an average of 6 units of blood (range, 0 to 26) before sclerotherapy. There were eight deaths during the first month, mainly from causes other than hemorrhage. Definitive control was achieved in 79% of 24 hospitalizations for acute hemorrhage in 22 patients in a report by Palani and coworkers (38) (rigid endoscope, general anesthesia, sodium morrhuate). Stray and associates (79) achieved hemostasis in 10 of 11 admissions for acute bleeding (single oblique channel or twin-channel fiberscope, paravariceal injections, polidokanol). Cessation of bleeding for at least 24 hours was reported by Alwmark and colleagues (80) for 95% of 72 patients with acute hemorrhage (rigid endoscope, paravariceal injections, polidokanol). Sclerotherapy was begun within 8 hours of admission. Kjaergaard and coworkers (81) reported similar results with 94% hemostasis in 29 patients (fiberoptic endoscope, paravariceal injections, polidokanol). Ten percent of the patients bled to death during a median follow-up of 17 months (range, 1 to 48). Sclerotherapy was begun during the first 24 hours. Terblanche and colleagues (46) have recently reported on 71 patients with acute variceal hemorrhage. Balloon tamponade in combination with sclerotherapy controlled bleeding in 95% of episodes in 71 patients.

Balloon tamponade and/or intravenous vasopressin was used in nearly all these reported series to stabilize a patient's hemodynamic condition before sclerotherapy was begun (35,38,53,63,79–81). A report by Lewis and associates (37) is an exception, although these investigators did fix a balloon in the cardia during injections. The report by Fleig and coworkers (39), noted above, concerned persistent hemorrhage that was unresponsive to tamponade. Here also, the authors achieved hemostasis in 92% of patients. Because other temporary methods for controlling hemorrhage also were used in most acute sclerotherapy series, the question arises as to whether some patients would have had no further bleeding without slcerotherapy. This question is difficult to answer on the basis of available data. However, Barsoum and colleagues (40) reported a trial that compared balloon tamponade with sclerotherapy in 50 patients who were assigned randomly to each group. A successful result was defined as the absence of hemorrhage for 1 month after treatment. Tamponade alone was successful in 42% of the patients, whereas sclerotherapy achieved a 74% success rate. Sclerotherapy was done with a rigid endoscope and general anesthesia. Although there was a high proportion of Child's C patients in the sclerotherapy group, mortality was the same for both groups. The author and his colleagues have performed sclerotherapy to stop acute spurting variceal hemorrhage in 23 patients by means of the technique described above. In 88% of patients, this approach stopped the hemorrhage during the procedure, and no further bleeding was detectable for 48 hours.

The incidence of recurrent bleeding during the follow-up period after sclerotherapy also is difficult to assess. A study by Terblanche and associates (96) compared acute injection therapy alone with acute injections plus a long-term series of injections. Reduction of the number and severity of bleeding episodes was demonstrated with the latter approach. However, the patients in each group were not evenly matched on the basis of several variables, and the numbers of patients were small. Other investigators have emphasized that rebleeding episodes and transfusion requirements are reduced significantly by a series of injection procedures (58,72,97). However, Hennessy and coworkers (45) questioned the usefulness of long-term sclerotherapy because of a rebleeding rate of 44% in their uncontrolled series, although they did conclude that sclerotherapy was effective for acute and emergent hemorrhage.

An important study by Clark and colleagues (53), published in 1980, reported a trial of sclerotherapy in 36 patients compared to a control group of 28 patients treated medically. Rebleeding occurred in one-third of patients in the sclerotherapy group and in more than two-thirds of those in the control group. The difference was statistically significant at various intervals of follow-up. At 1 year, survival was 65% in the sclerotherapy group as compared to only 46% in the control group. This difference, however, was not statistically significant. In an extension of this report by Macdougal and associates (98), the rebleeding rate for patients in the sclerotherapy group (n = 51) was 43% as compared to 75% for patients in the control group (n = 56), a statistically significant difference. Overall, the risk for bleeding was reduced threefold by sclerotherapy for each month of follow-up. Most remarkable was that survival at 1 year for patients in the treatment and control groups was 75% and 58%, respectively, a statistically significant difference. The authors thought that this improvement in survival was related to the ability to obliterate all variceal channels. A similarly favorable effect on mortality was demonstrated by Goodale and coworkers (60), who compared survival in 48 Child's B and C patients who underwent sclerotherapy to the outcome for a similar group of nontreated patients described by Graham and Smith (1).

The results of other studies, some preliminary in nature, appear to support these conclusions. Results at 2-week follow-up in a study that compared sclerotherapy with medical management included a decrease in the number of episodes of bleeding and transfusion requirements as well as reduction of mortality in the treatment group (99). However, the differences were not statistically significant, the numbers of patients in each group were small and the follow-up period was short. Hemostasis was maintained in 89% of 76 patients at 1-week follow-up in another study (80). After an initial injection series, the procedure was repeated at intervals of 3 to 6 months. However, hemostasis was maintained in 40% of patients at 6 months but in only 24% of them at 1 year. Assessment of these results was complicated by the fact that 30% of the patients had died by 1 year. Liver failure was the most common cause of death in Child's C patients, but hemorrhage was most commonly the cause in Child's B patients. Hedberg and colleagues (73) reported "no bleeding from varices after the third treatment week in patients followed up to 14 months."

Other preliminary reports disagree with these conclusions. A study by Trudeau and coworkers (100) found that sclerotherapy did not favorably influence transfusion requirements or survival in a group of 16 Child's C patients as compared to the transfusion requirements and survival that characterize the natural course of variceal bleeding in such patients, as described by Graham and Smith (1). A later report by these investigators concluded that sclerotherapy reduced loss of blood in Child's C patients but that it did not favorably influence survival (101). Cello and associates (76) compared sclerotherapy with esophageal transection and reanastomosis in a small num-

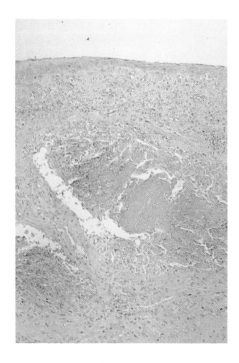

Fig. 8. Photomicrograph shows an organizing thrombus in a varix 9 weeks after the initial session of sclerotherapy.

ber of poor-risk patients and concluded that sclerotherapy was superior to transection and reanastomosis. There was no rebleeding in surgically treated patients, but mortality was 83%. By contrast, rebleeding occurred in one-third of injected patients, and mortality was 67%.

It is difficult to assess the overall effect of sclerotherapy because many variables are involved. However, it appears that sclerotherapy has a favorable effect on transfusion requirements, both in the early acute period and during an extended follow-up period. However, a substantial number of treated patients still experience further episodes of hemorrhage, perhaps about 40% of them. Some data indicate that there is a favorable influence in regard to survival, but final judgment on this point awaits additional studies.

A few reports of postmortem studies of the esophagus after sclerotherapy are available (70,71,82,102). Characteristic changes that occur in the first few days after injection include thrombus formation and an intense inflammatory response in the region. The inflammation subsides and the thrombus becomes well organized after a few weeks (Fig. 8). Fibrosis follows, but it is uncertain when this change begins. One study (82) found fibrosis as early as 2 weeks after the first injection. Another report (102) indicated that several months had elapsed before fibrosis appeared. An increase in the number and diameter of veins in the deep layers of the esophagus also was demonstrated by the latter investigation. This increase was taken as evidence that blood was being shunted away from the intrinsic plexus. Evans and coworkers (70) reported on an autopsy series of eight patients who had undergone intravariceal injections of tetradecyl sulfate and had died after varying periods of follow-up. They found that thrombosis of varices was present by 24 hours. The onset of fibrosis was at 1 month, which was intermediate to the onset reported in the two earlier investigations.

SCLEROTHERAPY IN VARICEAL HEMORRHAGE DUE TO PORTAL VEIN OBSTRUCTION

Variceal bleeding in children most often is due to obstruction of the portal vein as a result of thrombosis, fibrosis or congenital malformation. Obstruction frequently is related to umbilical vein catheterization in infancy. The success of surgical shunting procedures depends on the size of the vessels to be used and, therefore, on the age of the patient. Fonkalsrud and colleagues (103) found that children who do not undergo surgical intervention frequently experience a decrease in the number of episodes of bleeding with increasing age. This decrease probably is a result of the development of other collateral venous channels. Because of this possibility, it would seem prudent to wait as long as is possible before resorting to surgical intervention.

Fearon and Sass-Kortsak (95) first reported a favorable outcome for sclerotherapy in children, and this result has been confirmed by other investigators (104). Lilly and coworkers (105) described a technique that requires a slotted rigid endoscope, general anesthesia and 5% sodium morrhuate. Six children were treated, four beginning at the time of active hemorrhage. There was no episode of rebleeding during the follow-up period, which ranged from 2 months to 3½ years. A pediatric fiberscope was used to make intravariceal injections of 5% ethanolamine in 21 children in another study (78). Only eight patients had portal vein obstruction. A small-diameter fiberscope was thought to be difficult to use if brisk bleeding was encountered. However, varices were obliterated in 18 patients after a mean of 3.5 procedures. No patient died of hemorrhage. Twenty-four percent of the group had recurrent hemorrhage by 1 month. The authors considered the patients as a homogeneous group and did not define the outcome for the extrahepatic group separately.

The author and his colleagues have performed sclerotherapy in eight patients with extrahepatic portal hypertension. Their average age was 21.8 years, and they had sustained an average of 7.6 bleeding episodes with a mean transfusion requirement of 23.5 units per patient. Six patients had previously undergone portosystemic shunt procedures. A mean of 5.5 sclerotherapy procedures was performed. The mean follow-up period was 24.4 months, during which time the average number of episodes of bleeding was 0.9, and the total mean transfusion requirement was 2.25 units. Bleeding in one patient proved difficult to control, and 11 procedures were performed. He sustained five episodes of bleeding during the follow-up period and required 12 transfusions. The results in this patient unfavorably influenced the mean figures for bleeding during the follow-up period. Overall, most patients with this type of portal hypertension have responded well to sclerotherapy.

COMPLICATIONS OF
SCLEROTHERAPY

The complication rate for endoscopic sclerotherapy as found in the literature ranges from 2% to 15% per patient (34,44,53,58,63,90,91). Terblanche and colleagues (46) encountered 22 major complications in 18 of 66 patients (27%) in a 5-year experience. Macdougal and associates (98) encountered complications in 21 of 107 patients who underwent 240 injection procedures. In a trial of prophylactic sclerotherapy, complications occurred in 12.5% of the sclerotherapy-treated group (n = 32) (41). A survey of the membership of the American Society for Gastrointestinal Endoscopy, which pertained to experience before 1981, revealed complication rates of 19% per patient and 9% per procedure (47). A later survey of the ASGE, which covered experience before 1982, showed decreases in these rates to 16.7% per patient and 6.4% per procedure (106). In the early Cleveland experience, a serious complication occurred in 2.4% of the procedures (63). The most recent determinations for our series are 12.3% per patient and 3.4% per procedure. In general, most serious complications occur early in a patient's course.

Substernal chest discomfort after sclerotherapy develops in about one-fourth to one-half of patients. This discomfort frequently is difficult to quantitate. It may be a mild "burning" sensation or severe "crushing" pain. Pain usually lasts 12 to 24 hours but may persist (60). Odynophagia, which may persist for several days, also may occur (60). Pain usually does not indicate necrosis or perforation. Perforation as a result of the chemical action of a sclerosant usually is more insidious and requires several days to 1 week to become fully developed. However, pain during and/or immediately after completion of a procedure can signify perforation as a result of instrument trauma. Two such cases were included in the report by Macdougal and associates (98). In one case, a rigid endoscope was used; in the other case, an unsuspected esophageal diverticulum was perforated. Chest pain or discomfort has been noted after intravariceal sclerotherapy (38,57,58,60,72). It also has occurred after paravariceal injections and combinations of the two methods (40,80). The etiologic basis of postprocedure pain is not certain. Whether it is related to the type of sclerosant or its concentration or to the pattern of injections is not clear. Harris and colleagues (83) assert that chest pain is more common when ethanolamine is used than when tetradecyl sulfate is used. However, it does occur with the latter as well. Some authors attribute severe chest pain to chemical mediastinitis, but there is no proof that such inflammation is the cause. In the author's experience, the discomfort does not correlate with other possible signs of mediastinitis, such as fever or pleural effusion. Gebhard and coworkers (107) have suggested esophageal spasm as a cause of the pain on the basis of a study of barium swallows in 11 patients after sclerotherapy. Esophageal spasm probably is the best explanation.

A low-grade rise in temperature occurs after sclerotherapy in 10% to 15% of patients, although fever was noted in almost one-half of the patients in a report by Hughes and colleagues (58). In most instances, the temperature increases slightly and then reaches a plateau, at which point it stabilizes for 24 to 48 hours. Barsoum and associates (108) have treated some febrile episodes with dexamethasone when sepsis was eliminated as a possibility. Because fever resolves spontaneously and without apparent sequelae in most cases, the use of dexamethasone seems unwarranted. Further, the issue of sepsis and bacteremia during and after sclerotherapy is not yet resolved. It does appear, however, that elevation of temperature after the procedure is not due exclusively to bacteremia or sepsis (109). Therefore, fever alone should not be an indication for antibiotic therapy. However, high-spiking temperature elevations are not a characteristic finding after sclerotherapy and are a cause for concern regarding the possibility of sepsis.

Pleural effusion may be found on chest roentgenograms in asymptomatic patients after sclerotherapy. This phenomenon occurred in more than one-half of the patients reported by Hughes and coworkers (58). There is no clear understanding of the cause of this complication. Infiltrates also may be seen on follow-up chest roentgenograms, and this finding may be a greater cause for concern in view of a recent report of serious pulmonary complications (110). Most effusions resolve with no apparent sequelae. Whether there is permanent subclinical damage to the lungs or pleura is unknown. In general, it is difficult to speculate on the long-range complications of sclerotherapy. Because many patients who have undergone this therapy have an underlying chronic, fatal illness that affects many organ systems, it is difficult to obtain long-term follow-up in a large group of patients.

Two patients have been described in whom acute respiratory failure developed after sclerotherapy; in most respects, the respiratory failure was similar to adult respiratory distress syndrome (110). This complication was mentioned, but not elaborated upon, in another report (111). Monroe and colleagues (110) described dyspnea, which was poorly responsive to administration of oxygen, along with bilateral alveolar infiltrates seen on chest roentgenograms. Sodium morrhuate was used, and the authors pointed out that this substance, which is not homogeneous, contains elements known to be toxic to the lungs. They were able to demonstrate transient increases in pulmonary artery pressure and lymph flow in an animal model with injections of sodium morrhuate, but no change in alveolar capillary permeability was found. It is logical to expect that pulmonary complications can result from sclerotherapy because an injected substance can be readily transported to the right side of the heart and lungs via the azygous system. The frequency at which such complications occur is not established. Potential long-term problems, such as pulmonary hypertension, have not been eliminated from consideration. Some agents may be more hazardous in this respect than others, but this possibility has not been confirmed.

The various reports of esophageal manometry in relation to sclerotherapy are somewhat conflicting. A decrease in lower esophageal sphincter pressure after sclerotherapy has been described (112). A decrease in the amplitude of contractions in the distal portion of the esophagus, a high percentage of simultaneous, nonpropulsive contractions and delayed clearance were found by manometry and radionuclide scanning in a study of 19 patients who had undergone from seven to 13 injection procedures (84). Other abstracts of studies described no

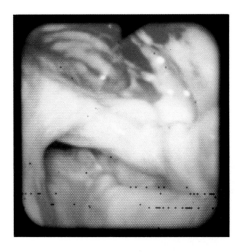

Fig. 9. Endoscopic view of an esophageal ulcer and a perforation 10 days after injections at this site to control acute bleeding.

serious alterations in esophageal motility (113). The abstract by Simon and colleagues (114) reported no alteration when manometry was done before and after sclerotherapy. It is possible that some techniques, for instance, paravariceal injection, or some sclerosing agents may have a greater effect on esophageal muscle. It would seem that some degree of damage to the neuromuscular plexus and esophageal musculature must result from sclerotherapy. However, the clinical implications of this possibility are unknown.

Esophageal stricture occurred after sclerotherapy in 3% of patients in the ASGE membership survey (47). This presumably is a direct action of the sclerosant, although a contribution from acid reflux has not been eliminated from consideration. Stricturing could be related to the type and concentration of agent used and to the method of injection. Paravariceal injection should, logically, result in a higher incidence of stricture than should other techniques. In one series, 31% of the patients had strictures when paravariceal injections of polidokanol were used (81). However, there are no data to support this reasoning, and strictures have occurred with virtually every agent and technique. Most strictures have been managed successfully with simple bougienage. Transient dysphagia after sclerotherapy also has been observed. Because this dysphagia usually resolves spontaneously, it probably is due to spasm and transient esophageal dysfunction.

Perforation of the esophagus occurs in about 1% to 2% of patients (47,106). Instrument perforation is rare when fiberoptic endoscopes are used, but this occurrence has been reported with the use of rigid instruments. Perforation related to the action of the sclerosant usually takes 5 to 7 days or longer to develop (Figs. 9 and 10). Symptoms may be minimal. For example, Carr-Locke and Sidky (115) reported on a patient with an esophageal-bronchial fistula that did not cause symptoms until 1 month after sclerotherapy. The concomitant use of corticosteroids for chronic active hepatitis may have been a contributing factor. Conservative management usually is indicated; such therapy consists of broad-spectrum antibiotics and chest tube drainage in some cases. Because

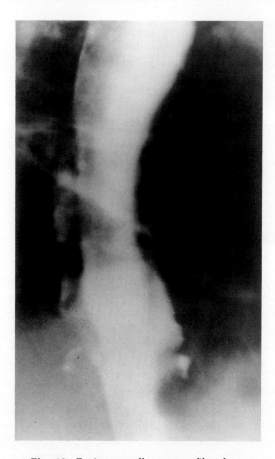

Fig. 10. Barium swallow x-ray film demonstrates esophageal necrosis and a localized perforation 10 days after sclerotherapy for acute bleeding.

perforations usually develop slowly, many wall off and remain localized. In time, even perforations that appear to be catastrophic by contrast study may heal.

Ulceration of the esophagus is a controversial issue. Many authors regard this as a complication. However, it is an extremely common finding after sclerotherapy (Fig. 11). Further, most ulcers heal, although a permanent but a clinically unimportant defect may remain (Fig. 12). An area of healed ulceration may, in fact, indicate an absence of variceal flow. However, serious ulceration and esophageal necrosis may occur, sometimes as the forerunner of perforation. Ulceration in a region of incomplete variceal thrombosis and fibrosis may lead to hemorrhage. Such bleeding may be impossible to control because further sclerotherapy may lead to additional tissue damage, and balloon tamponade and direct surgical intervention would be contraindicated in an area of necrosis. Therefore, it sometimes is difficult to draw a line between an inconse-

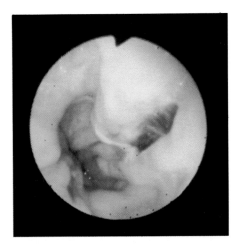

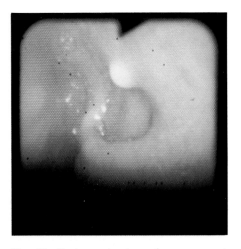

Fig. 11. Endoscopic view of an ulcer at the site of injection 5 days earlier.

Fig. 12. Endoscopic view of a permanent defect in the esophageal wall due to previous ulceration after six sessions of sclerotherapy.

quential or even beneficial ulceration and one that should be considered a complication.

As with perforation, ulcers appear after about 5 to 7 days (71). It is possible that some agents or techniques are more ulcerogenic than others. No ulceration was observed in one report on 53 patients who received 122 intravariceal injections of ethanolamine, thrombin and cefazolin (73). However, other investigators have described ulcers with the use of ethanolamine (58). Little difference in local toxicity among various agents was found in one animal study (116). Trudeau and associates (117) found that a solution of 1% sodium tetradecyl sulfate plus 33% ethanol was somewhat less ulcerogenic than other solutions, but in general they did not find much difference among the various agents tested. Brooks and Galambos (118) compared a variety of sclerosants in their patients and noted that each solution produced ulceration. Also, they concluded that serious ulceration occurred more frequently in patients classified as having Child's C liver disease. This point has not been considered in other investigations.

Ulceration was the most common complication in the 1981 ASGE survey, accounting for 42% of all complications (47). Sanowski and coworkers (119) noted ulcers in 57% of patients. Exudate adherent to injected varices also was found in one-third and erosions in 14% of the patients. In the author's series, yellowish, plaquelike lesions occurred in 45% of the patients and actual ulceration was found in 30% of them (Fig. 13), (63).

Small ulcers probably are not a common source of recurrent bleeding after sclerotherapy, although the opposite view has been proposed, as supported by three instances in a small experience (120). However, large ulcers may be the source of serious blood loss, especially if nearby variceal vessels have been inadequately treated.

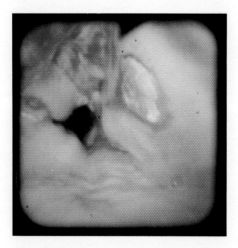

Fig. 13. Endoscopic view of yellowish plaques at the sites of injections 5 days earlier.

The pathogenesis of large ulcers is not entirely clear. Because all agents appear to be capable of inducing ulcers, it is more likely that technique or perhaps the concentration of the agent(s) is responsible. Aside from intravariceal as opposed to paravariceal injection, ulceration might be in large measure related to the amount of active agent deposited at one location, either because of an excessive number of injections in a small area or because of fewer injections with a concentrated agent. The most serious ulcers in the author's series occurred in two patients in whom it was necessary to control active hemorrhage with the technique described above. By design, this technique results in the concentration of a large amount of the active agent in a small tissue volume to induce an inflammatory reaction. If this explanation is correct, the elements that lead to serious ulceration remain under the control of endoscopists; one must consider the tissue density of the active agent produced by injections.

The second most common complication in the survey of 1981 was hemorrhage (47). In the second survey of the ASGE, the frequency of this complication decreased by 28%, but there was an interesting reciprocal increase in the rate of ulceration (106). One can speculate that better control of hemorrhage was achieved at the expense of increased damage to the esophagus.

Intramural hematomas have been induced by sclerotherapy, in one case complicated by bacteremia and death and in another case by perforation (38,83). No coagulopathy, particularly disseminated intravascular coagulation, was found by Gardner and Brooks (121) in a study in which injections consisted of 5% sodium morrhuate, 100 units of thrombin, 2 ml of cefazolin and 50% dextrose. The partial thromboplastin time was transiently prolonged after injection in the series by Hedberg and associates (73). Goodale and coworkers (60) reported two episodes of portal vein thrombosis. One patient had received a prolonged infusion of vasopressin, but there were no extenuating circumstances in the second patient. This complication also was reported by Barsoum and colleagues (108) in one patient. A patient in whom a bleeding duodenal varix developed during sclerotherapy has been described (122). This bleeding varix also was managed with injection sclerotherapy. The eyes of patients and personnel should be protected from accidental contact with sclerosants (123,124).

Data regarding the occurrence of bacteremia during or after sclerotherapy are conflicting. Fourteen episodes of bacteremia in 11 patients were documented by Cohen and colleagues (109). There was a predominance of oropharyngeal flora, and most positive cultures were obtained within the first 5 minutes after a procedure. Fever and abnormalities on chest roentgenograms after the procedure did not correlate with bacteremia. Camara and colleagues (69), however, documented bacteremia in 5% of their patients (40 procedures, 18 patients). Brayko and coworkers (125) found positive blood cultures in five of nine sclerotherapy sessions. A high proportion of the cultures were positive for *Pseudomonas aeruginosa*, which they related to contamination of the endoscopy equipment, especially the water bottle. With better disinfecting techniques, no positive cultures were found. However, Lange and associates (126) found a cumulative increase in the rate of septicemia associated with sclerotherapy but found no relation to instrument sterility or the lack of it. It would appear that bacteremia does occur, as would be anticipated with sclerotherapy, but the incidence of this complication is not clearly established. The sources are the expected ones, namely, the endoscopy equipment and the mouth flora. Although antibiotic prophylaxis does not appear to be indicated for all patients according to available data, it would be prudent to consider this measure for patients with prosthetic heart valves.

CONCLUSION

A number of new strategies for the management of variceal hemorrhage are now in various stages of development. It is safe to assume that the picture will change in the next few years; it is certain that some techniques will be discarded. Endoscopic sclerotherapy is one of the most promising of the "new" ideas. Despite the flurry of activity and interest, there is much to be learned in the area of technique. New complications will surely be recognized. Although sclerotherapy appears to be beneficial in sparing the need for transfusion, its overall effect on the course of patients with variceal hemorrhage is less certain. Varices are within easy reach for endoscopists, making it attractive to think and hope that the problem of hemorrhage can be successfully attacked by this direct approach. Time will tell.

REFERENCES

1. Graham DY, Smith JL: The course of patients after variceal hemorrhage. *Gastroenterology* 80:800–809, 1981.
2. Krook H: Circulatory studies in liver cirrhosis. *Acta Med Scand Suppl* 318:1–160, 1956.

3. Reynolds TB, Ito S, Iwatsuki S: Measurement of portal pressure and its clinical application. *Am J Med* 49:649–657, 1970.

4. Viallet A, Marleau D, Huet M, et al: Hemodynamic evaluation of patients with intrahepatic portal hypertension. Relationship between bleeding varices and the portohepatic gradient. *Gastroenterology* 69:1297–1300, 1975.

5. Palmer ED, Brick IB: Correlation between the severity of esophageal varices in portal cirrhosis and their propensity toward hemorrhage. *Gastroenterology* 30:85–90, 1956.

6. Baker LA, Smith C, Lieberman G: The natural history of esophageal varices. A study of 115 cirrhotic patients in whom varices were diagnosed prior to bleeding. *Am J Med* 26:228–237, 1959.

7. Dagradi AE: The natural history of esophageal varices in patients with alcoholic liver cirrhosis: An endoscopic and clinical study. *Am J Gastroenterol* 57:520–540, 1972.

8. Beppu K, Inokuchi K, Koyanagi N, et al: Prediction of variceal hemorrhage by esophageal endoscopy. *Gastrointest Endosc* 27:213–218, 1981.

9. Resnick RH, Chalmers TC, Ishihara AM, et al: A controlled study of the prophylactic portacaval shunt; a final report. *Ann Intern Med* 70:675–688, 1969.

10. Jackson FC, Perrin EB, Smith AG, et al: A clinical investigation of the portacaval shunt. II. Survival analysis of the prophylactic operation. *Am J Surg* 115:22–42, 1968.

11. Conn HO, Lindenmuth WW, May CJ, et al: Prophylactic portacaval anastomosis. *Medicine (Baltimore)* 51:27–40, 1972.

12. Smith JL, Graham DY: Variceal hemorrhage: A critical evaluation of survival analysis. *Gastroenterology* 82:968–973, 1982.

13. Smith-Laing G, Scott J, Long RG, et al: Role of percutaneous transhepatic obliteration of varices in the management of hemorrhage from gastroesophageal varices. *Gastroenterology* 80:1031–1036, 1981.

14. Bengmark S, Börjesson B, Hoevels J, et al: Obliteration of esophageal varices by PTP. A follow-up of 43 patients. *Ann Surg* 190:549–554, 1979.

15. Freeman JG, Lishman AH, Cobden I, et al: Controlled trial of terlipressin ('glypressin') versus vasopressin in the early treatment of oesophageal varices. *Lancet* II:66–68, 1982.

16. Conn HO: Hazards attending the use of esophageal tamponade. *N Engl J Med* 259:701–707, 1958.

17. Conn HO, Simpson JA: Excessive mortality associated with balloon tamponade of bleeding varices: A critical reappraisal. *J Am Med Ass* 202:587–591, 1967.

18. Pitcher JL: Safety and effectiveness of the modified Sengstaken-Blakemore tube: A prospective study. *Gastroenterology* 61:291–298, 1971.

19. Hunt PS, Korman MG, Hansky J, et al: An 8-year prospective experience with balloon tamponade in emergency control of bleeding esophageal varices. *Dig Dis Sci* 27:413–416, 1982.

20. Novis BH, Duys P, Barbezat GO: Fiberoptic endoscopy and the use of the Sengstaken tube in acute gastrointestinal hemorrhage in patients with portal hypertension and varices. *Gut* 17:258–263, 1976.

21. Orloff MJ, Bell RH Jr, Hyde PV, et al: Long-term results of emergency portacaval

shunt for bleeding esophageal varices in unselected patients with alcoholic cirrhosis. *Ann Surg* 192:325–340, 1980.

22. Jackson FC, Perrin EB, Felix WR, et al: A clinical investigation of the portacaval shunt. V. Survival analysis of the therapeutic operation. *Ann Surg* 174:672–701, 1971.

23. Resnick RH, Iber FL, Ishihara AM, et al: A controlled study of the therapeutic portacaval shunt. *Gastroenterology* 67:843–857, 1974.

24. Conn HO: Therapeutic portacaval anastomosis: To shunt or not to shunt. *Gastroenterology* 67:1065–1071, 1974.

25. Reuff B, Degos F, Degos JD, et al: A controlled study of therapeutic portacaval shunt in alcoholic cirrhosis. *Lancet* I:655–659, 1976.

26. Reynolds TB, Donovan AJ, Mikkelsen WP, et al: Results of a 12-year randomized trial of portacaval shunt in patients with alcoholic liver disease and bleeding varices. *Gastroenterology* 80:1005–1011, 1981.

27. Warren WD, Millikan WJ Jr, Henderson JM, et al: Ten years portal hypertensive surgery at Emory. *Ann Surg* 195:530–542, 1982.

28. Hassab MA: Nonshunt operations in portal hypertension without cirrhosis. *Surg Gynecol Obstet* 131:648–654, 1970.

29. Sugiura M, Futagawa S: Further evaluation of the Sugiura procedure in the treatment of esophageal varices. *Arch Surg* 112:1317–1321, 1977.

30. Osborne DR, Hobbs KEF: The acute treatment of haemorrhage from oesophageal varices: A comparison of oesophageal transection and staple gun anastomosis with mesocaval shunt. *Br J Surg* 68:734–737, 1981.

31. Johnston GW: Six years' experience of oesophageal transection for oesophageal varices, using a circular stapling gun. *Gut* 23:770–773, 1982.

32. Lebrec D, Poynard T, Hillon P, et al: Propranolol for prevention of recurrent gastrointestinal bleeding in patients with cirrhosis, a controlled study. *N Engl J Med* 305:1371–1374, 1981.

33. Rector WG, Reynods TB: Propranolol in the treatment of cirrhotic ascites. (abstract) *Hepatology* 2:678, 1982.

34. Johnston GW, Rodgers HW: A review of 15 years' experience in the use of sclerotherapy in the control of acute haemorrhage for oesophageal varices. *Br J Surg* 60:797–800, 1973.

35. Terblanche J, Northover JMA, Bornman P, et al: A prospective evaluation of injection sclerotherapy in treatment of acute bleeding from esophageal varices. *Surgery* 85:239–245, 1979.

36. Soehendra N, de Heer K, Kempeneers I, et al: Sclerotherapy of esophageal varices: Acute arrest of gastrointestinal hemorrhage or long-term therapy? *Endoscopy* 15:136–140, 1983.

37. Lewis JW, Chung RS, Allison JG: Injection sclerotherapy for control of acute variceal hemorrhage. *Am J Surg* 142:592–595, 1981.

38. Palani CK, Abuabara S, Kraft AR, et al: Endoscopic sclerotherapy in acute variceal hemorrhage. *Am J Surg* 141:164–168, 1981.

39. Fleig WE, Stange EF, Ruettenauer K: Emergency endoscopic sclerotherapy for bleeding esophageal varices: A prospective study in patients not responding to balloon tamponade. *Gastrointest Endosc* 29:8–14, 1983.

40. Barsoum MS, Bolous FI, El-Rooby AA, et al: Tamponade and injection sclero-therapy in the management of bleeding oesophageal varices. *Br J Surg* 69:76–78, 1982.

41. Paquet KJ: Prophylactic endoscopic sclerosing treatment of the esophageal wall in varices—A prospective controlled randomized trial. *Endoscopy* 14:4–5, 1982.

42. Sugawa C, Okumura Y, Lucas CE, et al: Endoscopic sclerosis of experimental esophageal varices in dogs. *Gastrointest Endosc* 24:114–116, 1978.

43. Jensen DM, Silpa ML, Tapia JI, et al: Comparison of different methods for endo-scopic hemostasis of bleeding canine esophageal varices. *Gastroenterology* 84:1455–1461, 1983.

44. Paquet KJ, Oberhammer E: Sclerotherapy of bleeding oesophageal varices by means of endoscopy. *Endoscopy* 10:7–12, 1978.

45. Hennessy TPJ, Stephens RB, Keane FB: Acute and chronic management of esopha-geal varices by injection sclerotherapy. *Surg Gynecol Obstet* 154:375–377, 1982.

46. Terblanche J, Yakoob HI, Bornman PC, et al: Acute bleeding varices. A five-year prospective evaluation of tamponade and sclerotherapy. *Ann Surg* 194:521–530, 1981.

47. Sivak MV Jr: Endoscopic injection sclerosis of esophageal varices: ASGE survey. (Letter to the editor) *Gastrointest Endosc* 28:41, 1982.

48. Reilly JJ Jr, Schade RR, Roh MS, et al: Esophageal variceal sclerosis. *Surg Gynecol Obstet* 155:497–502, 1982.

49. Butler H: The veins of the oesophagus. *Thorax* 6:276–296, 1951.

50. Grobe JL, Kozarek RA, Sanowski RA, et al: Esophageal venography during endo-scopic variceal sclerosis. (abstract) *Gastrointest Endosc* 28:132, 1982.

51. Barsoum MS, Khattar NY, Risk-Allah MA: Technical aspects of injection sclerotherapy of acute oesophageal variceal haemorrhage as seen by radiography. *Br J Surg* 65:588–589, 1978.

52. Silvis SE, Sievert CE Jr, Wong N, et al: The disappearance of sodium morrhuate from a variceal injection site with and without compression. (abstract) *Gastrointest Endosc* 29:167, 1983.

53. Clark AW, Westaby D, Silk DBA, et al: Prospective controlled trial of injection sclerotherapy in patients with cirrhosis and recent variceal hemorrhage. *Lancet* II:552–554, 1980.

54. Williams KGD, Dawson JL: Fiberoptic injection of oesophageal varices. *Br Med J* 2:766–767, 1979.

55. Westaby D, Macdougall BRD, Melia W, et al: A prospective randomized study of two sclerotherapy techniques for esophageal varices. *Hepatology* 3:681–684, 1983.

56. Lewis J, Chung RS, Allison J: Sclerotherapy of esophageal varices. *Arch Surg* 115:476–480, 1980.

57. Kirkham JS, Quayle JB: Oesophageal varices: Evaluation of injection sclerotherapy without general anesthesia using the flexible fiberoptic gastroscope. *Ann R Coll Surg Engl* 64:401–405, 1982.

58. Hughes RW Jr, Larson DE, Viggiano TR, et al: Endoscopic variceal sclerosis: A one-year experience. *Gastrointest Endosc* 28:62–66, 1982.

59. Brooks WS Jr: Adapting flexible endoscopes for sclerosis of oesophageal varices. (abstract) *Lancet* I:266, 1980.

60. Goodale RL, Silvis SE, O'Leary JF, et al: Early survival after sclerotherapy for bleeding esophageal varices. *Surg Gynecol Obstet* 155:523–538, 1982.

61. Wang KP, Yang P, Hutcheon DF, et al: A new method of injection sclerotherapy of esophageal varices. *Gastrointest Endosc* 29:38–40, 1983.

62. Takase Y, Ozaki A, Orii K, et al: Injection sclerotherapy of esophageal varices for patients undergoing emergency and elective surgery. *Surgery* 92:474–479, 1982.

63. Sivak MV Jr, Stout DJ, Skipper G: Endoscopic injection sclerosis (EIS) of esophageal varices. *Gastrointest Endosc* 27:52–57, 1981.

64. Cooper WM: Clinical evaluation of sotradecol, a sodium alkyl sulfate solution, in the injection therapy of varicose veins. *Surg Gynecol Obstet* 383:647–652, 1946.

65. Blenkinsopp WK: Comparison of tetradecyl sulphate in sodium with other sclerosants in rats. *Br J Exp Pathol* 49:197–201, 1967.

66. Reiner L: The activity of anionic surface active compounds in producing vascular obliteration. *Proc Soc Exp Biol Med* 62:49–54, 1946.

67. Silpa ML, Jensen DM, Machicado GA, et al: Efficacy and safety of agents for variceal sclerotherapy. (abstract) *Gastrointest Endosc* 28:152–153, 1982.

68. Gibbert V, Feinstat T, Burns M, et al: A comparison of the sclerosing agents sodium tetradecyl sulfate and sodium morrhuate in endoscopic injection sclerosis of esophageal varices. (abstract) *Gastrointest Endosc* 28:147, 1982.

69. Camara DS, Gruber M, Barde CJ, et al: Transient bacteremia following endoscopic injection sclerotherapy of esophageal varices. *Arch Intern Med* 143:1350–1352, 1983.

70. Evans DMD, Jones DB, Cleary BK, et al: Oesophageal varices treated by sclerotherapy: A histopathological study. *Gut* 23:615–620, 1982.

71. Ayres SJ, Goff JS, Warren GH: Endoscopic sclerotherapy for bleeding esophageal varices: Effects and complications. *Ann Intern Med* 98:900–903, 1983.

72. Novis B, Bat L, Pomerantz I, et al: Endoscopic sclerotherapy of esophageal varices, *Isr J Med Sci* 19:40–44, 1983.

73. Hedberg SE, Fowler DL, Ryan RLR: Injection sclerotherapy of esophageal varices using ethanolamine oleate. A pilot study. *Am J Surg* 143:426–431, 1982.

74. Smith PM, Jones DB, Rose JDR: Simplified fibre endoscopic sclerotherapy for oesophageal varices. *J R Coll Physicians London* 16:236–238, 1982.

75. Yassin YM, Sherif SM: Sclerotherapy of oesophageal varices using the fiberoptic endoscope. *J R Coll Surg Edinburgh* 26:328–334, 1981.

76. Cello JP, Crass R, Trunkey DD, et al: Endoscopic sclerotherapy versus esophageal transection in Child's class C patients with variceal hemorrhage. Comparison with results of portacaval shunt. Preliminary report. *Surgery* 91:333–338, 1982.

77. Lilly JR: Endoscopic sclerosis of esophageal varices in children. *Surg Gynecol Obstet* 152:513–514, 1981.

78. Stamatakis JD, Howard ER, Psacharopoulos HT, et al: Injection sclerotherapy for oesophageal varices in children. *Br J Surg* 69:74–75, 1982.

79. Stray N, Jacobsen CD, Rosseland A: Injection sclerotherapy of bleeding oesophageal and gastric varices using a flexible endoscope. *Acta Med Scand* 211:125–129, 1982.

80. Alwmark A, Bengmark S, Börjesson B, et al: Emergency and long-term transesophageal sclerotherapy of bleeding esophageal varices. A prospective study of 50 consecutive cases. *Scand J Gastroenterol* 17:409–412, 1982.

81. Kjaergaard J, Fischer A, Miskowiak J, et al: Sclerotherapy of bleeding esophageal varices. Long-term results. *Scand J Gastroenterol* 17:363–367, 1982.

82. Helpap B, Bollweg L: Morphologic changes in the terminal oesophagus with varices, following sclerosis of the wall. *Endoscopy* 13:229–233, 1981.

83. Harris OD, Dickey JD, Stephenson PM: Simple endoscopic injection sclerotherapy of oesophageal varices. *Aust NZ J Med* 12:131–135, 1982.

84. Sauerbruch T, Wirsching R, Leisner B, et al: Esophageal function after sclerotherapy of bleeding varices. *Scand J Gastroenterol* 17:745–751, 1982.

85. Gertsch P, Loup P, Diserens H, et al: Endoscopic noninvasive manometry of esophageal varices: Prognostic significance. *Am J Surg* 144:528–530, 1982.

86. Mosimann R: Nonaggressive assessment of portal hypertension using endoscopic measurement of variceal pressure. Preliminary report. *Am J Surg* 143:212–214, 1982.

87. McCormack T, Smallwood RH, Walton L, et al: Doppler ultrasound probe for assessment of blood-flow in oesophageal varices. *Lancet* I:677–678, 1983.

88. Matthew JS, Jensen DM, Tapia JI, et al: Portal pressure measurement via endoscopy. (abstract) *Gastrointest Endosc* 29:190, 1983.

89. Crafoord C, Frenckner P: New surgical treatment of varicous veins of the oesophagus. *Acta Oto-Laryngol* 27:422–429, 1939.

90. Moersch HJ: Further studies on the treatment of esophageal varices by injection of a sclerosing solution. *Ann Otol Rhinol Laryngol* 50:1233–1244, 1941.

91. Patterson CO, Rouse MO: The sclerosing therapy of esophageal varices. *Gastroenterology* 9:391–395, 1947.

92. Samson PC, Foree L: Direct injection of esophageal varices through the esophagoscope. *West J Surg Obstet Gynecol* 50:73–77, 1942.

93. Macbeth R: Treatment of oesophageal varices in portal hypertension by means of sclerosing injections. *Br Med J* 2:877–880, 1955.

94. Kempe SG, Koch H: Injection of sclerosing solutions in the treatment of esophageal varices. *Acta Oto-Laryngol Suppl* 118:120–129, 1954.

95. Fearon B, Sass-Kortsak A: The management of esophageal varices in children by injection of sclerosing agents. *Ann Otol Rhinol Laryngol* 68:906–915, 1959.

96. Terblanche J, Northover JMA, Bornman P, et al: A prospective controlled trial of sclerotherapy in the long term management of patients after esophageal variceal bleeding. *Surg Gynecol Obstet* 148:323–333, 1979.

97. Sivak MV Jr, Williams GW: Endoscopic injection sclerosis (EIS) of esophageal varices: Analysis of survival and transfusion requirement. (abstract) *Gastrointest Endosc* 27:129, 1981.

98. Macdougall BRD, Westaby D, Theodossi A, et al: Increased long-term survival in variceal haemorrhage using injection sclerotherapy. Results of a controlled trial. *Lancet* I:124–127, 1982.

99. Larson AW, Chapman DJ, Radvan G, et al: Esophageal variceal sclerotherapy (EVS): Acute phase results of a prospective controlled trial. (abstract) *Gastrointest Endosc* 28:136, 1982.

100. Trudeau W, Gibbert V, Young W, et al: Child's C patients receiving endoscopic injection sclerosis of bleeding esophageal varices fare no better than patients receiving conventional therapy. (abstract) *Gastrointest Endosc* 28:148, 1982.

101. Trudeau W, Prindiville T, Gibbert V, et al: Endoscopic injection sclerosis in Child's C patients with bleeding gastroesophageal varices. (abstract) *Gastrointest Endosc* 29:168, 1983.

102. Hunt BL, Mitros FA, Lewis JW: Histologic changes in esophagus after injection sclerotherapy. (abstract) *Gastrointest Endosc* 28:137, 1982.

103. Fonkalsrud EW, Myers NA, Robinson MJ: Management of extrahepatic portal hypertension in children. *Ann Surg* 180:487–493, 1974.

104. Granditsch G, Schilling R, Wodak E: Sclerotherapy of cardia varices in a small child by means of a flexible gastroscope. *Z Kinderchir Grenzgeb* 30:283–285, 1980.

105. Lilly JR, Van Stiegmann G, Stellin G: Esophageal endosclerosis in children with portal vein thrombosis. *J Pediatr Surg* 17:571–575, 1982.

106. Sivak MV Jr: Unpublished survey in conjunction with ASGE Postgraduate Course, Chicago, May 1982.

107. Gebhard RL, Ansel HJ, Silvis SE: Origin of pain during variceal sclerotherapy. (abstract) *Gastrointest Endosc* 28:131, 1982.

108. Barsoum MS, Mooro HAW, Bolous FI, et al: The complications of injection sclerotherapy of bleeding oesophageal varices. *Br J Surg* 69:79–81, 1982.

109. Cohen LB, Korsten MA, Scherl EJ, et al: Bacteremia after endoscopic injection sclerosis. *Gastrointest Endosc* 29:198–200, 1983.

110. Monroe P, Morrow CF Jr, Millen JE, et al: Acute respiratory failure after sodium morrhuate esophageal sclerotherapy. *Gastroenterology* 85:693–699, 1983.

111. Califano NA: Endoscopic sclerosis of varices. (abstract) *Gastrointest Endosc* 29:160, 1983.

112. Ogle SJ, Kirk CJC, Bailey RJ, et al: Oesophageal function in cirrhotic patients undergoing injection sclerotherapy for oesophageal varices. *Digestion* 18:178–185, 1978.

113. Larson GM: Esophageal motility after injection sclerotherapy. (abstract) *Gastrointest Endosc* 29:164, 1983.

114. Simon C, Cohen L, Scherl E, et al: Esophageal motility and symptoms after endoscopic injection sclerotherapy. (abstract) *Gastrointest Endosc* 29:192, 1983.

115. Carr-Locke DL, Sidky K: Broncho-oesophageal fistula: A late complication of endoscopic variceal sclerotherapy. *Gut* 23:1005–1007, 1982.

116. Shepherd MM, Lee RG, Bowers JH: Local toxicity of sclerosing agents used in canine esophagus. (abstract) *Gastrointest Endosc* 29:188, 1983.

117. Trudeau W, Prindiville T, Gibbert V, et al: An update on the safety of sclerosing agents used in endoscopic injection sclerosis. (abstract) *Gastrointest Endosc* 29:168, 1983.

118. Brooks WS, Galambos JT: Sclerotherapy of esophageal varices: Postinjection ulceration. (abstract) *Gastrointest Endosc* 29:191, 1983.

119. Sanowski RA, Kozarek RA, Brayko C, et al: Esophageal variceal sclerotherapy (EVS): Course and complications. (abstract) *Gastrointest Endosc* 29:193, 1983.

120. Ayres SJ, Goff JS, Warren GH, et al: Esophageal ulceration and bleeding after flexible fiberoptic esophageal vein sclerosis. *Gastroenterology* 83:131–136, 1982.

121. Gardner EC, Brooks WS Jr: Absence of disseminated intravascular coagulation with endoscopic sclerosis of esophageal varices. *Gastrointest Endosc* 28:67–69, 1982.

122. Sauerbruch T, Weinzierl M, Dietrich HP, et al: Sclerotherapy of a bleeding duodenal varix. *Endoscopy* 14:187–189, 1982.

123. Bullimore DW: Sclerotherapist's eye. (Letter to the editor) *Gastrointest Endosc* 28:271, 1982.

124. Bat L, Shemesh E, Niv Y, et al: More about sclerotherapist's eye. (Letter to the editor) *Gastrointest Endosc* 28:271, 1982.

125. Brayko CM, Kozarek RA, Sanowski RA: Bacteremia during esophageal variceal sclerotherapy: Its cause and prevention. (abstract) *Gastrointest Endosc* 29:159–160, 1983.

126. Lange S, Laughlin B, Hughes RW, et al: Septic complications of variceal hemorrhage and ethanolamine sclerotherapy of varices. (abstract) *Gastrointest Endosc* 29:191, 1983.

3

Endoscopic Removal of Foreign Bodies

Patrick G. Brady

Ingestion of a foreign body may result in significant morbidity and mortality, with an estimated 1500 deaths related to this problem in the United States each year (1). Chevalier Jackson (2) published the classic article on management of foreign bodies of the esophagus with a rigid endoscope in 1937. This series was based on an analysis of 3266 cases. Rigid esophagoscopy under general anesthesia remained the procedure of choice for removal of esophageal foreign bodies until the past decade. Likewise, surgical removal via gastrotomy has been the standard therapy for foreign bodies and bezoars that failed to pass through the pylorus spontaneously. The first reports (3,4) of removal of gastrointestinal foreign bodies with a flexible fiberoptic endoscope appeared in 1972. Since then, improvements in flexible fiberoptic endoscopes and the development of foreign body forceps and snares designed for use with these instruments have made fiberendoscopic removal the procedure of choice for dealing with retained gastrointestinal foreign bodies. The literature is now replete with case reports and small series of fiberendoscopic removal of foreign bodies. However, information regarding general guidelines as well as detailed techniques, such as those established by Jackson for use with rigid endoscopes, are largely lacking for fiberendoscopic removal of foreign bodies. In this chapter, I will discuss these topics in relation to my personal experience as well as the literature.

ANATOMIC CONSIDERATIONS

A consideration of anatomic structures is essential to a proper understanding of the outcome of ingestion of foreign bodies. When a foreign body becomes impacted, it usually does so at areas of physiologic or pathologic narrowing.

Before entering the esophagus, the object must pass through the hy-popharynx. Pointed objects, such as small bones, may become impacted at this level, usually at the valleculae or in the piriform sinuses. These areas can be seen with a forward-viewing endoscope but are best evaluated by direct or indirect laryngoscopy.

There are four areas of physiologic narrowing in the esophagus. The first area is at the cricopharyngeal muscle, usually 15 cm from the incisor teeth. The cricopharyngeus and the few centimeters of the cervical segment of the esophagus immediately below it are a frequent site of impaction of foreign bodies (5–7). For this reason, when dealing with foreign bodies, it is important to pass a fiberoptic endoscope through the cricopharyngeus and into the esophagus under direct visual guidance to avoid further impaction or actual penetration of the esophageal wall by the foreign body as it is pushed distally by the instrument. Other areas of physiologic narrowing are at the aortic arch and the left main stem bronchus, which are 23 and 27 cm, respectively, from the incisor teeth. Objects that impact at the level of the aortic arch may pene-trate the esophageal wall, resulting in the formation of an aortoesophageal fistula. This catastrophic complication may present with a small herald bleed only to be followed at a later date by a massive, exsanguinating hemorrhage (6). The final area of narrowing lies at the level of the lower esophageal sphinc-ter, which is located just proximal to the esophagogastric junction.

Smaller, nonpointed foreign bodies usually lodge only transiently at points of physiologic narrowing in the esophagus. Failure of blunt objects (2.0 cm or less in width) to pass through the esophagus spontaneously should raise suspi-cion of stenosis or a motility disorder.

Once a foreign body has passed down the esophagus and entered the stomach, it usually continues through the remainder of the gastrointestinal tract without difficulty. The pylorus, the retroperitoneal, fixed angles of the duodenum, the ileocecal valve and the anus are potential levels at which ob-struction can occur. Common anomalies, such as Meckel's diverticulum, or less common ones, such as annular pancreas or duodenal diaphragm, may provide sites of impaction (8). Pathologic processes, such as benign and malignant strictures and tumors, and prior surgical intervention predispose to impaction. Bowel in a hernia sac also provides a potential site of impaction (9).

TYPES OF FOREIGN BODIES

Foreign bodies can be divided into two basic groups. Substances foreign to the gastrointestinal tract comprise the first group and include inorganic objects, such as coins, toys, nails and safety pins. This group will be referred to as true foreign bodies. It accounts for most foreign bodies found in children but fewer of those encountered in adults, with the exception of specific high-risk groups. A subgroup of true foreign bodies are those of iatrogenic origin, which are being seen with increasing frequency. Such foreign bodies include dental instruments, parts of nebulizers, tubes, prosthetic devices and biopsy instruments, for example, small-bowel capsules that have been inadvertently swallowed or lost in the gastrointestinal tract (10–13). True foreign bodies should be characterized as sharp or dull, pointed or blunt and toxic or nontoxic. Their length and width should be measured. These features along with the location of a true foreign body determine whether endoscopic removal is indicated.

Food-related foreign bodies constitute the second major group. They are most frequently found in older adults, who often have a history of preexisting gastrointestinal disease. This category includes impaction of food boluses in the esophagus, bones and phytobezoars. Medication may lodge in the esophagus, particularly in patients with an underlying motility disorder or stenosis. Although this occurrence usually presents as "pill esophagitis," hydrophilic colloid may cause obstruction of the esophagus by the bolus and present in an identical fashion to impaction of a food bolus.

PATIENT PROFILE

In most instances, ingestion of true foreign bodies probably occurs in children, particularly those between 1 and 5 years of age, who swallow them accidentally (14). Fortunately, most ingested true foreign bodies are small, blunt and nontoxic, for example, coins and small toys. Therefore, removal of foreign bodies in younger children is infrequently necessary. Occasionally, however, sharp, pointed or toxic foreign bodies may be ingested, and such objects can be safely removed with a flexible fiberoptic endoscope (15).

Five groups of adults are most prone to ingest foreign bodies or to suffer from impaction of food boluses. The five groups are persons with esophageal disease, alcoholism, psychopathologic disorders, mental retardation and prisoners (16,17). Impaction of a food bolus in the esophagus strongly suggests underlying esophageal disease. In a review of 18 patients who presented with esophageal impaction of food boluses, the author and his colleagues (16) found that 72% of the patients had a history of a documented esophageal stricture or long-standing dysphagia. Endoscopic evaluation showed that 78% of these patients had either an esophageal stricture or other serious esophageal disease directly responsible for the impaction (Table 1). Although 28% of the patients

TABLE 1. Endoscopic Findings in 18 Patients with Esophageal Impaction of Food Boluses

	Number	Percentage
Esophageal stricture	12	67
Squamous cell papilloma	1	6
Carcinoma	1	6

TABLE 2. Social History in Adults with Foreign
Bodies

Social History	True Foreign Body (20)	Food Bolus Impaction (38)
Alcohol abuse	7	6
Prisoner	9	1
Psychiatric disorders	11	—
Suicide attempts	6	—

wore dentures, in the author's experience, the underlying esophageal disease
contributed more to the development of impaction than did the dentures (16).
Dentures may, however, interfere with normal oral sensation and in this fashion contribute to the inadvertent ingestion of bones or such objects as toothpicks (17).

Adults who ingest true foreign bodies as opposed to those with impaction of
food boluses usually are younger and have no history of gastrointestinal disease, although they frequently have significant social histories (Table 2). Prisoners and persons with psychiatric disorders may intentionally swallow a
foreign body for the secondary gains associated with hospitalization and medical attention. Such patients also may ingest another foreign body during hospitalization in hopes of prolonging it. Therefore, it is necessary to keep such
patients under observation to avoid this problem.

CLINICAL PRESENTATION

Patients who have swallowed a foreign body may present with a wide range of
signs and symptoms. Many patients are fully aware of what has transpired and
give a clear history of the ingestion episode, including an exact description of
the foreign body. However, some patients are unaware that they have ingested
a foreign body and present with symptoms relating to a complication. A careful
history is helpful in arriving at a correct diagnosis in cases that are not obvious.
Esophageal foreign bodies may cause odynophagia, dysphagia or complete
esophageal obstruction with regurgitation and sialorrhea. A history of sudden
onset of odynophagia or dysphagia after eating or drinking should suggest the
possibility of impaction of a bone, aluminum can poptop, swizzle stick or
toothpick in the esophagus (17–19). Acute esophageal obstruction in a patient
with underlying esophageal disease suggests impaction of a food bolus at a
narrowed area in the lumen. Younger children and psychotic patients may be
unable to give an adequate history, and a high index of suspicion must be
exercised in such patients when there are signs and symptoms of esophageal
injury. Infants and younger children may present only with refusal to take
feedings or with chronic pulmonary aspiration.

Retained gastric foreign bodies may be completely asymptomatic, or they may present with subtle symptoms, for example, early satiety, long before such complications as obstruction, perforation and hemorrhage occur. The combination of pain and fever suggests perforation, which may be free and associated with peritoneal signs or confined with minimal or no abdominal signs. A history of unexplained hair loss associated with abdominal symptoms should raise suspicion of a trichobezoar.

Delays of weeks, or rarely years, may occur before a patient presents with symptoms relating to ingestion of a foreign body. A long-standing foreign body may result in free perforation, confined perforation with abscess formation or injury to adjacent solid organs or vascular structures due to migration of the object (20). Toxic foreign bodies may be ingested, particularly by children, resulting in either acute or chronic toxic reactions. Copper, lead and nickel poisoning have been reported after retention of metallic foreign bodies (21,22). Small alkaline disk batteries may cause corrosive injury, resulting in perforation (23,24). Yellow or orange wax crayons may contain paranitroaniline, a dye that can produce methemoglobinemia (25). At the time of presentation, an effort should be made to determine whether the ingested foreign body is potentially toxic.

Physical examination is important in assessing a patient's general condition and in detecting complications. Subcutaneous emphysema is an indication of perforation of the esophagus or hypopharynx. Large gastric foreign bodies rarely are palpable, and definitive diagnosis usually requires radiographic confirmation.

RADIOGRAPHIC EVALUATION

After a thorough history and physical examination have been completed, the first diagnostic study that should be obtained is a plain radiograph. Plain films of the neck, chest and abdomen should be taken in the posteroanterior and lateral projections to localize the positions of radiopaque foreign bodies. Lateral films of the neck are particularly important in recognizing bone fragments impacted in the cervical segment of the esophagus, which are obscured by the cervical spine in posteroanterior projections (Fig. 1). When a flat foreign body, such as a coin, is detected on an x-ray film of the chest, the question arises as to whether it is located in the upper portion of the esophagus or in the trachea. If the object is impacted in the trachea, it orients itself in a sagittal plane, whereas it is oriented in the frontal plane when it is in the esophagus. More than one foreign body may be present, even when a patient gives a history of ingesting only one foreign body, and additional foreign bodies should be carefully looked for on plain radiographs (Fig. 2).

Perforation may be manifest on plain radiographs in a number of ways. Esophageal perforation may result in subcutaneous air, particularly in the cervical and supraclavicular areas, pneumomediastinum, pleural effusion and,

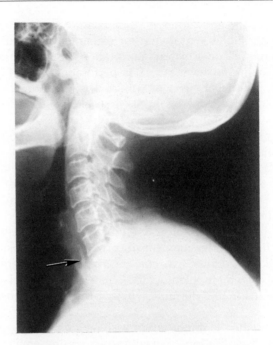

Fig. 1. A chicken bone impacted in the cervical portion of the esophagus. The bone was not seen in the posteroanterior projection because of the overlying cervical spine. On close observation, the bone is recognizable (arrow) in the lateral projection.

occasionally, pneumothorax. Gastric or duodenal perforation may present with free air under the diaphragm or with retroperitoneal air if the perforation is in the fixed duodenum. Mediastinal or retroperitoneal air may dissect widely in either direction, making it difficult to determine the exact site of perforation. In addition the foreign body may be clearly seen projecting beyond the wall of the viscus in the absence of other radiographic signs of perforation (Fig. 3). Finally, a soft-tissue mass, indicating confined perforation with local abscess formation, may be detected.

Many foreign bodies, such as glass, wood, plastics and meat boluses, are not radiopaque. Some thin, metallic foreign bodies, particularly aluminum bottle and can tops, cannot be seen on plain radiographs (18). Some foreign bodies may be composed of both radiopaque and radiolucent materials, leading to an underestimation of the size of the object on plain radiographs. Under these circumstances, particular attention must be given to the history, and a duplicate foreign body should be obtained and examined, if possible. Careful examination of soft-tissue films may be helpful. Under these circumstances, xeroradiography, well developed for mammography, is an excellent technique

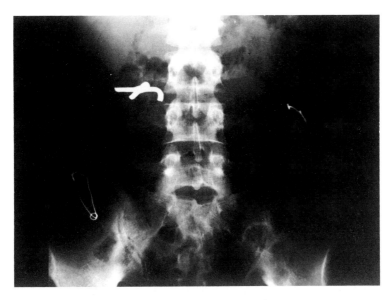

Fig. 2. A number of foreign bodies in a patient admitting to the ingestion of only one object.

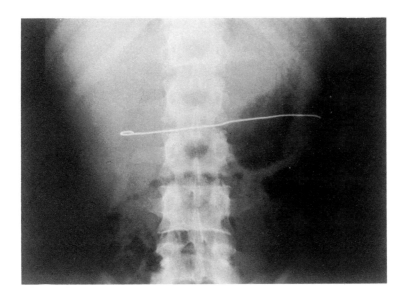

Fig. 3. An elongated, narrow foreign body (wire) whose sharp end is clearly seen projecting beyond the gastric wall. The hooked end has passed through the pylorus into the duodenum.

for visualizing the soft tissues of the neck and may clearly show foreign bodies not evident on a plain film (26).

Contrast studies may be required for detecting and evaluating radiolucent foreign bodies or for determining whether perforation has occurred and, if so, the site of the perforation. However, these studies are not required in all instances of ingestion of radiolucent foreign bodies and in some circumstances are contraindicated. When a patient presents with a history consistent with impaction of a food bolus and sialorrhea, the foreign body usually is located at or just below the cricopharyngeal muscle. A barium swallow adds little to the diagnosis, may result in aspiration and will render endoscopic removal more difficult. Therefore, barium studies should be avoided under these circumstances, and endoscopic removal should be done immediately after plain radiographs have been obtained because the latter alert the endoscopist to the presence of bone fragments.

In the case of a lower esophageal radiolucent foreign body, a barium esophagogram has the potential advantage of confirming the presence, size and exact location of the object. However, the disadvantage of coating the object with barium, thus obscuring its borders and compounding the difficulty of endoscopic extraction, remains. In practice, most lower esophageal impactions of food boluses are studied with barium before referral to an endoscopist takes place. If barium is used, it should be given slowly and in small sips to avoid aspiration. A thin suspension of barium is preferable because any residual may be removed by suction applied through a small esophageal tube or the channel of a flexible endoscope. The use of a cotton ball impregnated with barium should be avoided because it adds one more foreign body that may require extraction.

Gastrografin is a water-soluble contrast agent that is extremely hypertonic. If it is aspirated, pulmonary edema results (19). It is the contrast agent of choice for localizing a site of perforation but should not be used in an obstructed esophagus because of the potential for aspiration. If esophageal perforation is highly suspected and a Gastrografin swallow fails to reveal it, barium may be used in an attempt to localize a site of leakage. Endoscopy is rarely useful in detecting a site of perforation unless the foreign body is impacted at the site. If a perforation cannot be demonstrated by contrast agents and the patient is afebrile with a normal white cell count, conservative therapy may be employed despite the presence of mediastinal or subcutaneous air. If a site of leakage has been identified, surgical drainage is indicated.

INDICATIONS FOR ENDOSCOPIC REMOVAL

Once a foreign body has been localized, a decision must be made regarding removal as opposed to observation. It has been estimated that 70% of ingested foreign bodies pass through the gastrointestinal tract spontaneously and that only 1% or less result in perforation (7,20,27). However, highly selected series have reported overall incidences of perforation as high as 8%, and the incidence of perforation may increase to as high as 35% if only sharp or pointed foreign bodies are considered (16,28,29).

Impaction of a large piece of meat at or just below the cricopharyngeus with anterior compression of the trachea that causes respiratory obstruction, the so-called cafe coronary, is a true emergency situation (30,31). Obstruction of the esophagus by a food bolus at lower levels also requires prompt attention because of the potential for aspiration and other complications, the exception being impaction of a food bolus in the lower third of the esophagus without associated bones. Spitz (14) reported that 72% of rounded objects initially found in the lower third of the esophagus passed into the stomach spontaneously.

From a consideration of these factors and the nature of the foreign body, general guidelines for endoscopic removal can be developed. Endoscopic removal is indicated for all esophageal foreign bodies. If high-grade obstruction is not present, a delay of 12 hours is reasonable when a rounded foreign body is demonstrated in the lower third of the esophagus because of the high rate of spontaneous passage into the stomach. If a meat bolus has impacted in the lower third of the esophagus, a delay to permit spontaneous passage allows softening of the bolus, making it virtually impossible to extract in one piece. This phenomenon must be taken into consideration when timing endoscopic intervention for removal of impacted meat boluses from the distal portion of the esophagus.

Sharp or pointed foreign bodies, such as toothpicks, safety pins and razor blades, should be removed endoscopically, even if they have entered the stomach, because of the increased potential for complications with such objects. Long, narrow objects, such as wires, may not be able to negotiate the fixed duodenal angles and therefore should be removed endoscopically, if possible. Murat and colleagues (32) recommend removal of foreign bodies more than 6 cm in length in children and more than 13 cm in length in adults. Gastric foreign bodies greater than 2 cm in diameter may not pass through the pylorus, although if they are rounded or blunt, a period of observation is both safe and worthwhile. The author has seen quarters and a Susan B.Anthony dollar pass spontaneously, even though these coins have a diameter of 2.5 cm. Toxic foreign bodies, such as alkaline button batteries, should be removed endoscopically, if possible.

Although endoscopic removal has been recommended if an ingested foreign body does not leave the stomach within 48 to 72 hours (33), the author believes that rounded or blunt gastric foreign bodies may be managed more conservatively and recommends a 2-week period of observation. Observation should be ended for prolonged delays in the duodenum of more than 6 days for blunt objects (32,34). Although the average time for an object to traverse the gastrointestinal tract is approximately 5 days, the time depends to a large degree on the size and shape of an object (14,35). Table 3 illustrates the time required for five

TABLE 3. Time for Passage of True Foreign Bodies

Description	Number of days
Piece of iron grating 2.5 × 5 cm	3
Single-edge razor blade	5
Two halves of broken razor blade	10
X-shaped metal object 2 × 4 cm	11
Opened paper clip	18
	Average 9.4

foreign bodies, initially localized beyond the pylorus, to traverse the gastrointestinal tract spontaneously.

INSTRUMENT SELECTION AND PREPARATION

Once a foreign body has been localized, the instruments required for its removal must be chosen. Hypopharyngeal foreign bodies are best removed under direct visual guidance with a laryngoscope and curved forceps, such as a Kelly clamp. A forward-viewing fiberoptic endoscope is the instrument of choice for removing esophageal and gastroduodenal foreign bodies because it possesses the following advantages when compared with a rigid endoscope: general anesthesia usually is not required, patient acceptance and comfort are greater, visualization and maneuverability are enhanced and otherwise inaccessible areas, such as the antrum and duodenum, can easily be evaluated.

Forward-viewing fiberoptic endoscopes with one or two channels are available. The two-channel endoscope has a number of theoretical advantages. It enables the operator to use two grasping instruments simultaneously, it has a larger diameter, which dilates the esophageal lumen before a foreign body is withdrawn through it, and it enables the operator to have one channel free for suction when a single foreign body forceps is in use. Thus far, these advantages remain theoretical, and no study has demonstrated superiority of a two-channel endoscope or a single large-channel endoscope over a standard instrument. In two series involving the removal of 28 true foreign bodies, the author has used a two-channel endoscope on four occasions (16,36,37). It was most useful for removing elongated gastric foreign bodies, which necessitated the simultaneous use of a grasping forceps to pull the object away from the gastric wall and a snare to grasp the end of the object firmly. In infants and younger children, an endoscope 9.5 mm or less in diameter should be used.

The use of a protective plastic overtube should be considered when sharp or pointed foreign bodies must be removed and when the endoscope must be passed several times, for example, for removing a soft meat bolus piecemeal (38,39). The overtube serves to protect the mucosa from injury during withdrawal of the foreign body or during repeated passages of the endoscope through the hypopharynx and esophagus. Overtubes may be purchased commercially or made from Tygon tubing approximately 2 mm larger in internal diameter than the outside diameter of an endoscope. For use in the stomach, an overtube should be at least 60 cm long, whereas shorter overtubes suffice for esophageal use. The end of an overtube should be beveled smooth to facilitate passage and to prevent trauma from sharp edges. The inside of the overtube should be liberally lubricated when in use to allow easy passage of the endoscope through it. The overtube is first loaded over the endoscope up to the control handle, the endoscope is then inserted in the usual manner and the overtube is advanced over it as needed. When a foreign body is being withdrawn, the overtube remains in place, thus protecting the mucosal surface (Fig. 4).

A variety of foreign body forceps are available for use with fiberoptic endoscopes (Fig. 5). Endoscopists who plan to remove foreign bodies should have several such forceps available for immediate use. Standard endoscopic biopsy forceps are not generally useful for removing foreign bodies, except for objects with a small central opening, through which closed biopsy forceps will pass but opened forceps will not (Fig. 6). Polypectomy snares are the most versatile instruments for removal of foreign bodies. It is helpful to have snares available in several shapes and sizes. Baskets are less frequently required but are helpful in extracting smooth, rounded objects and meat boluses. Flat, metallic foreign bodies can be grasped with an alligator or similar forceps as well as with a snare. Available coin-grasping forceps are inferior to these instruments because they provide a weak grasp of the foreign body, which is therefore liable to fall off at points of anatomic narrowing. A Kelly clamp and laryngoscope should always be available when extraction of a foreign body is attempted for use in retrieving any object that is inadvertently dropped in the hypopharynx.

Proper preparation for removal of foreign bodies is essential for success. Preparation should include preliminary radiographic evaluation, as previously described. If there has been a delay of several hours or more between the initial radiographs and endoscopy, repeat plain films should be taken to ensure that the location of the radiopaque foreign body has not changed. Duplication of the foreign body and simulation of removal with a model are highly desirable. It is particularly important to test the available grasping forceps on a duplicate of the foreign body to determine which instrument is best suited in a particular case. This approach shortens the procedure time and helps ensure success. Foreign bodies should be removed promptly when indicated. However, endoscopists have time to review the literature regarding experience with similar cases if they are not familiar with extraction of the type of foreign body that is encountered.

Careful explanation of the procedure to the patient and adequate premedication allay anxiety and enhance cooperation. Atropine is useful in patients with esophageal obstruction and sialorrhea. It should be given in a dose of at least 0.6 mg in adults. The author has used meperidine and diazepam for sedation, with good results. Both medications can be given intravenously immediately before the procedure, allowing titration to the desired degree of sedation. The

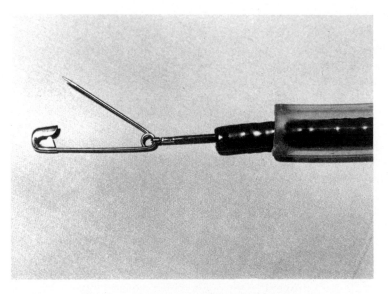

Fig. 4a. An opened safety pin grasped firmly with a foreign body forceps before withdrawal through an overtube.

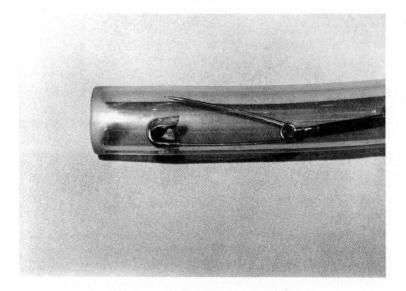

Fig. 4b. The safety pin has now been totally withdrawn into the overtube to avoid exposing mucosal surfaces to its sharp point.

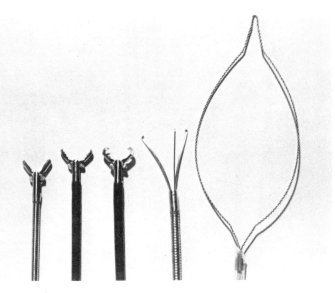

Fig. 5. A variety of instruments for removal of foreign bodies is available. From left to right are pictured a rubber-clad forceps, an alligator forceps, a rat-toothed forceps, a three-pronged forceps and a polypectomy snare.

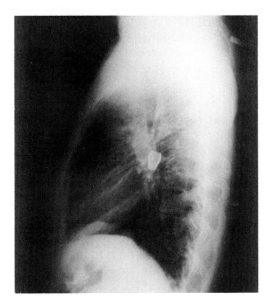

Fig. 6a. A nebulizer tip impacted in the midportion of the esophagus.

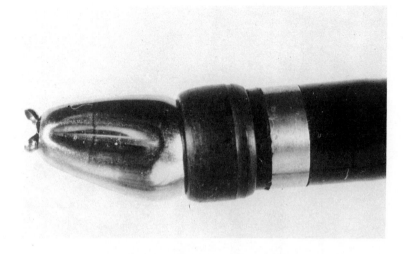

Fig. 6b. A method for removal of the nebulizer tip is demonstrated. The closed forceps easily passed through the central opening, but the opened forceps would not.

effect of meperidine can be readily reversed by naloxone, but no uniformly effective antagonist of diazepam is available. Although general anesthesia is rarely necessary for removal of foreign bodies with fiberoptic endoscopes, it may be required in younger children or uncooperative psychotic patients.

TECHNIQUES OF REMOVAL

ESOPHAGEAL FOREIGN BODIES

Safe extraction of an esophageal foreign body requires an adequate preliminary evaluation and the selection of proper equipment, including a grasping forceps or snare, as described in previous sections. The endoscope should be passed through the hypopharynx and cricopharyngeus under direct visual guidance to avoid inadvertently striking a foreign body and causing penetration of the esophageal wall. Extraction of a foreign body, once it has been located, requires good visibility, firm grasp of the object and removal without force. When grasped, most objects can be pulled back to the tip of the endoscope, and then the object and endoscope can be gently removed simultaneously. If the diameter of the object is smaller than the diameter of the endoscope, the tip of the instrument will offer some protection to the mucosa during withdrawal by keeping the lumen patent proximal to the foreign body. Pointed foreign bodies, such as bones and pins, should be withdrawn with the point trailing because advancing points perforate but trailing points do not (2). Objects with a sharp edge, such as half of a double-edged razor blade, should be extracted with the aid of an overtube to prevent mucosal laceration. Particular attention must be given to removal of a foreign body through the hypopharynx because loss of an object in this area may result in its aspiration. The endoscopist should have a curved clamp available to assist in extraction and should position the patient in the left lateral position with his or her head down. A Foley catheter should not be used to extract esophageal foreign bodies blindly. This technique is potentially hazardous because the lack of visual control makes perforation more likely if the object is sharp and because the lack of a firm grasp increases the likelihood of pulmonary aspiration.

Commonly encountered esophageal foreign bodies are impactions of meat boluses, safety pins and coins. Each of these types of foreign body will be considered in greater detail.

Meat Bolus Impactions

Impaction of a meat bolus in the esophagus is a common problem in older adults and frequently is associated with underlying esophageal stenosis (16). Suggestions for dealing with this problem have included pushing the bolus into the stomach blindly with a bougie, using a digestive agent and administering glucagon. Blind pushing of the bolus should not be attempted. The high incidence of underlying esophageal disease increases the probability of perforation with this method.

Enzymatic digestion of a meat bolus with papain, commercially available as Adolph's meat tenderizer, may be effective (38,39). However, this technique has two major drawbacks. First, an unsuccessful attempt renders subsequent endoscopic removal difficult because a snare or grasping forceps simply cuts through the softened bolus. Secondly, and more importantly, papain may digest the esophageal wall as well as the bolus. This effect is more likely to occur if there has been mucosal trauma from a bone fragment, if the integrity of the underlying mucosa is lost, as in peptic esophagitis, or if the bolus has been in place long enough to cause ischemia of the wall. Two deaths related to the use of papain have been reported. Anderson and colleagues (40) reported a perforation and subsequent death resulting from the use of a papain solution (caroid). Holsinger and associates (41) reported that a patient given papain 8 hours after the initial impaction of a meat bolus died. In the latter report, 27 patients had been treated successfully before perforation was encountered in the 28th patient. For these reasons, the use of papain in any form is not recommended.

Glucagon may be useful in the management of impaction of meat boluses in the lower two-thirds of the esophagus (42). Exogenous glucagon has an inhibitory effect on the lower esophageal sphincter, and this agent also is known to be helpful in overcoming smooth muscle spasm during radiologic examinations of the alimentary tract. The recommended dose is 1 mg intravenously, but smaller doses may be effective. The medication should be given slowly to avoid the side effects of nausea and vomiting. An unsuccessful trial of gluca-gon does not interfere with subsequent endoscopic removal. Glucagon also may be used at the time of endoscopy to relieve spasm in the lower portion of the esophagus, improving visualization.

If a meat bolus does not pass spontaneously or after a trial of glucagon, endoscopic removal is the procedure of choice. If endoscopy is performed within several hours of impaction, it usually is possible to remove the entire bolus in one piece with a snare or Dormia basket. If there has been a delay in endoscopy or if the patient has received papain, the bolus will be soft, neces-sitating piecemeal removal in small fragments. Because the piecemeal ap-proach can only be accomplished with several passages of an endoscope, the use of an overtube is advantageous (43).

Two additional endoscopic techniques may be useful in certain situations. If an endoscope can be worked around the meat bolus and the distal segment of the esophagus is found to be normal, the instrument can be withdrawn prox-imal to the bolus, which can then be gently pushed into the stomach. This method is contraindicated if bone fragments are present or if more than minimal resistance is encountered. If the bolus is soft and fragmented, the proximal end of a standard nasogastric tube may be passed alongside the endoscope and advanced over the foreign body under direct visual guidance. With the application of suction, large quantities of food can be removed with the endoscope left in place while the nasogastric tube is passed repeatedly (44). Because the proximal end of a nasogastric tube may have sharp edges, round-ing off the edges with an emory board helps avoid inadvertent mucosal injury.

Sharp and Pointed Foreign Bodies

Pointed foreign bodies include toothpicks, nails, needles and bones. These objects should be removed with the sharp point trailing to avoid mucosal laceration or perforation. If the object is pointed at both ends (toothpick), the proximal sharp end must be completely covered by the grasping forceps (Fig. 7). If the object has a single pointed end and is directed cephalad, it can be carried into the stomach and turned so that the pointed end trails before it is removed.

At least four techniques have been successfully used to extract opened safety pins from the esophagus and stomach. Griswold and coworkers (45) reported recovering an opened safety pin from the stomach by inserting the closed biopsy forceps through the hole in the spring and opening it. The safety pin was then withdrawn with the point trailing under direct visual guidance. No trauma resulted. In removing an opened safety pin from the esophagus with the point directed cephalad, the pin should be grasped, carried into the stomach and turned so that the pointed end trails during removal. Safety pin closure has been successfully accomplished with a snare before extraction (46). This maneuver is difficult and should be practiced with an identical safety pin before endoscopy is begun. The use of an overtube provides an added degree of safety with all pointed foreign bodies, particularly large safety pins. Success-ful removal of a safety pin through an overtube has been reported (47). The

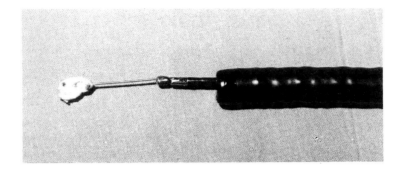

Fig. 7. This homemade blowgun dart made from a straight pin was accidentally swallowed. The point of the pin was grasped and completely covered by an alligator forceps, allowing safe withdrawal.

specific technique selected depends on the size of the safety pin, its position in the esophagus or stomach and the experience and preference of the endoscopist.

Coins

Coins, washers, buttons and other flat foreign bodies frequently are encountered in children and occasionally are seen in adults. Coins cannot be removed with the standard endoscopic biopsy forceps because the small jaws of this instrument easily slip off the metallic surface. However, coins can easily be removed when necessary by use of an alligator forceps, a snare or a specially designed coin-grasping forceps (48). Once firmly grasped, the coin and endoscope are removed simultaneously under direct visual guidance. In the esophagus, the coin should be rotated so that it lies in the coronal plane. This plane represents the widest diameter of the cervical segment of the esophagus and the hypopharynx, and it facilitates passage through these structures without the use of undue traction or loss of the object at points of anatomic narrowing.

GASTRODUODENAL FOREIGN BODIES

The techniques described for the removal of esophageal foreign bodies are generally applicable for gastric foreign bodies. The snare is the most versatile grasping instrument employed for the removal of gastric foreign bodies (49,50), but grasping forceps and Dormia baskets also are useful. Pointed objects, such as needles and pins, that are embedded in or penetrating the gastric wall may be removed by endoscopy alone, provided that free perforation or local abscess formation has not occurred (49,51,52).

Duodenal foreign bodies are more difficult to remove than are gastric foreign bodies because of the limited space for maneuvering, the fixed angles of the duodenum and the inability to use an overtube in this area. Despite these limitations, successful endoscopic removal of foreign bodies from the duodenum has frequently been reported (35,53). Intravenous glucagon (0.25 mg) may be administered during removal of a foreign body from the stomach or duodenum to relax the area and to obtain better visualization.

Elongated Foreign Bodies

Long, narrow objects, such as opened paper clips and stiff pieces of wire, are associated with a high incidence of perforation because they are unable to negotiate the fixed curves of the duodenum. In a series of 40 episodes of foreign body ingestion, two of the three perforations that were encountered involved wires longer than 13 cm (Fig. 3) (16). When such a foreign body is encountered, early endoscopic extraction is indicated. The snare is the grasping instrument of choice in this situation, regardless of whether the elongated object lies in the stomach (49–51) or the esophagus (54) or straddles the pylorus. If the end of the object is impacted against the gastric wall, preventing capture, changing the patient from a left lateral to a supine position usually frees the end of the object so that it can be snared. Alternatively, a two-channel endoscope may be used, allowing the endoscopist to pull the elongated object away from the gastric wall with a grasping forceps and simultaneously snare it, making use of the second instrument channel. The snare should be placed close to the cephalad end of the object so that during withdrawal, the long axis of the object may align itself with the long axis of the esophagus (Fig. 8). The object should be extracted under direct visual guidance and maintained at a distance no greater than 3 cm from the end of the endoscope. If the object is elongated and stiff, it may be difficult to withdraw through the hypopharynx. Manual extraction with a Kelly clamp, in which the patient's head is tilted backward and the neck is moved forward to create a straight passage from the cervical portion of the esophagus to the mouth, is a useful technique.

Razor Blades

Razor blades are commonly ingested objects that have sharp edges. In most instances, razor blades are swallowed by adults who have psychiatric disorders or who are prisoners. Either injector blades or double-edged blades that have been broken in half may be swallowed. The blades frequently are wrapped in toilet or tissue paper to protect the mouth and tongue during swallowing. Razor blades pass rapidly through the esophagus and usually are found in the stomach or small bowel at the time of presentation.

Injector razor blades may be removed with a snare by use of the previously described techniques. A broken double-edged blade must be removed with the aid of an overtube (37). This type of razor blade should not be removed from the duodenum because presently available overtubes are not suitable for use in this area and because unprotected withdrawal in essence places a handle on a sharp instrument, risking laceration and perforation. Surprisingly enough, swallowing razor blades is not associated with a high incidence of perforation (55), and therefore endoscopists must be absolutely certain that removal can be safely accomplished before undertaking the procedure.

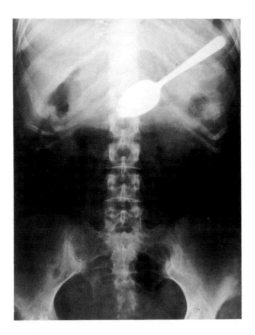

Fig. 8a. A plain abdominal radiograph demonstrates a spoon in the stomach.

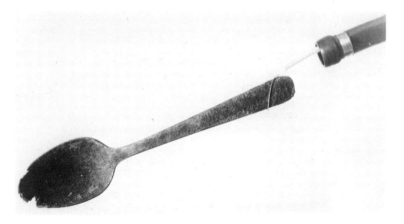

Fig. 8b. A snare has been placed correctly for removal of this elongated foreign body.

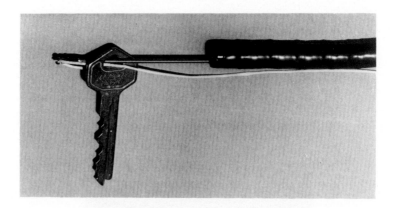

Fig. 9a. Removal of a foreign body that has a large opening. A biopsy forceps and a silk line have been inserted through the opening in the key.

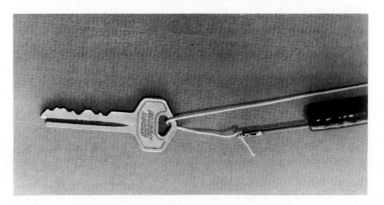

Fig. 9b. After withdrawal of the forceps, the line has been regrasped to form a complete loop. The endoscope and key may now be withdrawn simultaneously.

MISCELLANEOUS FOREIGN BODIES

A technique has been described for the removal of large objects that have a hole or a large central opening, for example, a ring or key (Fig. 9) (56). This technique entails grasping a line (silk thread or umbilical tape) with a biopsy forceps that has been passed through the biopsy channel of an endoscope. The forceps is then retracted into the end of the biopsy channel, and the line is brought along the outside of the endoscope. The entire apparatus is passed into the stomach, and the forceps is inserted through the hole in the foreign body under direct visual guidance. The forceps is then opened, and the line is released. After the forceps has been closed, it is retracted through the hole, leaving the line behind. Finally, the free end of the line is grasped and retracted into the biopsy channel to form a closed loop that holds the foreign body. The entire assembly is withdrawn together. This technique is useful for large objects with a hole that cannot be grasped with a foreign body forceps or snare.

GASTRIC BEZOARS

Gastric phytobezoars usually are found in patients with disorders of gastric motility. Surgical vagotomy and diabetic autonomic neuropathy are the most common causes of altered gastric motility encountered in practice. Both disorders are associated with delayed gastric emptying of solids. When accompanied by the ingestion of vegetable matter, such as citrus fruits, celery and vegetable or fruit skins and seeds, delayed gastric emptying of solids may result in the eventual formation of a gastric phytobezoar. Gastric outlet obstruction, although associated with delayed emptying, is rarely a cause of phytobezoar formation.

A persimmon bezoar (diospyrobezoar) results from the ingestion of unripened persimmons. These berries contain a juice that has large amounts of pectin and gum; these components of the juice form a coagulum when gastric acid is encountered. Unripe persimmons are one of the few materials that can form a bezoar in a normal stomach after a single ingestion. Persimmon bezoars are encountered less frequently than are other phytobezoars.

Trichobezoars, or hair balls, form in the stomachs of habitual hair swallowers, usually young women with otherwise normal stomachs. Trichobezoars are associated with a high incidence of complications, including gastric outlet obstruction, perforation and bleeding.

The type of therapy employed for a gastric bezoar depends on the type of bezoar encountered. Phytobezoars usually require endoscopy for a definitive diagnosis. At the time of initial endoscopy, mechanical fragmentation with a biopsy forceps or snare, followed by a liquid diet, results in resolution of the bezoar, in most cases within 48 hours (57,58). Alternatively, mechanical disruption of the bezoar may be achieved with a Water Pik adapted to the biopsy channel of an endoscope (59). The resultant water jet can be directed at the bezoar under visual guidance.

A variety of other nonsurgical methods have been successful in the management of gastric phytobezoars. Examples are enzymatic dissolution and the use of metoclopramide to restore normal gastric emptying. Cellulase is an enzyme that is capable of dissolving plant cellulose, and it has been used successfully to manage gastric phytobezoars (60). Cellulase usually is given with meals in a dose of 75 mg dissolved in water. Direct endoscopic injection of cellulase into a bezoar through a polyethylene catheter also has been employed with success after therapy with oral cellulase had failed (61). Acetylcysteine also may be injected directly into a phytobezoar under endoscopic guidance. This approach is useful if the plant material is held together by viscous mucus, but it has no effect on a tightly compacted bezoar with little or no mucous component.

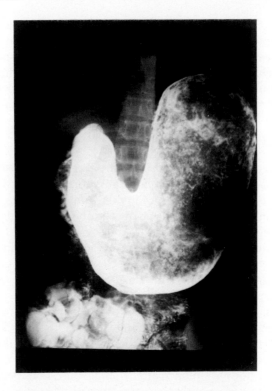

Fig. 10. A radiograph of a large trichobezoar that formed a cast of the stomach
and proximal portion of the duodenum.
The intertwined hair could not be removed by endoscopic methods.

Papain has been employed successfully in the management of persimmon
bezoars but not of other types of phytobezoars (62). The use of papain should
be reserved for persimmon bezoars that are resistant to mechanical disruption
because papain is a proteolytic enzyme that has an ulcerogenic potential in the
esophagus and stomach.

Once a phytobezoar has resolved, therapy must be instituted to prevent
recurrence. Therapy should include a low-fiber diet, eliminating such foods as
citrus fruits and stringy vegetables, which are frequent components of phytobezoars. Also, an attempt should be made to correct any underlying motility
disorder with metoclopramide, bethanecol or a combination of the two agents.

Small trichobezoars may be removed endoscopically with a foreign body
forceps or snare. Large trichobezoars cannot be removed with endoscopic
methods because the entwined hair prevents fragmentation of the large bezoar
into small components suitable for removal (Fig. 10). Because no dissolving
agent is useful in this situation, large trichobezoars must be removed surgically.

RECTAL AND COLONIC FOREIGN BODIES

Rectal and colonic foreign bodies can be divided into two major groups: those that have been ingested and those that have been inserted through the anal canal. As has been discussed previously, foreign bodies that have been swallowed may pass through the upper gastrointestinal tract only to become impacted in the colon, most frequently at the level of the ileocecal valve or in the rectosigmoid. Inserted foreign bodies may include large and bizarre objects, such as bottles, fruits and light bulbs. Such large objects can be extracted only after the anal canal has been relaxed by local or general anesthesia. Large objects are best removed with the use of large-caliber rigid instruments, provided that they have not migrated too far proximally. If such a large object lies proximal to the rectum, the patient may be sedated and kept on bed rest until it passes spontaneously into the rectum, where extraction may be attempted.

Ingested and small inserted foreign bodies are suitable for removal with flexible fiberoptic colonoscopes. A partial list of objects removed from the colon with these instruments includes dental prostheses, dental instruments, safety-pins, rubber tubing and water-filled balloons (63–65). Most ingested foreign bodies that have passed through the ileocecal valve traverse the colon without difficulty and should be managed conservatively. Indications for removal include prolonged hangup at the ileocecal valve, obstruction, confined perforation and the presence of an elongated or pointed foreign body. Confined perforation or fistula formation does not appear to be a contraindication to endoscopic removal, as indicated by closure of a colocutaneous fistula after removal of a foreign body in one report (66). Biopsy, pronged polyp grasping and special foreign body forceps may all be useful in removing colonic foreign bodies, but the polypectomy snare is the most versatile instrument, and it has been used in most cases to date. Although most reports of removal of colonic foreign bodies describe individual cases, Viceconte and colleagues (63) have recently reported successful extraction of 18 foreign bodies from 15 patients ranging in age from 15 months to 84 years, indicating that this procedure can be consistently applied to properly selected cases.

COMPLICATIONS AND RESULTS

Diagnostic esophagogastroduodenoscopy is a safe procedure, having a complication rate of only 1.3 per 1000 cases (67). As a general rule, therapeutic procedures have a higher complication rate than do diagnostic procedures; however, the vast majority of reports on fiberendoscopic removal of foreign bodies mention no complications caused by the procedure. Classen and associates (68), in a review of removal of foreign bodies from 186 patients at four German institutions, reported only one instance of esophageal perforation and no other complications. The potential complications of fiberendoscopic removal of foreign bodies include perforation, hemorrhage, impaction of the foreign body and pulmonary aspiration.

The success rate of fiberendoscopic removal of foreign bodies is high but, again, the exact frequency is difficult to determine because most reports desribe only a few cases. In addition, many reports deal specifically with techniques and thus discuss only successful removal. In the author's most recent experience with 40 separate episodes of ingestion of foreign bodies, an overall successful removal rate of 84% was achieved (16). The rate of successful management depended to some degree on the type of foreign body being removed, being 92% for esophageal impactions of food boluses and 76% for true foreign bodies.

More data must be prospectively collected on fiberendoscopic management of gastrointestinal foreign bodies before the exact frequency of complications and success rates for removal of various types of foreign body can be defined. Complications will be reduced to a minimum and success enhanced with proper planning, including a dry run. The available data, despite their limitations, do indicate that fiberendoscopic removal of gastrointestinal foreign bodies is a safe and useful procedure that can prevent foreign body-induced complications, obviate the need for general anesthesia and surgical intervention in most cases and reduce the need for or duration of hospitalization. It is the procedure of choice when removal of a gastrointestinal foreign body is deemed advisable.

REFERENCES

1. DeVaneson J, Pisani A, Sharma P, et al: Metallic foreign bodies in the stomach. *Arch Surg* 112(5):664–665, 1977.

2. Jackson C, Jackson CL: *Diseases of the Air and Food Passages of Foreign Body Origin.* Philadelphia, Saunders, 1937.

3. Maimon HN, Milligan FD: Removal of a foreign body from the stomach. *Gastrointest Endosc* 18:163–164, 1972.

4. Gelzayd EA, Jetly K: Fiberendoscopy: Removal of a retained sewing needle from the stomach. *Gastrointest Endosc* 18:161–162, 1972.

5. Bakara A, Bikhazi G: Oesophageal foreign bodies. *Br Med J* 1:561–563, 1975.

6. Nandi P, Ong GB: Foreign body in the oesophagus: A review of 2394 cases. *Br J Surg* 65:5–9, 1978.

7. Haglund S, Haverling M, Kuylenstierna R, et al: Radiologic diagnosis of foreign bodies in the oesophagus. *J Laryngol Otol* 92:1117–1125, 1978.

8. Kassner EG, Rose JS, Kottmeier PK, et al: Retention of small foreign objects in the stomach and duodenum. *Radiology* 114:683–686, 1975.

9. Macmanus JE: Perforations of the intestine by ingested foreign bodies. *Am J Surg* 53:393–402, 1941.

10. Brady PG, Johnson WF: Removal of foreign bodies: The flexible fiberoptic endoscope. *South Med J* 70:702–704, 1977.

11. Strohecker JS, Brady PG: Ileoscopy: Removal of a foreign object with the flexible fiberoptic endoscope. *Am J Proctol Gastroenterol Colon Rectal Surg* 31:12–17, 1980.

12. Madsen JE Jr, Boone WT, Livstone EM: Endoscopic removal of a dental instrument from the stomach. *Am J Gastroenterol* 66:377–379, 1976.

13. DeLuca RF, Ferrier JP, Wortzel EM: Polypectomy snare extraction of foreign bodies from the esophagus. Two interesting cases. *Am J Gastroenterol* 66:374–376, 1976.

14. Spitz L: Management of ingested foreign bodies in childhood. *Br Med J* 4:469–472, 1971.

15. Ament ME, Christie DL: Upper gastrointestinal fiberoptic endoscopy in pediatric patients. *Gastroenterology* 72:1244–1248, 1977.

16. Vizcarrondo FJ, Brady PG, Nord JH: Foreign bodies of the upper gastrointestinal tract. *Gastrointest Endosc* 29:208–210, 1983.

17. Cockerill FR III, Wilson WR, Van Scoy RE: Traveling toothpicks. *Mayo Clin Proc* 58:613–616, 1983.

18. Rogers LF, Inqini JP: Beverage can pull-tabs: Inadvertent ingestion or aspiration. *J Am Med Ass* 233:345–348, 1975.

19. Gelfand DW: Complications of gastrointestinal radiologic procedures: I. Complications of routine fluoroscopic procedures. *Gastrointest Radiol* 5:293–315, 1980.

20. Perelman H: Toothpick perforation of the gastrointestinal tract. *J Abdom Surg* 4:51–53, 1962.

21. Rivers AB, Davison HL: Foreign bodies in the stomach. *Ann Intern Med* 4:742–751, 1931.

22. Lacroix J, Morin CL, Collin P: Nickel dermatitis from a foreign body in the stomach. *J Pediatr* 95:428–429, 1979.

23. Blatnik DS, Toohill RJ, Lehman RH: Fatal complication from an alkali battery foreign body in the esophagus. *Ann Otol* 86:611–615, 1977.

24. Votteler TP, Nash JC, Rutledge JC: The hazard of ingested alkaline disc batteries in children. *J Am Med Ass* 249:2504–2506, 1983.

25. Alexander WJ, Kadish JA, Dunbar JS: Ingested foreign bodies in children. *Prog Pediatr Radiol* 2:256–285, 1969.

26. Doust BD, Ting YM, Chuang V: Detection of aspirated foreign bodies with xeroradiography. *Radiology* 111:725–727, 1974.

27. Ziter FMH: Intestinal perforations in adults due to ingested opaque foreign bodies. *Am J Gastroenterol* 66:382–385, 1976.

28. Miller SF: Foreign body ingestions. *Am Fam Physician* 11:123–126, 1975.

29. Rosch W, Classen M: Fiber endoscopic foreign body removal from the upper gastrointestinal tract. *Endoscopy* 4:193–197, 1972.

30. Rosenow EC III: Foreign body aspiration. *Postgrad Med* 49:164–167, 1971.

31. Haugen RK: The cafe coronary: Sudden deaths in restaurants. *J Am Med Ass* 186:142–143, 1963.

32. Murat J, Vuillard P, Petua J, et al: A propos de 108 observations de corps étrangers deglutis du tube digestif a l'exclusion de l'oesophage. *Lyon Chir* 65:379–388, 1969.

33. Waye JD: Removal of foreign bodies from the upper intestinal tract with fiberoptic instruments. *Am J Gastroenterol* 65:557–559, 1976.

34. Pellerin D, Fortier-Beaulieu M, Guegnen J: The fate of swallowed foreign bodies: Experience of 1250 instances of sub-diaphragmatic foreign bodies in children. *Prog Pediatr Radiol* 2:286–302, 1969.

35. Manegold BC, Mennicken C: Gastrointestinal foreign bodies. *Excerpta Med Int Congr Ser* 555:79–85, 1981.

36. Brady PG: Removal of gastrointestinal foreign bodies with the fiberoptic endoscope. *J Ky Med Ass* 76:431–433, 1978.

37. Witzel L, Scheurer V, Muhlemann A, et al: Removal of razor blades from stomach with fiberoptic endoscope. *Br Med J* 2:539, 1974.

38. Robinson AS: Meat impaction in the esophagus treated by enzymatic digestion. *J Am Med Ass* 181:1142–1143, 1962.

39. Hargrove MD Jr, Boyce HW Jr: Meat impaction of the esophagus. *Arch Intern Med* 125:277–278, 1970.

40. Anderson HA, Bernatz PE, Grandlay JH: Perforation of the esophagus after use of a digestant agent. *Ann Otol Rhinol Laryngol* 68:890–896, 1959.

41. Holsinger JW Jr, Fuson RL, Sealy WC: Esophageal perforation following meat impaction and papain ingestion. *J Am Med Ass* 204:188–189, 1968.

42. Ferrucci JT, Long JA: Radiologic treatment of food impaction using intravenous glucagon. *Radiology* 125:25–28, 1977.

43. Rogers BHG, Kot C, Meiri S, et al: An overtube for the flexible fiberoptic esophagogastroduodenoscope. *Gastrointest Endosc* 28:256–257, 1982.

44. McCray RS: Foreign body endoscopy. *Gastrointest Endosc* 27:236–237, 1981.

45. Griswold FC, Haislip CE, Gardner JR: Removal of an intragastric foreign body using the flexible fiberoptic esophagoscope. *Gastrointest Endosc* 19:194–195, 1973.

46. Altman AR, Gottfried EB: Intragastric closure of an ingested open safety pin. *Gastrointest Endosc* 24:294–295, 1978.

47. Spurling TJ, Zaloga GP, Richter JE: Fiberendoscopic removal of a gastric foreign body with overtube technique. *Gastrointest Endosc* 29:226–227, 1983.

48. Larkworthy W, Jones RTB, Mahoney M, et al: Removal of ingested coins utilizing fibre-endoscopy and special forceps. *Br J Surg* 61:750–752, 1974.

49. DeGerome JH: Snare extraction of a gastric foreign body. *Gastrointest Endosc* 20:73–74, 1973.

50. Olsen H, Lawrence W, Bernstein R: Fiberendoscopic removal of foreign bodies from the upper gastrointestinal tract. A simple and consistent method using a snare. *Gastrointest Endosc* 21:58–60, 1974.

51. Sartory A, Trabant G: Endoscopic extraction of a perforating paperclip from the stomach. *Endoscopy* 10:217–218, 1978.

52. Schwartz JT, Graham DY: Toothpick perforation of the intestines. *Ann Surg* 185:64–66, 1977.

53. Manegold BC: Endoscopic foreign body removal including suture extraction, in Demling L, Koch H (eds): *Operative Endoscopy Past and Future*. Baltimore, University Park Press, 1977, pp. 119–127.

54. Kline MM: Endoscopic snare in removal of an esophageal foreign body. *Gastrointest Endosc* 20:165–166, 1974.

55. Johnson WE: On ingestion of razor blades. *J Am Med Ass* 208:2163, 1969.

56. Dunkerly RC, Schull HJ, Avant G: Fiberendoscopic removal of large foreign bodies from the stomach. *Gastrointest Endosc* 21:170–171, 1974.

57. McKechnie JC: Gastroscopic removal of a phytobezoar. *Gastroenterology* 62:1047–1051, 1972.

58. Brady PG: Gastric phytobezoars consequent to delayed gastric emptying. *Gastrointest Endosc* 24:159–161, 1978.

59. Madsen R, Skibba RM, Galvan A, et al: Gastric bezoars. A technique of endoscopic removal. *Dig Dis Sci* 23:717–719, 1978.

60. Pollard HB, Block GE: Rapid dissolution of phytobezoar by cellulase enzyme. *Am J Surg* 116:933–936, 1968.

61. Gold MH, Patterson TE III, Green GI: Cellulase bezoar injection: A new endoscopic technique. *Gastrointest Endosc* 22:200–202, 1976.

62. Dann D, Rubin S, Passman H, et al: The successful medical management of a phytobezoar. *Arch Intern Med* 103:598–601, 1959.

63. Viceconte G, Viceconte GW, Bagliolo G, et al: Endoscopic removal of foreign bodies in large bowel. *Endoscopy* 14:176–177, 1982.

64. Sorenson RM, Bond JH Jr: Colonoscopic removal of a foreign body from the cecum. *Gastrointest Endosc* 21:134–135, 1975.

65. Wolf L, Geraci K: Colonoscopic removal of balloons from the bowel. *Gastrointest Endosc* 24:41, 1977.

66. Vemula NR, Madariaga J, Brand DL, et al: Colonoscopic removal of a foreign body causing colocutaneous fistulas. *Gastrointest Endosc* 28:195–196, 1982.

67. Silvis SE, Nebel OT, Rogers BHG, et al: Endoscopic complications: Results of the 1974 American Society for Gastrointestinal Endoscopy survey. *J Am Med Ass* 235:928–930, 1976.

68. Classen M, Farthmann EF, Seifert E, et al: Operative and therapeutic techniques in endoscopy. *Clin Gastroenterol* 7:741–763, 1978.

4

Endoscopic Placement
of Intestinal Tubes

Jeffrey L.Ponsky

Therapeutic intubation of the alimentary tract is well established and widely practiced. Indications for intubation include intestinal decompression, diversion of secretions, intestinal stenting and provision of enteral alimentation. Historically, tubes placed for these purposes have been passed through the nose or rectum and positioned blindly or under radiographic guidance. Such placement may be laborious and difficult and occasionally is unsatisfactory. Manipulation and placement by fiberoptic endoscopy has added a new dimension to intestinal intubation.

UPPER INTESTINAL INTUBATION

Long tubes frequently are used for intestinal decompression. Such tubes often are weighted with mercury at the tip and depend on normal peristalsis to carry them distally. Passage from the stomach occasionally is delayed or impossible, even with fluoroscopic guidance. A gastroscope may be used to grasp the tip of a tube directly and advance it into the small intestine. This maneuver can be accomplished by tying a loop of a silk suture around the tip of the tube and grasping it with a forceps passed through the biopsy channel of the endoscope. The forceps may then direct the tube into the duodenum or more distal small bowel (Fig. 1). The endoscope must be removed with care to avoid inadvertent removal of the adjacent tube. The same method may be employed to guide a tube through a gastroenterostomy or Billroth II anastomosis to deliver distal alimentation into the efferent limb or for selective decompression of the afferent loop.

94

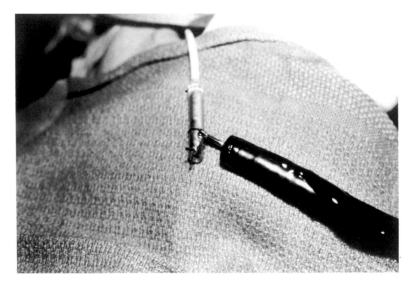

Fig. 1. An intestinal tube with a suture tied at its tip is directed with a forceps passed through an endoscope.

COLONIC DECOMPRESSION

Sigmoid volvulus may be reduced by sigmoidoscopy. Flexible fiberoptic sigmoidoscopes and colonoscopes have been used effectively in this situation (1). It usually is desirable to place a large-bore tube through the area of the reduced volvulus to maintain the reduction and to allow complete decompression of the colon. An endoscope may be used to guide the tube into the correct position. This maneuver can be accomplished by tying a long suture to the end of the tube and passing it through the biopsy channel of the endoscope in a retrograde fashion. The endoscope is then introduced to the desired level, and the suture is pulled further in a retrograde fashion to lead the tube alongside the endoscope into the colon. The endoscope is then removed, leaving the tube and the suture in place (2, 3). This technique has been described by several authors for use in the upper and lower bowel (Fig. 2a and 2b).

Colonoscopes have been used successfully to decompress massive colonic distention, such as seen in pseudoobstruction of the colon (4–6). The instrument is carefully inserted with minimal insufflation of air, and decompression by suction is achieved. Recurrent distention may necessitate repeating the procedure at intervals; however, insertion of a large-bore tube into the sigmoid colon, as described above, may maintain the decompression.

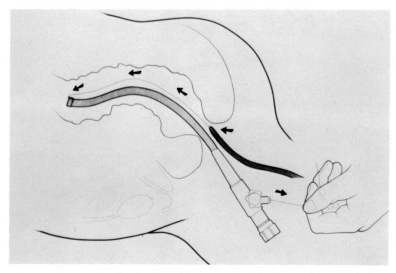

a

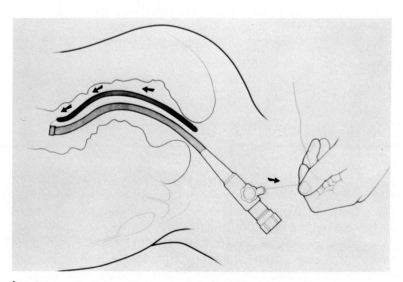

b

Fig. 2. A suture passed retrograde through the biopsy channel of an endoscope (a) is used to pull an intestinal tube into position in the colon (b).

PERCUTANEOUS ENDOSCOPIC GASTROSTOMY

Gastrostomy has long been an accepted means of providing enteral alimentation in patients who are unable to swallow. Unfortunately, this procedure has required laparotomy and, often, general anesthesia in poor-risk patients. Percutaneous endoscopic gastrostomy allows the creation of a feeding gastrostomy without the need for laparotomy or general anesthesia, and this procedure has been used in infants, children and adults, with low morbidity (7–10).

TECHNIQUE

Before the procedure is begun, a catheter is prepared. The flared distal end of a 16 French mushroom catheter is cut off (Fig. 3). A suture is placed in the tube at this site and threaded through a tapered intravenous catheter. The. tubing is stretched to allow the cannula to fit snugly over it, creating a dilator-type end (Fig. 4). The suture is knotted as it exits the intravenous cannula. A piece of soft rubber tubing approximately 3 cm in length is prepared, and small holes are cut in its side. This tubing is passed over the end of the catheter and positioned so that it comes to lie immediately behind the mushroom tip of the catheter (Fig. 5). A similar rubber bolster is prepared for use at the end of the procedure.

Feedings are withheld for 8 hours before the procedure, and a single parenteral dose of an antibiotic that offers prophylaxis against oral flora is given. The patient is placed in the supine recumbent position. This position is main-

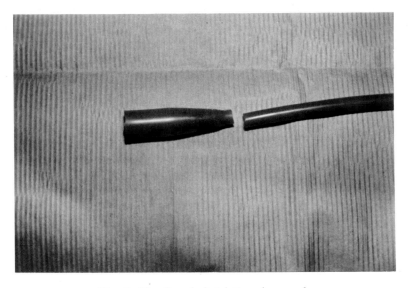

Fig. 3. The flared distal tip of a mushroom catheter is cut off.

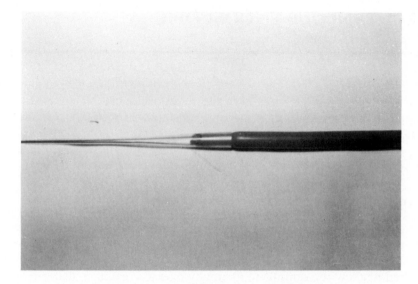

Fig. 4. The end of the tube is stretched, and a tapered intravenous catheter is slipped over it to create a dilator-like end.

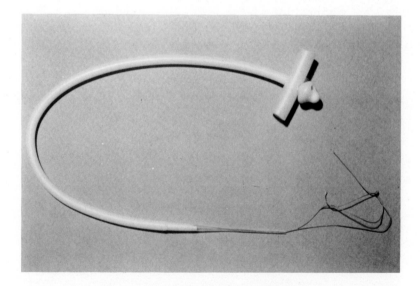

Fig. 5. The percutaneous gastrostomy catheter is completely assembled with the internal bolster and suture attachment.

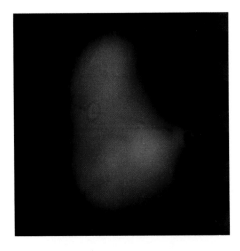

Fig. 6. With the room lights dimmed, the light of the endoscope transilluminates the abdominal wall, allowing visualization of the site for gastrostomy.

tained throughout the procedure, and an assistant must continuously monitor the airway and frequently suction the posterior part of the pharynx to avoid aspiration. The posterior part of the pharynx is anesthetized in the usual fashion with a topical agent. Intravenous sedation also is administered.

The abdomen is prepared and draped in a sterile fashion. Shaving should be minimal and limited to the left upper quadrant. A gastroscope is introduced, and the stomach is inspected. Air is then insufflated to distend the stomach fully. This maneuver causes the liver and colon to be displaced away from the stomach and allows the gastric wall to come into direct contact with the abdominal wall. The room lights are dimmed, and the assistant inspects the abdominal wall as the gastroscope is moved through the body of the stomach. The light of the gastroscope will be seen to transilluminate the abdominal wall (Fig. 6), and a site for the gastrostomy is chosen in the left upper quadrant at a point approximately two-thirds of the distance from the umbilicus to the left costal margin (Fig. 7). Good transillumination at this site helps ensure that the stomach and abdominal walls are in direct contact at this point. Finger pressure is applied to the selected area by the assistant as the endoscopist observes the indentation of the interior of the stomach (Fig. 8). This maneuver helps the endoscopist identify the site where puncture of the stomach will occur. Several milliliters of local anesthetic are infiltrated into the abdominal skin at the selected site, and an incision approximately 0.5 cm in length is made in the skin with a number 11 scalpel blade. Before making an attempt at puncture of the stomach, the endoscopist passes the polypectomy snare through the biopsy channel of the endoscope. He or she may open it and position it over the place where the puncture will occur (Fig. 9).

The assistant now thrusts a tapered intravenous cannula through the previously made incision and into the gastric lumen. If the endoscopist has positioned the snare appropriately, the needle will pass into the center of the open snare loop. If the snare has not been so positioned, the endoscopist must loop the snare wire around the needle (Fig. 10). The snare is then closed around the needle catheter, and the stylet of the catheter may be removed. A long silk

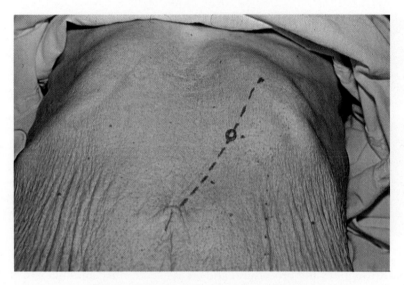

Fig. 7. The site chosen for puncture is approximately two-thirds of the distance from the umbilicus to the left costal margin.

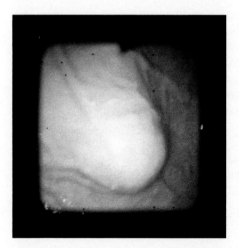

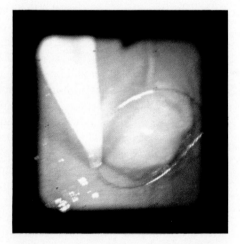

Fig. 8. Indentation of the gastric wall is noted as finger pressure is applied to the abdomen. This indentation is the site where puncture will take place.

Fig. 9. The snare is opened over the point where puncture will take place.

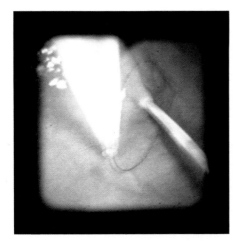

Fig. 10. The snare is looped around the intravenous cannula.

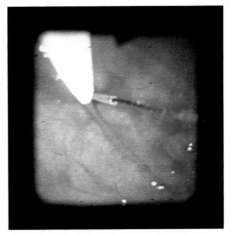

Fig. 11. The silk suture passes through the cannula into the stomach.

suture, at least 60 inches in length, is passed by the assistant through the catheter into the stomach. The endoscopist will see the suture pass from the catheter into the stomach (Fig. 11). After several inches of suture have been passed into the stomach, the snare is loosened and allowed to slip from around the catheter down around the silk suture (Fig. 12). The snare is then tightened once again to capture the silk suture (Fig. 13).

The endoscope, snare and suture are then removed from the patient, making no attempt to pull the suture into the biopsy channel of the instrument. The silk suture is allowed to run freely at the abdominal entry point, and after the

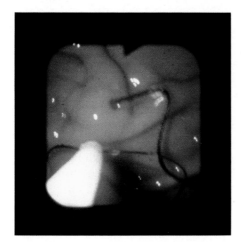

Fig. 12. The snare is loosened and allowed to slide down around the silk suture.

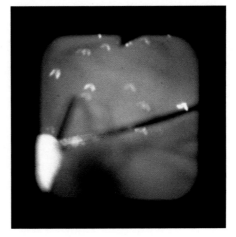

Fig. 13. The snare is tightened to capture the silk suture.

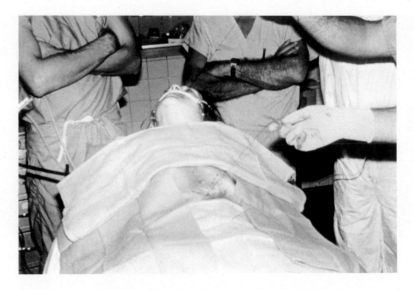

Fig. 14. The silk suture enters the abdominal wall and exits from the patient's mouth.

silk is out of the patient's mouth, the catheter used to puncture the stomach may be removed from the abdominal wall by carefully pulling it off the silk suture. At this point in the procedure, the silk suture can be seen to enter the patient's abdominal wall and exit the patient's mouth (Fig. 14).

The suture at the end of the previously prepared gastrostomy tube is tied securely to the silk suture that is exiting the patient's mouth. The tube is lubricated, and the assistant begins pulling on the abdominal end of the silk suture. The gastrostomy tube will progress, in a retrograde fashion, down through the mouth, esophagus and stomach (Fig. 15). The dilator-like end of the tube will exit the abdominal wall as traction is applied to the silk suture (Fig. 16). Pull is continued on the silk suture until the rubber tube emerges from the skin. If resistance is encountered, it always is due to an inadequate skin incision; in such instances, the incision should be enlarged before further pull is applied. Traction is continued until 5 or 6 inches of the tube have been pulled from the abdomen (Fig. 17).

The gastroscope is then reinserted, and the mushroom tip of the catheter is identified. It often is located at the esophagogastric junction or just inside the stomach (Fig. 18). The endoscopist then directs the assistant to pull the catheter from the abdominal wall. The pulling is continued under direct endoscopic vision until the rubber crossbar behind the mushroom head of the catheter is in contact with the gastric mucosa (Fig. 19). Excessive tension should be avoided because it causes necrosis of the interposed gastric and abdominal walls with early extrusion of the tube. The gastroscope may now be removed. The second rubber crossbar is applied on the outside of the tube and pushed down until it

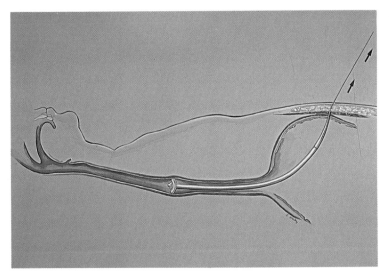

Fig. 15. The tube passes, in a retrograde fashion, down the esophagus and stomach and out the abdominal wall.

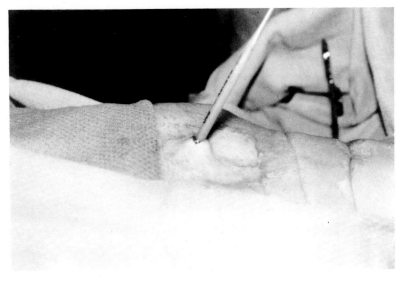

Fig. 16. The dilator-like end of the catheter exits the abdominal wall.

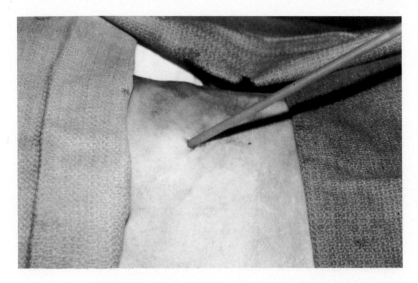

Fig. 17. Traction is continued until 5 or 6 inches of the tube have been pulled from the abdomen.

just meets the skin. Sutures are then placed into the skin under the crossbar and tied to the crossbar and to the catheter (Fig. 20). A "Christmas tree" adapter is applied to the distal end of the gastrostomy tube, and the procedure is complete (Fig. 21). Thus, the gastric and abdominal walls are held in close contact by the opposing rubber bolsters (Fig. 22). Feedings are begun the following day.

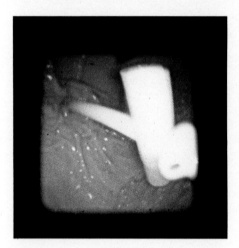

Fig. 18. The mushroom tip of the catheter is positioned in the stomach before being completely pulled into place.

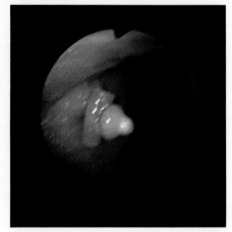

Fig. 19. The catheter is pulled from the abdomen until the rubber bolster comes in contact with the gastric mucosa.

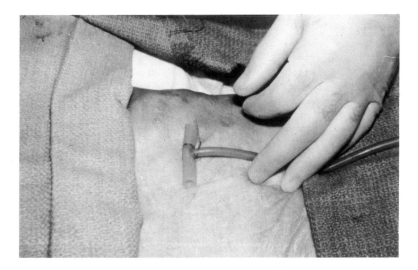

Fig. 20. The external bolster is applied and sutured in place.

Removal of the gastrostomy tube at a later date may be indicated because of improvement in the patient's condition or deterioration of the tube. Removing the tube is quite easy and merely requires a gentle, steady pull. The tube will diminish in diameter as it stretches and comes out of the stomach (Fig. 23). The inner crossbar remains in the stomach and is harmlessly passed in the stool (Fig. 24). If the tube is not replaced, the opening in the abdominal wall will

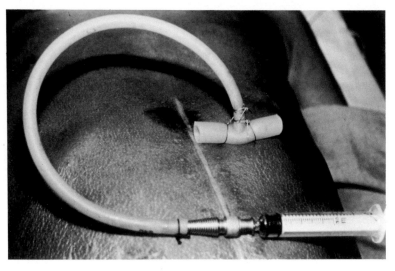

Fig. 21. A "Christmas tree" adapter is applied to the end of the catheter.

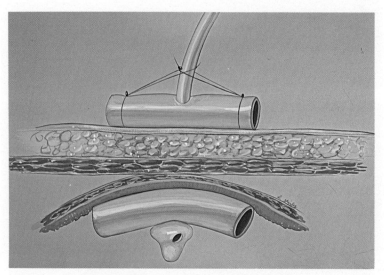

Fig. 22. The opposing bolsters hold the gastric and abdominal walls in close contact.

close within several hours (Fig. 25). When replacement with a new catheter is desired, a urinary balloon catheter or another mushroom catheter may be used. In the latter instance, the mushroom tip must be deformed with a stylet during insertion and then allowed to return to its usual form once it is inside the gastric lumen (Fig. 26). An inner crossbar is not required when a catheter is being replaced.

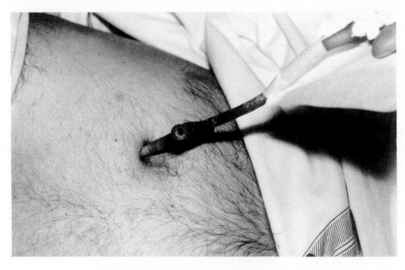

Fig. 23. Steady traction narrows the catheter, allowing its removal.

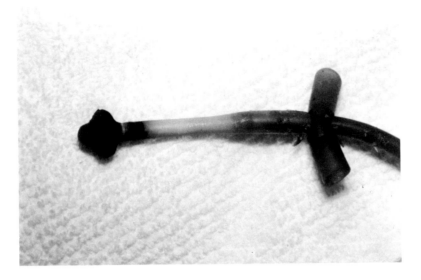

Fig. 24. The tip of a gastrostomy catheter removed after 18 months. The inner crossbar remains in the stomach and is passed in the stool.

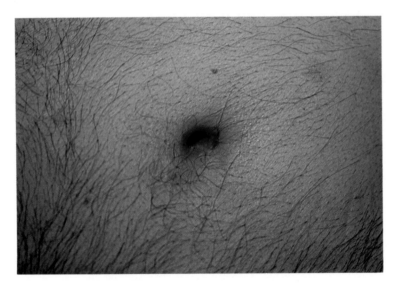

Fig. 25. The small opening in the abdominal wall after removal of the catheter will close rapidly.

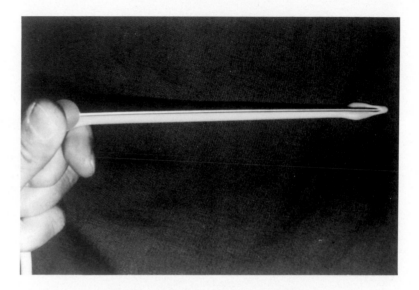

Fig. 26. A stylet is used to straighten a new mushroom catheter while it is being reinserted through an established gastrostomy tract.

PERCUTANEOUS ENDOSCOPIC JEJUNOSTOMY

Although gastrostomy feedings are satisfactory in providing enteral alimentation in most patients, there are some patients in whom gastroesophageal reflux and resultant aspiration pneumonia present a serious problem. In such patients, continuous jejunal feedings are preferable to intermittent gastric bolus feedings. Percutaneous endoscopic jejunostomy is a modification of percutaneous gastrostomy that allows continuous jejunal feedings in combination with gastric decompression (11).

TECHNIQUE

A catheter is prepared before the procedure is begun. The catheter is similar to that used for percutaneous gastrostomy; however, modifications are made in it to allow simultaneous jejunal feeding and gastric decompression. A small hole is cut in the side of the mushroom head of the catheter, and the distal end of a long Silastic feeding tube with a weighted tip is passed through this hole and the adjacent rubber bolster (Fig. 27). The Silastic feeding tube lies parallel to the gastrostomy tube until several centimeters from the end of the larger tube, where a small incision is made and the smaller feeding tube enters the larger gastrostomy tube. A stitch is placed through both tubes, and the common tube

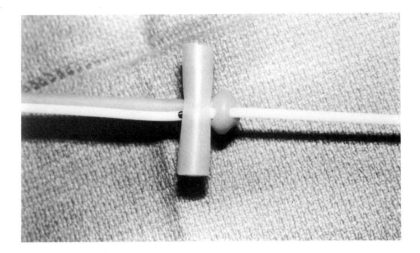

Fig. 27. A Silastic feeding tube is passed through a side hole in the mushroom head of the catheter and through the adjacent bolster.

is directed into the tapered intravenous catheter in the usual fashion (Fig. 28). The completed catheter consists of a gastrostomy tube and an adjacent, longer, jejunal feeding port (Fig. 29).

The procedure is carried out in a manner identical to that used for percutaneous gastrostomy. After the gastrostomy tube has been pulled out of the abdominal wall, the weighted end of the jejunal tube will still be at the patient's

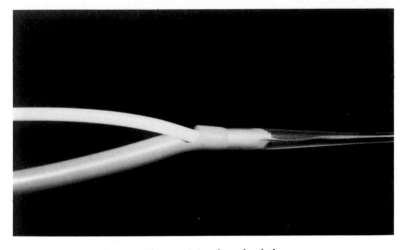

Fig. 28. The conjoined end of the gastrostomy and jejunostomy tubes fits snugly into a tapered intravenous catheter.

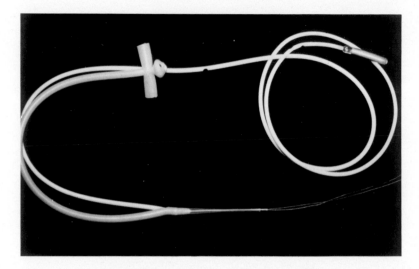

Fig. 29. The completed catheter for percutaneous endoscopic jejunostomy is shown.

mouth (Fig. 30). A silk suture is tied in a small loop around the weighted tip of the catheter to aid in its manipulation. The silk suture is then grasped with a foreign body forceps through the biopsy channel of the endoscope. The instrument is then reinserted into the stomach, carrying the weighted tube with it. Once the instrument has entered the stomach, the endoscopist directs the assistant to apply traction to the gastrostomy tube in the usual fashion until its

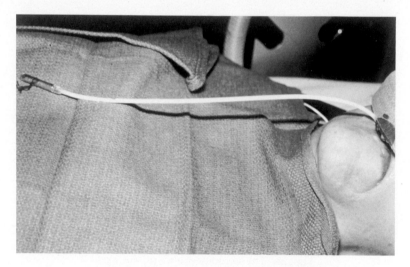

Fig. 30. The jejunal feeding tube remains at the patient's mouth after the gastrostomy portion has been pulled into the stomach.

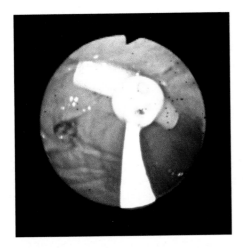 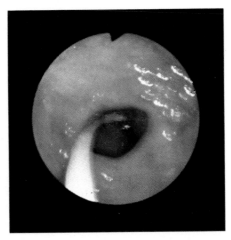

Fig. 31. The gastrostomy portion of the tube is pulled up until the rubber bolster is in contact with the gastric mucosa.

Fig. 32. The weighted tip of the jejunal catheter is deposited into the duodenal bulb.

rubber crossbar is in contact with the gastric mucosa (Fig. 31). The weighted tip of the jejunal tube is then deposited into the duodenal bulb (Fig. 32). The gastroscope may then be removed. The common end of the two tubes is next transected, and adapters are applied to each tube. Immediate feeding may be begun via the jejunal tube, while gastric decompression, by constant drainage, may be accomplished via the gastrostomy port (Fig. 33). A radiograph may be obtained to ensure that the jejunal tube is on its way into the small bowel.

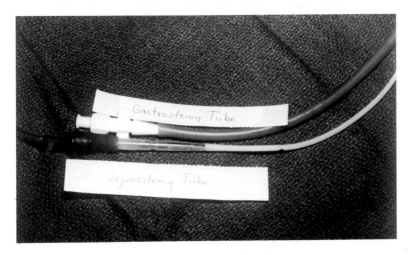

Fig. 33. Adapters are applied to the gastric and jejunal ports to allow continuous feeding in concert with gastric decompression.

COMMENT

Therapeutic gastrointestinal intubation is a useful clinical tool. Physicians have endeavored for years to expand the applications of such tubes but have been limited by the difficulty encountered in directing them to the desired point or by the consistent need for the tube to exit the patient's mouth or nose. Advances in flexible fiberoptic endoscopy have allowed precise positioning of gastrointestinal tubes and, more recently, have obviated the need for open laparotomy in the placement of feeding gastrostomies and jejunostomies. Creation of such enteral access is preferable to long-term nasoenteral intubation, which may predispose to gastroesophageal reflux, apsiration pneumonia and unsightly cosmetic deformities of the nasal cartilage.

Complications of percutaneous gastrostomy and jejunostomy include minor skin infection around the tube, early extrusion of the catheter, gastrocolic fistula and separation from the abdominal wall with resultant peritonitis. Skin infections have rarely occurred since the introduction of a preoperative dose of an intravenous cephalosporin. When skin infections do occur, they are easily managed with a small incision at the exit site of the tube to allow drainage of purulent material. Gastrocolic fistula has occurred as a result of pinching of the colon between the gastric and abdominal walls. Fortunately, this complication is rare and has been effectively managed by removing the tube. The fistulas have closed spontaneously within several days. Percutaneous gastrostomy also has been safely performed in patients who have previously undergone abdominal operations, including partial gastrectomy. Only complete esophageal obstruction has been a contraindication. The overall morbidity associated with percutaneous gastrostomy has been very low (less than 10%). No mortality directly related to the procedure has been reported. Some catheters have served for up to two years before becoming so worn that they have had to be replaced.

Endoscopically directed intubation of the alimentary tract is safe and extremely effective. Wider application of these techniques will certainly be forthcoming.

REFERENCES

1. Ghazi A, Shinya H, Wolff W: Treatment of volvulus of the colon by colonoscopy. *Ann Surg* 183:263–265, 1976.

2. Keller RT: A technique of intestinal intubation with the fiberoptic endoscope. *Gut* 14:143–144, 1973.

3. Chung RS: A technique for rapid intubation of the sigmoid and left colon. *Surg Gynecol Obstet* 157:279–282, 1983.

4. Nivatvongs S, Vermeulen F, Fang D: Colonoscopic decompression of acute pseudo-obstruction of the colon. *Ann Surg* 196:598–600, 1982.

5. Strodel WE, Nostrant TT, Eckhauser FE, et al: Therapeutic and diagnostic colonoscopy in nonobstructive colonic dilatation. *Ann Surg* 197:416–421, 1983.

6. Groff W: Colonoscopic decompression and intubation of the cecum for Ogilvie's syndrome. *Dis Colon Rectum* 26:503–506, 1983.

7. Gauderer MWL, Ponsky JL: A simplified technique for constructing a feeding gastrostomy. *Surg Gynecol Obstet* 152:82–85, 1981.

8. Gauderer MWL, Ponsky JL, Izant RH Jr: Gastrostomy without laparotomy: A percutaneous endoscopic technique. *J Pediatr Surg* 15:872–875, 1980.

9. Ponsky JL, Gauderer MWL: Percutaneous endoscopic gastrostomy: A nonoperative technique for feeding gastrostmy. *Gastrointest Endosc* 27:9–11, 1981.

10. Ponsky JL, Gauderer MWL, Stellato T: Percutaneous endoscopic gastrostomy: Review of 150 cases. *Arch Surg (Chicago)* 118:913–914, 1983.

11. Ponsky JL, Aszodi A: Percutaneous endoscopic jejunostomy. *Am J Gastroenterol* 79:113–116, 1984.

5

Endoscopic Management of Vascular Abnormalities

Albert M. Waitman
Dov Z. Grant
Frank Chateau

The ability to diagnose and manage vascular abnormalities of the gastrointestinal tract has been markedly enhanced over the past 25 years (1). With advances in techniques for radiologic and endoscopic diagnosis, it became apparent that such lesions were a common cause of gastrointestinal hemorrhage. Jensen (2), for example, found that 5% of cases of severe upper gastrointestinal bleeding were caused by such vascular malformations, as were 35% of cases of severe colonic bleeding. However, what constituted appropriate therapy for such lesions remained uncertain.

HISTORICAL BACKGROUND

For many years, it was recognized that there is a subset of patients with both acute and chronic gastrointestinal bleeding in whom an obvious source could not be readily demonstrated. Many such patients were elderly persons who had undergone a number of barium studies and even exploratory surgery in an unsuccessful attempt to locate a bleeding site (1).

It was not until the advent of modern angiographic techniques that bleeding was demonstrated to occur from a variety of vascular abnormalities in the gastrointestinal tract in many such patients. In 1960, Margulis and colleagues (3) reported on a patient who had cryptogenic bleeding for 20 years until mesenteric angiography revealed a bleeding vascular lesion in the colon. With further refinements, such as serial magnification techniques, it became possible to visualize smaller vessels than could be demonstrated by conventional studies (4).

114

Despite the availability of the newer radiologic techniques, the problem of locating such areas at operation remained. With general anesthesia, they tended to blanch and were difficult to find. Once a section of gut had been removed and processed for pathologic examination with the blood drained from it, the vascular lesions became even more elusive in the fixed state. With the development of rubber cast silicone techniques, demonstration of such lesions on pathologic examination became feasible (5, 6).

Direct visualization of bleeding gastrointestinal vascular lesions by means of endoscopy was first described by Bartelheimer and associates (7) in 1972.

NOMENCLATURE AND DESCRIPTION

The nomenclature and description of such lesions in the literature vary considerably. The most common description is that of fernlike vessels, but there are markedly different references to other characteristics, such as size, configuration of borders (sharp as opposed to blunted) and whether a round pale halo is seen around the lesions (8). The fernlike configuration is caused by feeding tributaries that enlarge as they reach the outer rim of such lesions, giving them an irregular appearance. The lesions usually are flat or only slightly raised. Some lesions have white flecks in the center, which may represent atheromatous plaques or ulcerations.

Although we have seen lesions with all these characteristics, we are not certain whether they represent appreciably different disease entities. Patients with lesions that have different characteristics do not have different bleeding patterns, and only the size and number of lesions have any prognostic implications.

The nomenclature is equally confusing. Variations in nomenclature result in part from lack of knowledge of the etiologic basis of such lesions and, as a consequence, numerous descriptive terms have been used (Table 1). Each nomenclature system has its advocates, but much of the discussion on terminology is semantic rather than scientific.

We consider a patient to have hereditary hemorrhagic telangiectasia (Osler-Weber-Rendu disease) if, in addition to gastrointestinal bleeding from arteriovenous malformations, there is either a family history of the disease or mucous membrane involvement. Otherwise, we make no differentiation in relation to the type of lesion. Although we segregate patients with this disease for statistical purposes, we have yet to find any meaningful difference between their clinical course and that of patients with other vascular lesions. Weaver and coworkers (9) have postulated that there is a spectrum of vascular lesions of the gastrointestinal tract, with those having an obvious pattern of inheritance at one pole and those that constitute an acquired subset at the other.

TABLE 1. Synonyms for Vascular Lesions Seen in the Colon

Telangiectasia
Vascular malformation
Angiectasia
Vascular ectasia
Angiodysplasia
Arteriovenous malformation
Arteriovenous fistula
Arteriovenous anastomosis
Arteriovenous shunt
Hemangioma
Angioma
Capillary hemangioma
Osler-Weber-Rendu disease

ETIOLOGIC BASIS

There is much speculation in the literature concerning the etiologic basis of such lesions. Most theories are based on clinical features. The average age of our patients has been in the eighth decade, and it has been suggested by us and other investigators that such lesions may represent a phenomenon of the aging process. It has been further postulated that vessels may become ectatic as a result of relative mesenteric ischemia during the aging process, resulting in arteriovenous shunting (10). Similar ischemia and shunting may be caused by cardiac disease. The high incidence of aortic valve disease in such patients has been noted (11–14). It is uncertain as to whether there is a direct cause and effect relationship between the two diseases or whether they represent separate entities that occur with increasing frequency in an aging population. Our experience has been that bleeding worsens a patient's cardiovascular status. Just as often, a failing cardiovascular system induces bleeding. Although it has been noted that correction of cardiovascular failure decreases bleeding, replacement of the aortic valve does not seem to prevent further bleeding. In three of our four patients with aortic valve prostheses, bleeding occurred after valve replacement. Weaver and colleagues (9) reported a similar experience with bleeding after valve replacement. Recurrent bleeding may be exacerbated by anticoagulation after valve replacement, and the use of porcine grafts that require less or no postoperative anticoagulation may alleviate some of this problem.

The high incidence of renal failure in such patients also has been used as a basis for explanations of the cause of the vascular lesions. Approximately one-half of our patients with renal failure had azotemia before the onset of gastrointestinal bleeding. Most of them had been on long-term hemodialysis and had undergone endoscopy for evaluation of chronic blood loss, at which point vascular lesions were discovered. In a similar proportion of patients, however, it seems that chronic, recurrent blood loss with resultant hypotension and anemia preceded progressive renal failure.

The locations of vascular anomalies also have been studied in an attempt to understand how they are formed. The most common locations are in the watershed areas of the gastrointestinal circulation: the cecum and the posterior wall of the stomach. The large number of anastomoses that occur in these areas may contribute to the formation of abnormal vessels. In addition, the posterior wall of the stomach is subjected to repeated barrages of food exiting from the esophagus, and this phenomenon may cause irritation of the mucosa overlying arteriovenous malformations and induce bleeding. The pressure in the cecum, which is the highest in the colon, may also have a role in precipitating hemorrhage.

LASER PHYSICS

Laser is an acronym for light amplification by the stimulated emission of radiation. First postulated by Albert Einstein (15), a laser is a source of very high intensity light energy. The light energy is converted to thermal energy on impact with tissue, and the resultant increase in the temperature of the tissue causes denaturation and coagulation. The depth of penetration in tissue of a laser beam is dependent on the wavelength of the laser and on the absorptive capacity of the tissue. The blue-green argon laser beam, which has a wavelength of 454.5 to 514.5 nm, is readily absorbed by blood and vascular lesions. The neodymium:YAG laser beam, which has a wavelength in the invisible near-infrared region, is not readily absorbed by blood and therefore penetrates tissue to greater depths than does an argon laser beam.

LASER THERAPY

Patients are premedicated with a 3 cm^3 gargle that consists of 2% tetracaine with 3 drops of simethicone. In most cases, intravenous sedatives are not used because of their tendency to blanch the vessels secondary to hypotension. If sedation is necessary, 25 mg of meperidine is given intravenously, the endoscope is passed and the effect of meperidine is reversed with 0.4 mg of naloxone administered intravenously. If serious intestinal spasm occurs, 1 mg of glucagon is administered intravenously.

We use an Olympus GIF-2T therapeutic endoscope for gastroscopy as well as colonoscopy. For lesions in the jejunum, we use an Olympus PCF. For redun-

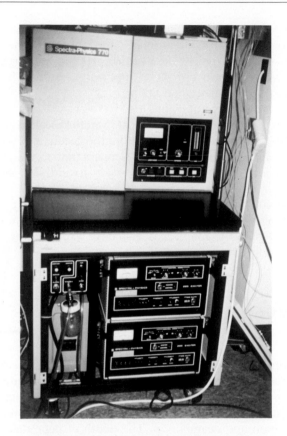

Fig. 1. A Spectra Physics 770 argon laser. The top right panel controls exposure and gas flow and also indicates the total time of exposure. A power meter is built in to regulate the application of energy.

dant colons, an Olympus LB-3W colonoscope is used to reach the cecum. The splinting device is then passed over the colonoscope. When the colonoscope is removed, the GIF-2T is passed through the splinting device.

The advantage of the Olympus GIF-2T is that it provides three channels of continuous use so that catheters do not have to be inserted and removed repeatedly from a single biopsy channel. With the Olympus GIF-2T, one channel is used for the laser fiber with coaxial carbon dioxide, a second for suction and the third for target water lavage. Target lavage is accomplished by attaching a foot-controlled Endopump (Frantz Medical) to the third channel. Thus, insufflation of air and carbon dioxide, suction, target water lavage and laser photocoagulation can all be carried out simultaneously.

When an endoscope is introduced, great care must be taken to avoid scraping the mucosa or creating artifacts due to trauma that may be mistaken for arteriovenous malformations. For gastroscopy, patients are fasted for 12 to 14 hours before the procedure is undertaken to ensure that the field is clear.

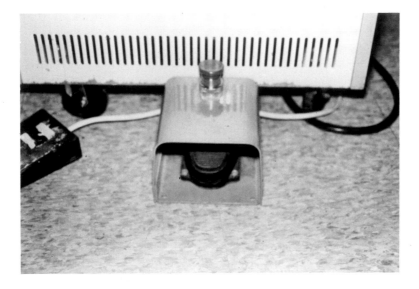

Fig. 2. The foot pedal that activates the laser. Note that the pedal is encased to prevent accidental contact. As a further precaution, the pedal must be depressed through two stages to fire the laser.

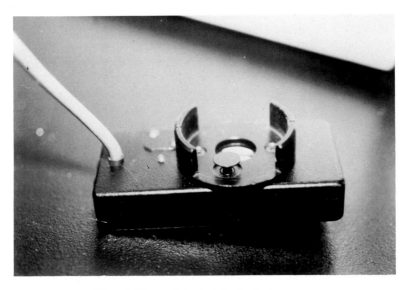

Fig. 3. The safety interlock that covers the endoscope eyepiece. When the foot pedal is depressed, a filter is inserted into the light path to prevent damage to the endoscopist.

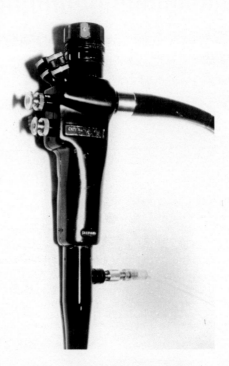

Fig. 4. A three-channel Olympus GIF-2T operating endoscope. The two top channels are for the laser fiber and for suction. Note the attachment of a water lavage catheter to the third channel at the bottom.

Before colonoscopy is begun, vigorous preparation is required so that residual stool does not obscure underlying arteriovenous malformations. Suctioning the stool may cause mucosal defects that mimic arteriovenous lesions. The theoretical risk of explosion with laser photocoagulation in the colon is minimized by vigorous preparation and by insufflation of carbon dioxide during the procedure.

A Spectra-Physics 770 argon laser with a 10-watt output at the fiber tip is used. The power output is regulated by a meter placed in the path of the partially diverted beam. The beam is transmitted through a single quartz fiberoptic waveguide encased in a polyethylene sheath 2.3 mm in diameter. This setup allows for coaxial transmission of carbon dioxide.

Exposure is accomplished by depressing a foot switch to fire the laser beam for a predetermined time interval, usually 1 second. The laser beam is focused by means of a modified microscope lens on the quartz fiberoptic waveguide

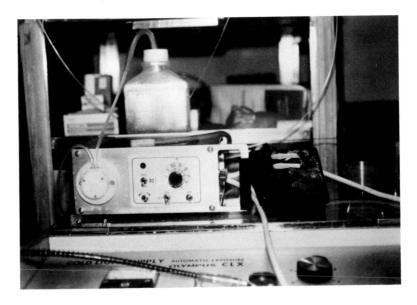

Fig. 5. A Frantz Endo-pump, which is attached to the third channel for water lavage. This pump may be activated by depressing the foot pedal. Various cassettes and dial settings regulate the rate of flow.

system that carries the energy to the tissue. The angle of divergence is 8 degrees. The spot size and the power density can be altered by varying the distance between the end of the fiberoptic system and the mucosa. When the waveguide is kept 1 to 2 cm from the mucosa, an area of approximately 0.2 cm in diameter can be treated. The calculated power density is approximately 250 watts per centimeter squared. A 1-second exposure at 6 to 8 watts creates a recognizable whitening of the mucosa, indicating that photocoagulation has taken place.

All bleeding arteriovenous malformations are treated with sequential 1-second pulses of 7.5 watts of argon laser energy applied under direct endoscopic guidance. If the lesions are not bleeding at the time of endoscopy, there are signs that may indicate which are the culpable areas. A clot at or near an arteriovenous malformation may be taken as an indication of recent hemorrhage, as may a small erosion in the lesion. If the lesion is so friable that gentle touching with the tip of the endoscope results in brisk bleeding, this finding strongly suggests that the lesion is the site of bleeding. Ease of bleeding also distinguishes arteriovenous malformations from artifacts. All arteriovenous malformations that satisfy the above-mentioned criteria are treated, even if they are not actively bleeding, as are all those that are greater than 5 mm in diameter.

Because most arteriovenous malformations are larger than the effective spot size of an argon laser, the periphery is treated in a circumferential pattern before the center is photocoagulated, resulting in edema of the wall and constriction of feeder vessels. If the center is treated first, intensive bleeding may occur from the feeder vessels.

Bleeding from arteriovenous malformations frequently occurs on first impact with the argon laser beam. If bleeding occurs, target water lavage and coaxial transmission of carbon dioxide can be used to wash away the overlying blood to permit visualization of the underlying vessels. This maneuver is best accomplished with the endoscope and laser beam perpendicular to the lesion.

Endoscopy should be repeated in 2 to 4 days to evaluate the completeness of coagulation. During repeat procedures, arteriovenous formations that were not seen a few days earlier may be visualized. There are many reasons for not visualizing all arteriovenous malformations at the time of the first procedure. The lesions may simply have been missed or after transfusion, the patient may be in a better state of hydration and have a higher hemoglobin level, thus making the area more visible. It also is possible that coagulation of arteriovenous malformations may cause more blood to be shunted into other areas, thus making the missed arteriovenous malformations more apparent. Therapy should not be considered complete until repeat endoscopy has failed to reveal additional bleeding sites and until the hemogram remains stable. Large lesions may have extensive transmural or submucosal anastomoses and may require more than one treatment.

If arteriovenous malformations are discovered serendipitously with no evidence of bleeding or anemia, they are not treated. Some endoscopists do not photocoagulate arteriovenous malformations unless they are actively bleeding or there is an adherent clot. We, however, perform laser photocoagulation on all serious lesions in patients with a history of gastrointestinal bleeding.

DIFFICULTIES IN DIAGNOSIS AND THERAPY

Arteriovenous malformations can be difficult to diagnose. Most patients undergo endoscopy during acute hemorrhage, when the hemoglobin level or blood pressure is low, making vascular lesions less visible. Visibility may be further diminished by administration of intravenous sedatives because the use of such agents lowers blood pressure and, consequently, causes blanching of arteriovenous malformations. We therefore recommend that patients with multiple bleeding episodes in whom no definitive diagnosis has been made undergo endoscopy without sedation at least once after they have received transfusions to restore the hemoglobin level to normal. This recommendation applies for patients with upper or lower gastrointestinal bleeding.

Another difficulty in diagnosing arteriovenous malformations is that they often are mistaken for artifacts due to trauma, such as that caused by endo-

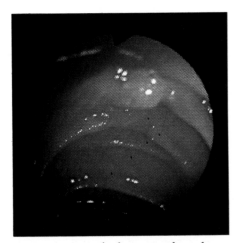

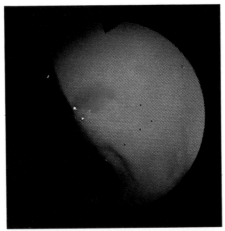

Fig. 6. A view of a large number of vascular malformations. The lesions on the thickened fold at the top have been photocoagulated. Note how easy it is to "miss" lesions located between and just under thick folds.

Fig. 7. The most common location for bleeding vascular lesions in the stomach is on the high posterior wall. The large lesion just under the cardioesophageal junction was seen only on retrovision of the endoscope, which can be seen passing through the cardioesophageal junction. This position makes it difficult to find such lesions as well as to position the laser fiber perpendicular to the site.

scopes, nasogastric tubes, suctioning and vigorous gastric lavage. It also may be difficult to differentiate arteriovenous malformations from small clots. In general, however, the artifacts produced by such trauma do not have the characteristic fernlike appearance of true vascular malformations.

If there is still uncertainty regarding the nature of a lesion, the precise location of the lesion should be noted and the patient should undergo repeat endoscopy at a later date. During endoscopy, great care must be taken to avoid trauma. Suctioning should be avoided, if possible. For adequate visualization of a stomach with large folds, maximal distention is essential. Distention may be enhanced by administration of glucagon, which also is helpful when small bowel endoscopy is used to search for arteriovenous malformations. Careful and copious lavage to remove any bile overlying the small bowel mucosa must be done to reveal additional lesions.

RESULTS OF COAGULATION

Relatively few studies have been reported on photocoagulation of arteriovenous malformations, and only small numbers of patients have been reported.

Howard and coworkers (16) found arteriovenous malformations in 26 pa-

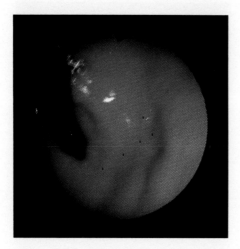

Fig. 8. The lesion is shown after successful photocoagulation. This 80-year-old woman has had no bleeding for 2½ years after the procedure.

tients with unexplained anemia or hematochezia in whom previous work-ups had been negative. Twenty-three patients underwent photocoagulation, with good results in 20 of them.

Jensen and Bown (17) reported on eight patients with arteriovenous malformations who had received more than 360 transfusions. A total of 395 arteriovenous malformations were treated in this series, and new lesions developed from 2 to 6 months after laser photocoagulation.

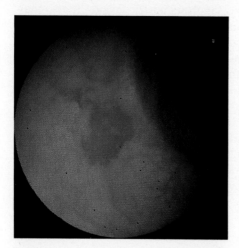

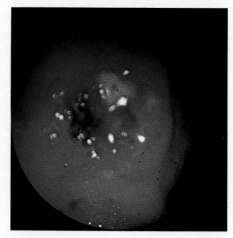

Fig. 9a. A large cecal arteriovenous malformation. Note the two central white flecks, which represent ulceration, and the streaming tributaries. These branches were treated by photocoagulation, and then the central vessel was photocoagulated.

Fig. 9b. The same lesion after photocoagulation.

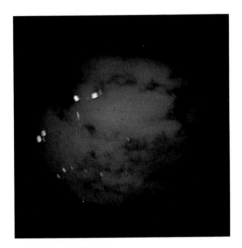

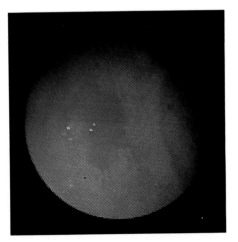

Fig. 10. Stool has been washed away with a water jet to reveal a large cecal vascular malformation at the top. Stool at the lower right might also be obscuring a lesion, and this stool must be washed away as well.

Fig. 11. A diffuse, blunted vascular lesion in the colon. Note the satellite vascular blushes.

Johnston (18) reported the use of neodymium:YAG photocoagulation in 22 patients with 440 angiomata. He noted good results in 19 patients; in the three remaining patients, massive hemorrhage occurred 7 to 16 days after laser photocoagulation.

Sudry and associates (19) treated 15 patients with gastrointestinal bleeding secondary to arteriovenous malformations. Ten patients required more than

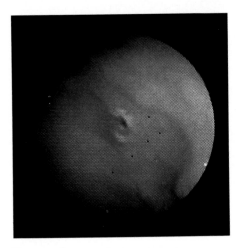

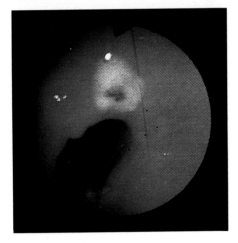

Fig. 12. The same lesion after photocoagulation.

Fig. 13. A large antral arteriovenous malformation in its healing phase. There is slight ulceration around the treated lesion.

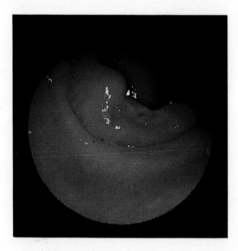

Fig. 14. A section of duodenal fold has been eroded after laser therapy; fibrosis is occurring.

one course of laser therapy, and rebleeding occurred in five patients after the completion of therapy.

Bowers and Dixon (20) found that transfusion requirements were markedly reduced in 13 patients 6 months after treatment with an argon laser.

We have used argon laser photocoagulation to treat more than 250 patients with arteriovenous malformations of the gastrointestinal tract. Preliminary evaluation of our data revealed a statistically significant reduction of transfusion requirements in most patients. Perforation or complications secondary to endoscopic laser photocoagulation did not occur in our series. Five of the more than 250 patients required surgical intervention for the continued bleeding after laser therapy.

OTHER TREATMENT MODALITIES

In the past, right hemicolectomy and/or partial gastrectomy had been performed in an attempt to terminate bleeding in such patients (21). Some of our patients had undergone "blind" right hemicolectomy as therapy for bleeding of unknown cause or location. Eleven of our patients had recurrent bleeding within 1 month after surgical intervention. Several series have been reported in which right hemicolectomy was the treatment of choice for arteriovenous malformations of the right portion of the colon. In the series reported by Boley (10), Richardson (22) and Tedesco (23) and their colleagues, 79 patients underwent right hemicolectomy for arteriovenous malformations diagnosed by colonoscopic or angiographic studies. The combined mortality in those reports was approximately 7%, with bleeding recurring in approximately 10% of cases.

Many angiographic techniques also have been used for this purpose; examples are injection of vasoactive substances, such as vasopressin, autologous clot injection and embolization (24).

More recently, endoscopic sclerosis with sodium morrhuate has been reported (25). Heater probes (26) as well as monopolar and bipolar coagulation also have advocates (27).

Although no double-blind, controlled studies have compared the effectiveness of various treatment modalities in the management of arteriovenous malformations, we believe that endoscopic laser photocoagulation is the treatment of choice for such lesions. There is no operative or anesthetic risk. In addition, laser photocoagulation is a no-touch technique and has the advantage of relatively easy access. A disadvantage of electrical coagulation is that the char built up over a lesion may be pulled off as the probe is withdrawn, resulting in massive bleeding.

Therapeutic angiographic techniques have several disadvantages: they are not readily repeatable, require the use of radiology suites, involve the administration of vasoactive drugs that have systemic side effects and have an inherent morbidity.

The apparent success of laser photocoagulation is dependent on many variables. We have found that the fewer the number of lesions, early control of the bleeding is more likely. Most bleeding occurs in readily accessible areas of the stomach, duodenum or colon, although bleeding occasionally occurs in areas that are beyond the reach of an endoscope or that are not readily accessible. We have encountered a few patients with hundreds of lesions scattered throughout the gastrointestinal tract, a situation that makes success unlikely with any form of treatment. We also have found that careful follow-up of patients with repeat prophylactic laser photocoagulation of new lesions diminishes the rate of recurrence of bleeding (28).

CONCLUSION

Arteriovenous malformations have become increasingly recognized as a cause of gastrointestinal bleeding. Fiberoptic endoscopy and advances in angiographic techniques have improved our ability to locate these sometimes elusive lesions in the gastrointestinal tract. Although various forms of therapy have been used, laser photocoagulation appears to be the procedure of choice because it has the highest degree of safety and efficacy. Careful endoscopic evaluation and adequate lavage with carbon dioxide allow visualization of arteriovenous malformations and facilitate their treatment. Adequate exposure of the endoscopic field through the use of coaxial carbon dioxide and target water lavage has markedly improved the endoscopic diagnosis and laser treatment of arteriovenous malformations of the gastrointestinal tract.

REFERENCES

1. Smith CR, Bartholomew LE, Cain JC: Heriditary hemorrhagic telangiectasia and gastrointestinal hemorrhage. *Gastroenterology* 44:1–6, 1963.

2. Jensen D: Laser, in Atsumi K, Nimsakul N (eds): *Proceedings of Laser—Tokyo '81*. Tokyo, Intergroup, 1981.

3. Margulis AR, Heinbecker P, Bernard HR: Operative mesenteric arteriography in the search for the site of bleeding in unexplained gastrointestinal hemorrhage. *Surgery* 48:534–539, 1960.

4. Baum S, Nusbaum M, Kuroda K, et al: Direct serial magnification arteriography as an adjuvant in the diagnosis of surgical lesions in the alimentary tract. *Am J Surg* 117:170–176, 1969.

5. Alfidi RJ, Hunter T, Hawk WA, et al: Corrosion casts of arteriovenous malformation. *Arch Pathol* 96:196, 1973.

6. Mitsudo SM, Boley SJ, Brandt LJ, et al: Vascular ectasia of the right colon in the elderly: A distinct pathological entity. *Hum Pathol* 10:585–600, 1979.

7. Bartelheimer W, Remmele W, Ottengann R: Colonoscopic recognition of hemangiomas in the colon ascendens. *Endoscopy* 4:109–114, 1972.

8. Rogers BHG: Electrocoagulation of vascular abnormalities of the large bowel, in Papp JP (ed): *Endoscopic Control of Gastrointestinal Hemorrhage*. Boca Raton, Florida, CRC Press, 1981, pp 145–181.

9. Weaver GA, Alpern HD, Davis JS, et al: Gastrointestinal angiodysplasia associated with aortic valve disease: Part of a spectrum of angiodysplasia of the gut. *Gastroenterology* 77:1–11, 1979.

10. Boley SJ, Sammortano R, Adams A: On the nature and etiology of vascular ectasias of the colon: Degenerative lesions of aging. *Gastroenterology* 72:650–660, 1977.

11. Heyde EC: Gastrointestinal bleeding in aortic stenosis. (Letter to the editor) *N Engl J Med* 259:196, 1958.

12. Schwartz BM: Additional notes on bleeding in aortic stenosis. (Letter to the editor) *N Engl J Med* 259:456, 1958.

13. William RC Jr: Aortic stenosis and unexplained gastrointestinal bleeding. *Arch Intern Med* 108:859–863, 1961.

14. Gelfond ML, Cohen T, Achert JJ, et al: Gastrointestinal bleeding in aortic stenosis. *Am J Gastroenterol* 71:30–38, 1979.

15. Einstein A: Zur Quantentheorie des Strahlung. *Phys Z* 18:121, 1917.

16. Howard OM, Buchanan JD, Hunt RH: Angiodysplasias of the colon. *Lancet* 2:16–19, 1982.

17. Jensen D, Bown S: Gastrointestinal angiomata in Fleischer D, Jensen D, Bright-Asare P (eds): *Therapeutic Laser Endoscopy in Gastrointestinal Disease*. Boston, Martinus Nijhoff Publishers, 1983, pp 151–159.

18. Johnston JH: Complications following endoscope laser therapy. *Gastrointest Endosc* 28:135, 1982.

19. Sudry P, Brunetaud JM, Paris JC, et al: Treatment of digestive angiomas with argon laser: about 15 cases (author's translation). *Gastroenterol Clin Biol* 5:426–432, 1981.

20. Bowers JH, Dixon JA: Argon laser photocoagulation of vascular malformations in the GI tract: Short term results. *Gastrointest Endosc* 28:126, 1982.

21. Bockus HL, Ferguson LK, Thompson C: Management of gastrointestinal hemorrhage of undetermined origin. *J Am Med Ass* 152:1228–1230, 1953.

22. Richardson JD, Max MH, Flint CM, et al: Bleeding vascular malformations of the intestine. *Surgery* 84:430–436, 1978.

23. Tedesco FJ, Griffin JW, Khan AQ: Vascular ectasia of the colon. *J Clin Gastroenterol* 2:233–237, 1980.

24. Reuter SR, Redman HC: *Gastrointestinal Angiography.* Philadelphia, Saunders, 1977, pp 237–245.

25. Young W, Gibbert V, Feinstat T, et al: The recurrent upper gastrointestinal bleeding in heridity hemorrhagic telangiectasia successfully treated by endoscopic sclerotherapy. *Gastrointest Endosc* 28:148, 1982.

26. Protell RL, Rubin CE, Auth DC, et al: The heater probe: A new endoscopic method for stopping massive gastrointestinal bleeding. *Gastroenterology* 74:257–262, 1979.

27. Rogers BHG: Endoscopic electrocoagulation of vascular abnormalities of the gastrointestinal tract in 51 patients. *Gastrointest Endosc* 28:142, 1982.

28. Brown SG, Storey DW, Swain CP, et al: Argon laser photocoagulation for upper gastrointestinal hemorrhage: Is technique the key to success? *Digestion* 22:294–301, 1981.

6

Endoscopic Management of Gastrointestinal Bleeding with Electrocoagulation

John P. Papp

Management of bleeding lesions in the upper gastrointestinal tract by use of endoscopy became feasible after the development of flexible fiberoptic endoscopes, which can reach into the duodenum. After a decade of endoscopy research, three modalities of electrocoagulation have become available: bipolar electrocoagulation, heater probe and monopolar electrocoagulation. This chapter will review the experimental studies that have been performed with each modality, discuss the techniques of application and review the clinical experience of American and European endoscopists.

BIPOLAR ELECTROCOAGULATION

Experiments in dogs comparing bipolar with monopolar electrocoagulation have shown reduced depth of injury (1,2). When compared with a 3-mm monopolar electrode, about twice as many applications and joules are required to stop bleeding with a bipolar probe (2). Machicado and colleagues (3), found that standard-sized canine esophageal ulcers stopped bleeding after 21 ± 1 applications with a bipolar probe. Fifteen percent of the ulcers were found to have transmural injury. In the same study, these investigators reported that 21 standard-sized canine duodenal ulcers stopped bleeding after 30 ± 4 applications, but 20% of them showed transmural injury. Johnston and associates (4) compared monopolar with bipolar electrocoagulation in the management of canine gastric ulcers. However, they used a model that was slightly different from that used by the above authors. Johnston and associates (4) did not use

130

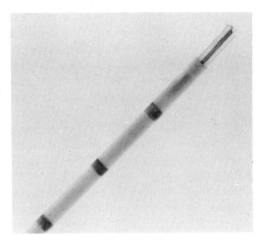

Fig. 1. A BICAP probe.

open-laparotomy canine models. They passed an endoscope per os into the dogs' stomachs. Monopolar electrocoagulation produced hemostasis in all 30 bleeding ulcers, with a mean of 16 applications for 0.5 second each. Sixteen ulcers demonstrated transmural injury. With a bipolar probe, a mean of 25 applications stopped the bleeding from standard-sized canine gastric ulcers in 29 of 30 cases. Five ulcers showed transmural injury. Johnston and associates (4) concluded that bipolar electrocoagulation produced less mucosal injury, was technically more difficult to use than monopolar electrocoagulation and was equally effective as monopolar electrocoagulation in producing hemostasis.

A new type of bipolar electrode has recently been developed. It is a circumactive, six-bipolar probe. The bipoles are longitudinal electrodes that are equally spaced along the sides and over the rounded tip of a cylindrical probe. The probe is called a BICAP hemostatic system. (ACMI, Stamford, Connecticut) (Fig. 1). The probe can be introduced through the larger biopsy channels of most endoscopes. The central opening allows fluid to be infused intermittently or constantly. Two probe sizes are available, 2.4 and 3.2 mm. Auth and coworkers (5) reported effective hemostasis in experimentally induced canine gastric ulcers with a limited depth of injury at a setting of 7 for 1 second.

An encouraging report by Verhoeven and colleagues (6) on the use of a BICAP probe was reported in 1981. Bleeding from 10 gastric ulcers and from four of five duodenal ulcers was stopped, with only one ulcer rebleeding in each group. Bleeding from two marginal ulcers also was stopped. Further experience of this group with a BICAP probe in 40 patients has resulted in initial hemostasis in 35 patients and failure in the remaining five patients. Nine of the 35 patients in whom initial hemostasis occurred rebled after 12 hours to several days later. Nine of the 40 patients eventually required surgical intervention. Six patients in this series died, four of them postoperatively. Lesions that were electrocoagulated with the BICAP probe included 30 gastric or duodenal ulcers, two Mallory-Weiss tears, five telangiectases, two lesions after polypectomy and one suture line bleeding after surgical intervention.

Risa and coworkers (7) were able to stop active bleeding from duodenal ulcers in only five of 12 patients. In four patients, the bleeding could not be stopped; rebleeding occurred in the remaining three patients. These investigators used a 2.3-mm BICAP probe. Of eight actively bleeding gastric ulcers, three showed no further bleeding after use of the probe, two continued to bleed and three rebled. Risa and coworkers (7) also were successful in stopping the bleeding from two marginal ulcers, one Mallory-Weiss tear and one telangiectasia. The results of this series were confirmed by a multicenter clinical trial reported by Gilbert and associates (8). A 2.4-mm probe was used. Of 15 gastric ulcers that showed immediate hemostasis, seven subsequently rebled. Of 14 duodenal ulcers, 11 stopped bleeding initially, but three rebled. In addition three of four stomal ulcers stopped bleeding as did three of four Mallory-Weiss tears, when a BICAP electrocoagulation probe was used. All six arteriovenous malformations were treated, and one rebled. Fifty percent of the gastric ulcers and 43% of the duodenal ulcers rebled or continued to bleed when a BICAP probe was used.

Contrary to the poor results noted above, Winklet and colleagues (9) reported complete success with a BICAP probe in 13 patients. The probe was used in this series to manage esophagitis, an ulcer in an esophageal hiatal hernia, Mallory-Weiss tears, gastritis, duodenitis, duodenal ulcers, a vascular malformation of the duodenum and a hemorrhagic adenocarcinoma of the stomach.

A modified bipolar probe with constant perfusion of distilled water at 20 ml per minute has been used by Yamamoto and associates (10). The probe measures 3.4 mm. Its electrodes are arranged in a square, equally spaced 0.5 mm apart, and are 2.4 mm in length and 1 mm in diameter. With 1 to 2-second pulses, the bipolar probe is directly applied to a bleeding vessel. Yamamoto and associates (10) found that a mean of three applications was effective in producing hemostasis in gastric and mesenteric serosal vessels. Subsequently, the probe has been used in 32 patients with gastrointestinal bleeding on 35 occasions. Sixteen gastric ulcers, eight duodenal ulcers, three stomal ulcers, four cases of gastric erosion, two gastric carcinomas, one Mallory-Weiss tear and one case of postbiopsy bleeding were successfully managed with a mean of 6.8 applications. Five patients rebled after 2 hours to 15 days later. Two of the five patients underwent repeat electrocoagulation, which was successful in producing hemostasis. The advantages of this technique are as follows: no adherence to tissue because of constant perfusion of distilled water, capability for applying the probe tangentially and vertically and limited depth of injury.

A "hot-squeeze" bipolar technique has recently been advocated by Mills and coworkers (11). This technique involves grasping a bleeding vessel, occluding its lumen, and then applying bipolar electrocoagulation to produce hemostasis. The hot-squeeze technique was compared with the BICAP, liquid and dry monopolar and heater probe techniques. Mills and coworkers (11) concluded that bond strengths (mean bursting pressure) was significantly better with their technique. A major disadvantage of this technique is that it requires great skill to grasp an actively bleeding vessel. These investigators recognized that such a maneuver is difficult, but they believe that a major advantage of the technique is that it enables the operator to seal large bleeding vessels more effectively than is possible with other thermal endoscopic methods.

HEATER PROBE

Application of a "hot iron" has been used for centuries to stop bleeding. Use of this technique to stop bleeding in the gastrointestinal tract was begun at the University of Washington in Seattle in the 1970s. Protell and colleagues (12) reported on the use of a heater probe delivered by means of an endoscope. A heater probe is a hollow aluminum cylinder with an inner coil. Its outer surface is coated with Teflon. The aluminum cylinder effectively transfers heat to tissue from its end or sides. Heater probes with a diameter of 3.2 or 2.4 mm are available. Such probes can be passed through the larger biopsy channels of most endoscopes. The probes reach operating temperature in less than 5 seconds. The temperature is preset at 140° or 150° C; the amount of energy in joules also is preset. Before a heater probe is used, the energy source can be set to produce 1 to 29 joules. Heat is produced by dissipation of electrical energy within the tip of the probe to the aluminum cylinder; the heat is then conveyed to the target tissue. Protell and colleagues (12) demonstrated the effectiveness of a heater probe in unoperated heparinized dogs. However, they were concerned about not being able to predict the depth of injury. Jensen and associates (13) reported less injury with a 3.2-mm probe when the energy setting was 15 joules and 12 applications were given. However, 13% of the canine bleeding gastric ulcers showed full-thickness injury. When these investigators switched to a higher pulse setting but fewer applications, 14 of 15 ulcers stopped bleeding and no full-thickness injury was noted. When a 2.4-mm probe was used at pulse settings of 15 and 20 joules, the results were similar and no full-thickness injury was noted.

A comparison of dry and liquid monopolar, bipolar (BICAP) and heater probes revealed that these instruments were equally effective at optimal pulse settings of 20, 70, 17 and 15 joules, respectively (13). Liquid and dry monopolar probes were found to cause full-thickness injury in more than 50% of experimentally induced canine ulcers. Swain and colleagues (14) reported that a heater probe was almost as effective as monopolar electrocoagulation but that the modest depth of injury that occurred with the heater probe made it the most promising instrument. The advantages of a heater probe are as follows: portability, absence of electrical hazard, coaxial channel for application of water jet, capability for controlling and presetting rate of pulses, minimal adherence to the base of an ulcer due to Teflon coating, effectiveness, low cost and capability for use at angles other than directly vertical.

MONOPOLAR ELECTROCOAGULATION

The term *coagulation* can mean fulguration or desiccation. *Fulguration* is defined as sparking of tissue to produce necrosis without a cutting effect. *Desiccation* is defined as necrosis caused by application of a surgical electrode to tissue in a manner that avoids a sparking or cutting effect. When a power source is activated, current flows from the active electrode to the target tissue and then through the patient's body to an electrode on the skin. Tissue necrosis is controlled by current density. There are many variables in the performance of electrocoagulation, but experience has shown that the most important variable is the amount of energy per application delivered to the target tissue. This variable is measured in joules.

Blackwood and Silvis (15), in 1971, reported attempts to quantitate the effects of electrocoagulation on canine stomach. They used a Bovie electrosurgical unit. The dogs underwent gastroscopy, and lesions were produced in the mucosa of the gastric body at various settings with a monopolar electrode. In their next study, Blackwood and Silvis (16) used a Cameron-Miller electrosurgical unit as the power source. They studied the effects of amperage and duration of application on the depth of tissue necrosis of the gastric mucosa in anesthetized dogs. An electric current strength of 400 to 425 milliamperes for 1 to 1.5 seconds resulted in mucosal necrosis and minimal muscle necrosis. By prolonging the application time to 2 seconds or increasing the current to 500 milliamperes, a significant increase in muscle necrosis could be produced. Repeating applications on the same area increased the depth of necrosis by 70% to 80%. Blackwood and Silvis (16) concluded that there would be difficulty in standardizing the technique of electrocoagulation.

The author and his coworkers (17) used a Cameron-Miller monopolar coagulator electrode and coagulator unit to produce lesions in canine gastric mucosa endoscopically via a gastrostomy; different power settings and duration of application were used. Contrary to the findings of Blackwood and Silvis (16), the size of an ulcer produced by electrocoagulation did not correlate with the depth of injury at higher settings of the Cameron-Miller coagulator unit. At settings from 5 to 6, the depth of injury could be limited to the submucosa when the mucosa was electrocoagulated for 1 to 7 seconds. Variable degrees of injury occurred at higher settings and at longer durations of application because coagulum formed around the monopolar electrode and because it was not possible to use the same electrode pressure for each lesion that was produced. Similarly, the author and his associates (18) produced esophageal and duodenal lesions by varying the power setting and duration of application. A setting of 6 or higher resulted in transmural injury. Further, although injury was limited to the duodenal mucosa with a current strength of 600 milliamperes at a setting of 5 for 1 second, when only the setting was changed, from 5 to 6, transmural injury occurred, indicating that depth of injury does not depend solely on amperage. Mucosal injury was produced in canine esophagus at settings of 4.5 to 5 for 1 second, but use of higher settings for 1 and 3 seconds resulted in transmural injury. It was concluded that electrocoagulation in the duodenal bulb was much safer than electrocoagulation in the esophagus.

Sugawa and colleagues (19) reported no transmural injury when a Cameron-Miller electrode and coagulator unit were used at settings of 5 and 7 for 5 to 7 seconds. Similarly, Mann and Mann (20), again with a Cameron-Miller electrode found no transmural injury in the esophagus or duodenum at settings of 5, 6 and 7 for 1, 3 and 5 seconds. The discrepency between the latter two reports and that of the author and his coworkers (18) relates to the use of different animal models. In addition, the pressure of application of the monopolar electrode on the mucosa may well have been different in these reports.

By means of an analog computer inserted between an electrosurgical generator and an active electrode, Piercey and colleagues (21) evaluated the efficacy and safety of monopolar electrocoagulation. The analog computer measured actual energy delivered to the target tissue and could be adjusted to deliver a predetermined amount of energy. A force gauge with a predetermined energy of 20 joules, was used to evaluate the effect of electrode pressure on depth of injury. Piercey and colleagues (21) concluded that despite analog computer assistance in controlling energy delivered during monopolar electrocoagulation of experimentally induced canine gastric ulcers, depth of injury was unpredictable and excessively deep.

TECHNIQUES

Electrocoagulation of bleeding upper gastrointestinal lesions cannot be achieved unless the stomach is free of blood and the patient's condition is stabalized. There are numerous ways of clearing the stomach of blood. I use an Edlich gastric lavage tube (Fig. 2). It is passed orally into the stomach. Two or more liters of iced saline may be used to remove blood, food and clots. The patient usually is placed in the left lateral decubitus position. Thereafter, sedation is achieved as necessary, with intravenous diazepam. Before sedation is instituted, an oral bite block is placed. The esophagus is inspected carefully to rule out esophageal varices, esophagitis, ulceration, tumor or Mallory-Weiss tear. Once the endoscope has entered the stomach, it is passed along the lesser curvature to the antrum, avoiding the gastric pool. Once the antrum and pylorus have been inspected, the endoscope is advanced into the duodenal bulb and second portion of the duodenum. If no lesion is seen and if the bile is clear yellow, the endoscope is withdrawn into the stomach to ascertain the cause of bleeding. Care must be taken not to occlude the suction channel while blood and fluid are being aspirated from the gastric pool. If I find an ulcer without stigmata of recent bleeding, endoscopic therapy is not necessary. However, if I observe active bleeding from a visible vessel (Fig. 3), a visible vessel without bleeding (Fig. 4), blood oozing from a clot in the base of an ulcer (Fig. 5) or a "red spot" (Fig. 6), I consider performing electrocoagulation because of the high risk for such lesions to continue to bleed or rebleed (22). Electrocoagulation should not be attempted if torrential bleeding is observed or if esophageal varices are encountered. The technique for applying a BICAP probe and the techniques of monopolar electrocoagulation described by Gaisford (23), Matek

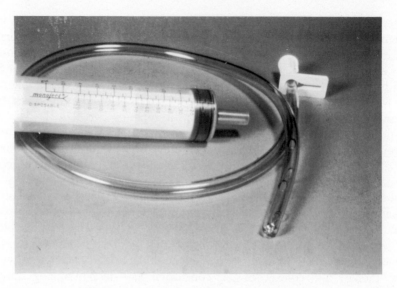

Fig. 2. An Edlich gastric lavage tube (36
French) and syringe.

and associates (24) and the author (25) are similar. The technique for applying a
heater probe is somewhat different.

A heater probe is applied to a vessel with firm pressure to coapt its walls.
Several applications of energy for 1 second may be required for producing
hemostasis. Firm pressure must be applied to the tip of the probe while energy
is being delivered. Fifteen joules is the usual amount of energy per application.
A coaxial channel is available for use to wash away blood and debris. The
possibility that a heater probe may stick to vessels has been noted by various
authors.

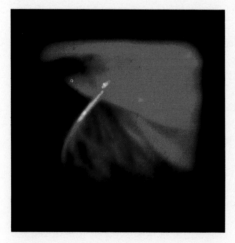

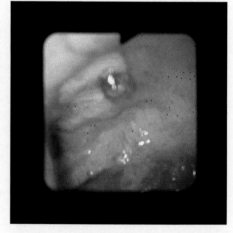

Fig. 3. An actively bleeding rim vessel in
an ulcer.

Fig. 4. A visible vessel with a diameter of
3 mm in a duodenal ulcer.

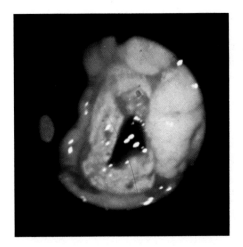
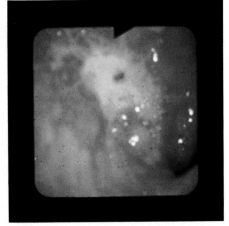

Fig. 5. A gastric ulcer with oozing from a clot in its base.

Fig. 6. A "red spot" in a duodenal ulcer.

The technique for applying a BICAP probe is an important aspect of the procedure. The electrode is placed within 2 to 3 mm of the vessel, and firm pressure is applied. Subsequently, the BICAP hemostatic source is activated at a setting of 9 for 2 seconds. This procedure is repeated until circumferential coagulation has occurred. The probe is then placed firmly on the vessel, and several applications are given until complete hemostasis has occurred.

Once a bleeding lesion is seen by Gaisford (23), he directs a jet of saline delivered through the electrode cannula to the lesion to allow precise identification of the bleeding vessel. If the vessel is 1 mm or less in diameter, he places a monopolar electrode on the vessel and applies pressure to coapt it. Simultaneously, he applies 1- to 2-second pulses of coagulation current. If a larger vessel is found, he applies current circumferentially until the bleeding has stopped. Subsequently, current may be applied directly to the vessel. Although the number of applications around and on a vessel vary for each lesion, from four to 10 are typically given.

Matek and colleagues (24) have modified the technique of the author (25). These investigators use simultaneously instillation of distilled water (electrohydrothermal electrode) via a monopolar electrode and high-frequency Electrotom-170 RF machine as the power source. Five holes are placed in the tip of the monopolar electrode, and distilled water is perfused at a rate of 20 to 40 ml per minute. Insufflation of carbon dioxide, saline and hydrogen peroxide through the probe was studied in standard-sized canine gastric ulcers. Distilled water proved to be most effective. At a setting of 6, the electrode is activated against the bleeding lesion, and distilled water is perfused simultaneously. In a few cases, current is continuously applied for as long as 180 seconds. Matek and colleagues (24) reported that the advantages of their technique are as follows: use of lower energy levels, capability for lengthening duration of coagulation to the therapeutic range to reduce depth of penetration, almost complete absence of charring at the bleeding site and improved visibility.

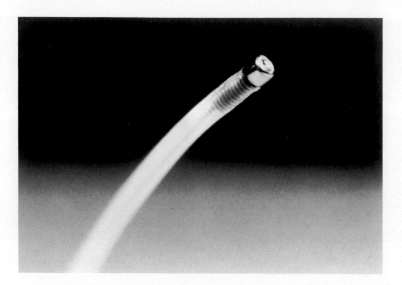

Fig. 7. A monopolar electrode.

A subsequent modification of this technique involved the incorporation of a spring mechanism in the monopolar electrode, allowing a virtually constant force of application to the bleeding site (26). Bleeding from 50 experimentally induced, standard-sized canine gastric lesions was successfully arrested by use of this technique at power settings of 6 to 8.

The author's (25) technique was described in 1976. Once endoscopic examination has demonstrated that a lesion is the site of bleeding, a Cameron-Miller monopolar electrocoagulation probe (Fig. 7) is passed down the biopsy channel and directed to within 2 to 3 mm of the vessel. Current is delivered for 2 to 3 seconds per application. Several applications may be necessary to stop bleeding as the electrode is moved circumferentially around the vessel. Although the electrode should be pressed firmly against the mucosa, it should yield with movement of the mucosa. The Cameron-Miller electrocoagulation unit (model 80-7910) usually is set at 5. If a coagulum accumulates around the electrode, the instrument must be withdrawn and cleaned. The author does not perform irrigation with the coagulation electrode, as do Gaisford (23) and Matek and associates (24).

If blood is oozing from a clot in the base of an ulcer, the clot is dislodged directly by the probe or electrocoagulated to the probe. The clot is then lifted off the ulcer, and the electrode is withdrawn into the biopsy channel, making the clot fall off. The base of the ulcer is then viewed, and therapy is directed at a specific bleeding point. In most instances, direct electrocoagulation of an artery results in further bleeding.

If an artery is actively bleeding, the patient and endoscope must be positioned so that the stream of blood is away from the endoscope. This maneuver may be difficult if a duodenal artery is bleeding but less difficult if a gastric artery is the bleeding point. As the electrode is advanced to a site near the visible vessel, it should not be activated while it is passing through blood; application of current in this setting would lead to accumulation of a coagulum, raising the impedance. The probe should be activated only when it is positioned firmly against the mucosa. Pressure should be applied firmly, but it should yield to movement of the mucosa. Once the bleeding has stopped, it is important to resist the temptation to coagulate the vessel directly. Coagulation should be performed circumferentially to ensure that adequate hemostasis has been achieved.

The amount of energy (joules) used to stop bleeding from a vessel depends on the impedance, the milieu around the vessel and how often the electrode is cleaned. The author and his colleagues (27) have used an analog computer in an attempt to quantitate the amount of energy that is required for arresting arterial bleeding. On average, four 2.5-second applications of 103 joules were needed to stop a bleeding 1-mm duodenal rim vessel at a setting of 5. Five 2-second applications at a setting of 5 were required for 2- and 3-mm, non-bleeding, visible vessels; the energy range was 63 to 105 joules. Five applications of approximately 2 seconds duration at a setting of 5 were used to electrocoagulate three arteriovenuos malformations; the energy range was 30 to 56 joules.

The author's (25) technique is based on the concept that monopolar electrocoagulation achieves hemostasis by producing coagulation in the submucosa. When heat energy is applied around a vessel, the surrounding tissue shrinks, narrowing the vessel. Simultaneously, the pressure of application coapts the vessel. These two events result in coagulation of the vessel and cessation of bleeding.

CLINICAL EXPERIENCE

Koch and coworkers (28) reported their experience with monopolar electrocoagulation performed with a high-energy output generator. These investigators described successful coagulation in 15 bleeding patients but also noted three perforations and one death. It is unclear from their report how much pressure was applied and for how long current was administered. Because of their report, enthusiasm in Europe for monopolar electrocoagulation was dampened during the early 1970s. Youmans and colleagues (29) reported the use of monopolar electrocoagulation performed with a cystoscope via a gastrostomy to produce hemostasis of a bleeding malignant ulcer and bleeding stress ulcers. This report prompted several research groups in the United States to look for ways of using monopolar electrocoagulation to control bleeding in the gastrointestinal tract.

Since the fall of 1971 at the Blodgett Memorial Medical Center, the author has evaluated 681 patients with acute upper gastrointestinal tract bleeding by endoscopy to determine the cause of the hemorrhage. Of 353 patients, 205 had duodenal ulcers, 176 had gastric ulcers (including 26 marginal ulcers) and 10 had esophageal ulcers. Fifty-two patients (20.4%) had actively bleeding duodenal ulcers. Of 176 gastric ulcers, 51 (28.9%) were actively bleeding (44 of 150 gastric ulcers and seven of 26 marginal ulcers). Two of 10 esophageal ulcers showed arterial bleeding. Obviously, a number of patients had several lesions. This experience is similar to that of the American Society for Gastrointestinal Endoscopy national study on upper gastrointestinal bleeding, which reported 29.8% actively bleeding duodenal ulcers and 22.5% actively bleeding gastric ulcers.

In an uncontrolled, but consecutive, series from 1971 to 1983, patients with upper gastrointestinal tract bleeding admitted to the Blodgett Memorial Medical Center underwent endoscopy within 12 hours after admission or, for patients already hospitalized, within 6 hours after the onset of bleeding. Early experience with this series has previously been reported (25, 30–33). No patient was excluded from consideration for endoscopic hemostasis because of severity of hemorrhage. About one-fifth of the patients bled after being treated in the hospital for other medical problems. A total of 119 patients underwent electrocoagulation on 123 occasions. In addition to the previously mentioned ulcer series, 16 of 48 patients with Mallory-Weiss tears had active arterial bleeding. Electrocoagulation was performed successfully in 14 patients and unsuccessfully in two patients. This experience was reported in part in 1980 (33). In addition to the above patients, treatment was successful in a micellaneous group of patients with the following lesions: two varices of the gastric fundus and eight arteriovenous malformations of the stomach and duodenum.

Electrocoagulation was unsuccessful in six patients with duodenal ulcers and in two patients with Mallory-Weiss tears because torrential bleeding obscured vision and because it was not possible to position the monopolar electrocoagulation probe near the bleeding vessels due to the angle of the probe and vessel. These eight patients received surgical treatment after endoscopy identified the site of bleeding. Of the remaining 111 patients, 12 rebled 4 hours to several days later (six patients with gastric and six with duodenal ulcers). Four patients underwent repeat electrocoagulation, which resulted in complete cessation of bleeding. Seven patients received surgical treatment, one of whom died of persistent bleeding. One patient suffered cardiac arrest preoperatively.

Multiple medical problems were a common occurrence, necessitating treatment in various intensive-care units. Despite the severity of their illnesses, only 10 of 119 patients died during the 1-year follow-up period. Many patients in this series were elderly, with the average age of those having gastric or duodenal ulcers being 63 and 69 years, respectively. Six patients died during hospitalization, including the single patient who died of persistent bleeding, noted above. The 5% mortality (six of 119 patients) is much lower than the experiences of other investigators (34), who have reported mortalities of 20% to 50% in patients aged 60 years or older with upper gastrointestinal tract bleeding. The remaining four deaths were due to carcinomatosis, and occurred several months later. It should be pointed out that the patients in this series had actively bleeding ulcers or Mallory-Weiss tears and were considered candidates/for surgical intervention. The operative approach would have been used in many cases if monopolar electrocoagulation had not been effective in stopping the bleeding. More than one-third of the patients were considered poor surgical risks, and more than one-fifth of the patients would not have been candidates for surgical intervention unless exsanguination was imminent. Neither morbidity nor mortality occurred as a result of electrocoagulation. There was no instance of aspiration, respiratory compromise, perforation or cardiac arrest during endoscopy. The number of days and cost of hospitalization were substantially reduced by the use of electrocoagulation, as evidenced by a retrospective analysis (32, 33).

In 1975, Sugawa and colleagues (19) reported treating six patients with monopolar electrocoagulation, achieving initial hemostasis in all cases. The patients had the following lesions: one Mallory-Weiss tear, one gastric ulcer, three cases of gastric erosion and one gastric polyp. Two patients rebled and required surgical intervention (one patient with gastric erosion and one with a gastric ulcer). Volpicelli and colleagues (35) were successful in achieving hemostasis with monopolar electrocoagulation in 12 patients: six patients with duodenal, five with gastric, and one with esophageal ulcers. The gastric ulcer in one patient rebled and electrocoagulation was repeated with no further bleeding. In 1979, Gaisford (23) reported a 92% success rate in achieving hemostasis with endoscopic monopolar electrocoagulation in 71 patients with upper gastrointestinal tract bleeding. Rebleeding occurred in six patients, with four gastric ulcers. Repeat electrocoagulation was successful in these four cases. In the remaining two patients, rebleeding from a Mallory-Weiss tear and a gastric leiomyosarcoma necessitated surgical intervention. The lesions in the 71 patients treated by Gaisford were as follows (some patients had more than one lesion): four esophageal ulcers, six Mallory-Weiss tears, two gastric varices, 29 gastric ulcers, six cases of gastric erosion, two gastric polyps, two gastric leiomyomas, three pyloric channel ulcers, 13 duodenal ulcers and eight jejunal ulcers. No complication was reported as a result of electrocoagulation.

In 1980, Hojsgaard and Wara (36) reported that bleeding had been stopped in 41 of 52 patients, a 79% success rate. Six patients had such massive bleeding that endoscopic hemostasis was impossible, and electrocoagulation was unsuccessful in five patients; surgical intervention stopped the bleeding in these five patients. Rebleeding occurred from 1 to 6 days after electrocoagulation in four patients with gastric ulcers and in three with duodenal ulcers. The electrocoagulated lesions in this series were as follows: 15 gastric ulcers, 10 prepyloric ulcers, 12 duodenal ulcers and nine anastomotic ulcers. One-fourth of the patients in this study were 78 years of age or older. Similar results were obtained when Wara and colleagues (37) combined monopolar electrocoagulation with cimetidine treatment.

When their series became larger, Wara and colleagues (38) again reported their experience with monopolar electrocoagulation in patients with gastroduodenal bleeding. Over a 1-year period, 69 consecutive patients with active bleeding, verified by endoscopy, were entered into this study. This larger series included the 52 patients described previously as well as 17 newer participants. Electrocoagulation was successful in all 17 additional patients. Nine of these 17 patients showed rebleeding, and repeat electrocoagulation was successful in six cases. Repeat coagulation was not considered in the remaining three patients. Neither morbidity nor mortality occurred as a result of elec-

trocoagulation. Wara and colleagues (38) concluded that endoscopic electrocoagulation is an effective treatment, especially if it is performed in quiescent
phases of massive gastrointestinal hemorrhage.

In a study reported by Fischer (39), monopolar electrocoagulation was successful in stopping the bleeding in 33 of 34 patients. Fischer used a Cameron-
Miller electrocoagulation probe. Several short applications of coagulation current were applied between irrigation periods; the duration of the current was
0.5 to 2 seconds, and a setting of 5 was used with the Valley Lab SSE-2 and
Neo-Med cautery units. All 34 patients underwent emergency endoscopy to
locate the site of upper gastrointestinal tract bleeding. The electrocoagulated
lesions included 16 duodenal ulcers, 11 gastric ulcers, three cases of gastric
erosion, one marginal ulcer, two Mallory-Weiss tears and one case of
duodenitis. The bleeding from one Mallory-Weiss tear could not be stopped
and was managed surgically. Fischer's previous operative mortality in patients
with acute upper gastrointestinal tract bleeding was approximately 20%. His
mortality was reduced to zero because using monopolar electrocoagulation
changed an emergency procedure to an elective one, if indicated. Combining
the numbers of patients in the series discussed previously (33–39) reveals that
monopolar electrocoagulation was successful in achieving hemostasis in 258 of
284 patients (91%). In nine patients, electrocoagulation was unsuccessful, and
surgical intervention became necessary. Rebleeding occurred in 28 patients
(approximately 10%), but repeat electrocoagulation stopped the bleeding in 11
of these patients.

CASE REPORTS

Case 1

A 66-year-old man had melena, hematochezia and hematemesis for the 4 days
preceding admission to another hospital. Despite medical treatment and transfusion of 4 units of blood, the patient became hypotensive and was transferred
to Blodgett Memorial Medical Center. He had been taking 10 aspirins per day
for headache for several days before the onset of melena. His medical history
included a myocardial infarction 4 years earlier and, more recently, angina
pectoris, diabetes mellitus and hypertension.

Upper gastrointestinal tract endoscopy with an Olympus GIF-1T was performed 12 hours after admission. Several units of blood had been given to
stabilize the patient's blood pressure. Hemorrhagic, erosive gastritis, duodenal
erosions and an actively bleeding vessel in a duodenal ulcer were seen. The
bleeding stopped after several 2.5- to 3-second applications of monopolar electrocoagulation with a Cameron-Miller electrode at a setting of 5 on a Cameron-
Miller coagulator unit. The patient was discharged 7 days later on a medical
program and has had no further bleeding for 1 year. He had received 19 units
of blood.

As reported in the ASGE survey in 1981, this patient's risk of death from
gastrointestinal bleeding was increased by the presence of multisystem disease, his age and the severity of bleeding, as manifested by hematochezia and

the number of units of blood that had to be given (40). Not only did electrocoagulation stop the bleeding, but subsequent medical management enabled the patient to avoid surgical intervention for which he was a poor risk.

Case 2

A 15-year-old girl was admitted to Blodgett Memorial Medical Center because of hematemesis and syncope. She had suffered from midepigastric pain for the 2 days preceding admission. For the past year, she had been taking 8 extra-strength aspirins per day for headache. In the emergency room, she was found to be hypotensive. The hemoglobin level was 9.6 gm.%.

Upper gastrointestinal tract endoscopy was performed in the emergency room after gastric lavage via an Edlich tube. Clots of blood and bright red blood were aspirated from the stomach. A 1.5-cm gastric ulcer with a visible, non-bleeding vessel was observed (see Fig. 4). The lesion was electrocoagulated without difficulty. In addition, numerous gastric and duodenal erosions were seen.

The patient also was treated with cimetidine and antacids. The bleeding had stopped. Several months later, upper gastrointestinal tract endoscopy was performed for evaluation of abdominal pain. No ulcer was found, but diffuse gastritis was encountered.

The patient's risk for rebleeding was greater than 50%. Because the visible vessel was electrocoagulated immediately, no further bleeding occurred and surgical intervention was obviated.

Case 3

A 39-year-old man had upper gastrointestinal tract bleeding 9 days after Nissen repair. The hemoglobin level had decreased from 15.6 to 11.1 g/dl in association with the the onset of melena. Near the angulus was a 1.5-cm gastric ulcer with an actively bleeding vessel close to its rim (see Fig. 3). Several applications of current with a BICAP probe, at a setting of 6 for 2 seconds and at a setting of 9 for 1 second, failed to stop the bleeding. Subsequently, 3-second applications of current with a Cameron-Miller monopolar electrode at a setting of 5.5 were successful in stopping the bleeding. No further bleeding occurred, and the patient was discharged a few days later on a medical program.

Vessels near the rim of an ulcer seem to be easier to electrocoagulate than those in other parts of an ulcer. If one is unable to stop bleeding with a BICAP probe, monopolar electrocoagulation should be tried.

Case 4

A 69-year-old woman with acute myocardial infarction, persistent pain and congestive heart failure was transferred to Blodgett Memorial Medical Center. She was started on heparin and streptokinase perfusion. During the initial hours of hospitalization, the patient had protracted vomiting. Twenty-four hours later, acute upper gastrointestinal tract bleeding occurred. Emergency endoscopy with an Olympus GIF-1T revealed an actively bleeding Mallory-

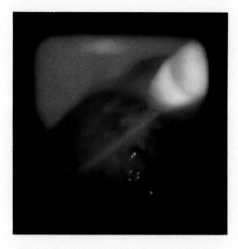

Fig. 8. Active bleeding from a Mallory-Weiss tear at the gastroesophageal junction. A monoplar electrode is seen approaching the bleeding site.

Weiss tear (Fig. 8). The bleeding stopped after the tear received several 2- to 3-second applications of current from a Cameron-Miller electrocoagulation probe at a setting of 5. The action of heparin was reversed by giving protamine sulfate. The patient died about 12 hours later. Autopsy confirmed that the bleeding lesion was a Mallory-Weiss tear and documented that death had occurred from a spontaneous rupture of the anterior wall of the heart with acute cardiac tamponade.

Although most Mallory-Weiss tears stop bleeding spontaneously, some tears require endoscopic or surgical treatment. In this instance, the bleeding had to be stopped immediately due to the precarious cardiovascular status of the patient. The approach used to electrocoagulate a Mallory-Weiss tear is different from the approach used for a bleeding ulcer. It is not possible to position an endoscope and probe at the correct angle to a Mallory-Weiss tear. At best, the probe can be positioned obliquely to the tear but usually is positioned parallel to it. The probe is placed in the tear as near as possible to the bleeding vessel but not directly on it. Only the inner aspects of the tear are coagulated; normal mucosa is not treated.

Case 5

A 77-year-old man presented to the emergency room at Blodgett Memorial Medical Center with complaints of nausea and hematemesis. The hemoglobin level was 9.6 g/dl. After several units of blood had been given, upper gastrointestinal tract endoscopy was performed with an Olympus GIF-1T. An 0.8-cm duodenal ulcer with a "red-spot" was found (see Fig. 6). As it was being observed, it began to pulsate and bleed actively. The vessel was immediately electrocoagulated with a Cameron-Miller monopolar electrode, and the bleeding stopped. The patient was discharged 5 days later on a medical program. He had received 8 units of blood.

Although red spots (small, retracted arteries) do not rebleed as often as do protruding, visible vessels, they do rebleed in approximately 5% to 10% of cases. Red spots should be treated immediately to prevent further bleeding.

ARTERIOVENOUS MALFORMATIONS

Electrocoagulation of arteriovenous malformations in the stomach and duodenum is accomplished by a technique similar to that used for arteries. The electrode is placed on the peripheral border of the malformation with moderate pressure and is moved circumferentially until a complete circle has been made. Several applications of current are given, but never on the same area. If the malformation measures greater than 1 cm, it may have to be treated a second time. The center of an arteriovenous malformation should never be electrocoagulated until its periphery has been treated; otherwise, torrential bleeding may occur.

I have treated eight patients with arteriovenous malformations. They were included in the series previously described (27) (see Clinical Experience). The duration of application ranged from 0.9 to 2.2 seconds. The current varied from 30 to 56 joules per application and was delivered with a Cameron-Miller coagulator unit at a setting of 5. Farup and colleagues (41) also used monopolar electrocoagulation successfully to treat gastric and duodenal arteriovenous malformations. Other investigators have used a hot biopsy forceps with success (42–44).

The author and his colleagues (45) have studied the effects of fulguration and electrocoagulation on canine colonic mucosa. Transmural injury was produced when applications that lasted more than 1 second were given at settings of 4.5 to 6 on a Cameron-Miller unit and at settings of 3 to 6 on a Valley Lab SSE 3. Several authors (33, 46, 47, 49, 50) have had excellent results in stopping the bleeding from arteriovenous malformations in the colon and have reported no morbidity or mortality.

THE VISIBLE VESSEL

The implications of the visible vessel were noted in the early 1970s, but this feature was overlooked as a major cause of rebleeding until the late 1970s and early 1980s. Foster and colleagues (22) defined the stigmata of recent bleeding from ulcers as consisting of fresh bleeding from a lesion, a fresh or altered blood clot or black slough adherent to a lesion (Fig. 9) and a vessel protruding from the base or margin of an ulcer (see Fig. 4).

In a prospective study, Storey and associates (48) followed up 47 patients

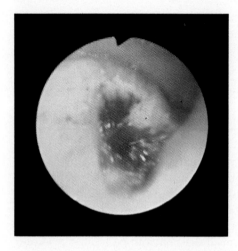

Fig. 9. A duodenal ulcer with black eschar in its base.

with ulcers and stigmata of bleeding. Nineteen of 34 patients (56%) with a visible vessel showed rebleeding, as compared to only one of 13 patients (8%) with other stigmata of bleeding. In 40 patients without stigmata, no further bleeding occurred. Eight of 16 nonbleeding, visible vessels rebled and four of 39 spots (10%) rebled in a study by Vallon and colleagues (49). Similar findings have been reported by Domschke and coworkers (50). Fifty-six percent of visible vessels rebled, whereas only 8% of oozing lesions, black spots and blood clots rebled. No rebleeding occurred in patients with ulcer disease and no stigmata. Swain and associates (51) reported similar findings. When a vessel is actively bleeding, it will continue to bleed or rebleed in 78% to 100% of cases (49, 52–54).

The author (55) has reported a prospective study of 32 patients who had bleeding ulcers with visible vessels in the upper gastrointestinal tract. Sixteen patients were assigned randomly to a control group and treated medically, and 16 patients underwent electrocoagulation immediately after the nonbleeding, visible vessels had been identified. In the control group, seven patients had gastric ulcers and nine had duodenal ulcers. Six of the vessels in the gastric ulcers and seven of the vessels in the duodenal ulcers rebled (81%). In the control group the vessels in the gastric ulcers were centrally located, whereas four of the vessels in the duodenal ulcers were centrally located and three were near the rim. The vessels rebled 4 hours to 20 days after medical treatment, with the vast majority rebleeding within 36 hours. By contrast, in the electrocoagulation group, the vessel in one fundal ulcer rebled 3 days after treatment; the vessels in the remaining 15 ulcers (93%) showed no further bleeding.

The average hospital stay for patients in the electrocoagulation group who were treated successfully was 8.3 days, which was similar to the average stay of the three patients in the control group whose bleeding stopped spontaneously. The patients in whom rebleeding occurred were hospitalized an average of 15.9 days. The cost of hospitalization for patients who successfully underwent electrocoagulation was, on the average, $1900 less than the cost for patients in whom rebleeding occurred (55). Monopolar electrocoagulation was found to be safe and effective in arresting bleeding and in stopping rebleeding as well as in reducing length and cost of hospitalization.

CONCLUSION

After more than 13 years of experimental and clinical evaluation, monopolar electrocoagulation has been found to be a safe, effective and inexpensive modality of treatment. Careful attention must be given to the technique of application. Although bipolar electrocoagulation causes less injury, it also is less effective in producing lasting hemostasis. Further experience with heater probes must accrue before their applications in the management of bleeding in the upper gastrointestinal tract can be ascertained.

REFERENCES

1. Moore JP, Silvis SE, Vennes JA: Evaluation of bipolar electrocoagulation in canine stomachs. *Gastrointest Endosc* 24:148–151, 1978.

2. Protell RL, Gilbert DA, Opie EA, et al: Computer-assisted electrocoagulation: Bipolar vs. monopolar in the treatment of experimental gastric ulcer bleeding. *Gastroenterology* 80:451–455, 1981.

3. Machicado GA, Jensen DM, Tapia JI, et al: Treatment of bleeding canine duodenal and esophageal ulcers with argon laser and bipolar electrocoagulation. *Gastroenterology* 81:859–865, 1981.

4. Johnston JH, Jensen DM, Mautner W: Comparison of endoscopic electrocoagulation and laser photocoagulation of bleeding canine gastric ulcers. *Gastroenterology* 82:904–910, 1982.

5. Auth DC, Gilbert DA, Opie EA, et al: The multipolar probe—A new endoscopic technique to control gastrointestinal bleeding. (abstract) *Gastrointest Endosc* 26:63, 1980.

6. Verhoeven AGM, Bartelsman JFWM, Huibregtse K, et al: A new multipolar coagulation electrode for endoscopic hemostasis, in *Stomach Diseases. Current Status. Proceedings of the 13th International Congress on Stomach Diseases.* Amsterdam-Oxford-Princeton, Excerpta Medica, 1981, pp 216–221.

7. Risa L, Miscusi G, Caruso C: L'elettrocoagulatore multipolare BICAP net trattament delle emmorragie digestive, in *Advances in Digestive Surgery and Endoscopy.* Rome, 1983, pp 117–123.

8. Gilbert DA, Verhoeven T, Jensen K, et al: A multicenter clinical trial of the BICAP probe for upper gastrointestinal bleeding. (abstract) *Gastrointest Endosc* 28:150, 1982.

9. Winklet WP, Comer G, McCray RS: Initial experience with BICAP mutipolar electrocautery in the control of upper gastrointestinal hemorrhage. (abstact) *Gastrointest Endosc* 29:169, 1983.

10. Yamamoto H, Hajiro K, Matsui H, et al: Endoscopic bipolar electrocoagulation: Development of a new bipolar coagulator for stopping gastrointestinal bleeding. *Gastroenterol Jpn* 17:75–79, 1982.

11. Mills TN, Swain CP, Dark JM, et al: The "hot squeeze" bipolar forceps. A more effective endoscopic method for stopping bleeding from large vessels in the gastrointestinal tract. (abstract) *Gastrointest Endosc* 29:184–185, 1983.

12. Protell RL, Rubin CE, Auth DC, et al: The heater probe: A new endoscopic method for stopping massive gastrointestinal bleeding. *Gastroenterology* 74:257–262, 1978.

13. Jensen DM, Tapia JI, Machicado GA, et al: Endoscopic heater and multipolar probes for treatment of bleeding canine gastric ulcers. (abstract) *Gastrointest Endosc* 29:151, 1982.

14. Swain CP, Mills TN, Shemesh E, et al: Which electrode? A consumer's guide to endoscopic electrocoagulation of upper gastrointestinal bleeding. (abstract) *Gastrointest Endosc* 29:187–188, 1983.

15. Blackwood WD, Silvis SE: Gastroscopic electrosurgery. *Gastroenterology* 61:305–314, 1971.

16. Blackwood WD, Silvis SE: Standardization of electrosurgical lesions. *Gastrointest Endosc* 21:22–24, 1974.

17. Papp JP, Fox JM, Wilks HS: Experimental electrocoagulation of dog mucosa. *Gastrointest Endosc* 22:27–28, 1975.

18. Papp JP, Fox JM, Nalbandian RM: Experimental electrocoagulation of dog esophageal and duodenal mucosa. *Gastrointest Endosc* 23:27–28, 1976.

19. Sugawa C, Shier M, Lucas CE, et al: Electrocoagulation of bleeding in the upper part of the gastrointestinal tract. *Arch Surg (Chicago)* 110:975–979, 1975.

20. Mann SK, Mann NS: Effect of monopolar electrocoagulation on esophagus, stomach, and duodenum in dogs. *Am J Gastroenterol* 71:568–571, 1979.

21. Piercey JRA, Auth DC, Silverstein FE, et al: Electrosurgical treatment of experimental bleeding canine gastric ulcers: Development and testing of a computer control and a better electrode. *Gastroenterology* 74:527–534, 1978.

22. Foster DN, Miloszewski KJA, Losowsky MS: Stigmata of recent haemorrhage in diagnosis and prognosis of upper gastrointestinal bleeding. *Br Med J* 1:473–477, 1978.

23. Gaisford WD: Endoscopic electrohemostasis of active upper gastrointestinal bleeding. *Am J Surg* 137:47–53, 1979.

24. Matek W, Fruhmorgen P, Kaduk B, et al: Modified electrocoagulation and its possibilities in control of gastrointestinal bleeding. *Endoscopy* 4:253–258, 1979.

25. Papp JP: Endoscopic electrocoagulation of upper gastrointestinal hemorrhage. *J Am Med Ass* 236:2076–2079, 1976.

26. Matek W, Fruhmorgen P, Kaduk B, et al: The healing process of experimentally produced bleeding lesions after hemostasis electrocoagulation with simultaneous instillation of water. *Endoscopy* 12:231–236, 1980.

27. Papp JP, Auth DC, Silverstein FE: Analog computer evaluation of monopolar electrocoagulation in patients having had UGI bleeding. (abstract) *Gastrointest Endosc* 26:73, 1980.

28. Koch H, Pesch HJ, Bauerle H, et al: Experimentelle Untersuchungen und Klinische Erfahrungen zur Electrokogulation Blutende Lasionen im oberen Gastrointestinaltrakt. *Fortschr Endosk* 10:67–71, 1972.

29. Youmans CR, Patterson M, McDonald DF, et al: Cystoscopic control of gastric hemorrhage. *Arch Surg (Chicago)* 100:721–723, 1970.

30. Papp JP: Endoscopic electrocoagulation in upper gastrointestinal hemorrhage: A preliminary report. *J Am Med Ass* 230:1172–1173, 1974.

31. Papp JP: Endoscopic electrocoagulation of actively bleeding arterial upper gastrointestinal lesions. *Am J Gastroenterol* 71:516–521, 1979.

32. Papp JP: *Endoscopic Control of Gastrointestinal Hemorrhage.* Boca Raton, Florida, CRC Press, 1981.

33. Papp JP: Electrocoagulation of actively bleeding Mallory-Weiss tears. *Gastrointest Endosc* 26:128–129, 1980.

34. Himal HS, Watson W, Jones CW, et al: The management of upper gastrointestinal hemorrhage. *Ann Surg* 179:489–493, 1972.

35. Volpicelli NA, McCarthy JD, Bartlett JD, et al: Endoscopic electrocoagulation: An alternative to operative therapy in bleeding peptic ulcer disease. *Arch Surg (Chicago)* 113:483–486, 1978.

36. Hojsgaard A, Wara P: Gastroduodenal haemorrhage treated by endoscopic electrocoagulation. *Ugeskr Laeg* 142:501–510, 1980.

37. Wara P, Hojsgaard A, Amdrup E: Endoscopic electrocoagulation combined with cimetidine: A pilot study of the applicability in active bleeding from gastroduodenal ulcer. *Acta Chir Scand* 146:431–434, 1980.

38. Wara P, Hojsgaard A, Amdrup E: Endoscopic electrocoagulation—An alternative to operative hemostasis in active gastroduodenal bleeding? *Endoscopy* 12:237–240, 1980.

39. Fischer M: Endoscopic electrocoagulation of bleeding upper gastrointestinal lesions. *Mil Med* 146:407–409, 1981.

40. Gilbert DA, Silverstein FE, Tedesco FJ, et al: The national ASGE survey on upper gastrointestinal bleeding. III. Endoscopy in upper gastrointestinal bleeding. *Gastrointest Endosc* 27:94–102, 1981.

41. Farup PG, Rosseland AR, Stray N, et al: Localized telangiopathy of the stomach and duodenum diagnosed and treated endoscopically. *Endoscopy* 2:1–6, 1981.

42. Sassaris M, Pang G, Hunter F: Telangiectasia of the upper gastrointestinal tract: Report of six cases and reviews. *Endoscopy* 15:85–88, 1983.

43. Weaver GA, Alpern HD, Davis JS, et al: Gastrointestinal angiodysplasia associated with aortic valve disease: Part of a spectrum of angiodysplasia of the gut. *Gastroenterology* 77:1–11, 1979.

44. Weingart J, Lux G, Elster K, et al: Recurrent gastrointestinal bleeding in Osler's disease successfully treated by endoscopic electrocoagulation in the stomach. *Endoscopy* 7;160–164, 1975.

45. Papp JP, Nalbandian RM, Wilcox RM, et al: Experimental evaluation of electrocoagulation and fulguration of dog colon mucosa. *Gastrointest Endosc* 25:140–141, 1979.

46. Nuesch HJ, Kobler E, Buhler H, et al: Angiodysplasien des Kolon—Diagnose und Therapie. *Schwiez Med Wochenschr* 109:607–611, 1979.

47. Tedesco FJ, Griffin JW Jr, Khan AQ: Vascular ectasia of the colon: Clinical, colonoscopic and radiographic features. *J Clin Gastroenterol* 2:233–237, 1980.

48. Storey DW, Bown SG, Swain CP, et al: Endoscopic prediction of recurrent bleeding in peptic ulcers. *N Engl J Med* 305:915–916, 1981.

49. Vallon AG, Cotton PB, Laurence BH, et al: Randomised trial of endoscopic argon laser photocoagulation in bleeding peptic ulcers. *Gut* 22:228–233, 1981.

50. Domschke W, Lederer P, Lux G: The value of emergency endoscopy in upper gastrointestinal bleeding: Review and analysis of 2014 cases. *Endoscopy* 15:126–131, 1983.

51. Swain CP, Bown SG, Salmon PR, et al: Nature of the bleeding point in massively bleeding gastric ulcers. (abstract) *Gastroenterology* 84:1327, 1983.

52. MacLeod IA, Mills PR, MacKenzie JF, et al: Neodymium yttrium aluminum garnet laser photocoagulation for major haemorrhage from peptic ulcers and single vessels: A single blind controlled study. *Br Med J* 286:345–348, 1983.

53. Rutgeerts P, Van Trappen G, Broeckaert L, et al: Controlled trial of Yag laser treatment of upper digestive hemorrhage. *Gastroenterology* 83:410–416, 1982.

54. Griffiths WJ, Neumann DA, Welsh JD: The visible vessel as an indicator of uncontrolled or recurrent gastrointestinal hemorrhage. *N Engl J Med* 300:1411–1413, 1979.

55. Papp JP: Endoscopic electrocoagulation in the management of upper gastrointestinal tract bleeding. *Surg Clin North Am* 62:797–806, 1982.

7

Laser Treatment of Bleeding Peptic Ulcers and Visible Vessels

Bergein F. Overholt

Physicians concerned with the treatment of upper gastrointestinal hemorrhage have increasingly recognized the potential of endoscopy to provide effective therapy for bleeding peptic ulcers. More recently, considerable attention has centered around the "visible vessel" in patients with bleeding peptic ulcers. By definition, the term refers to a vessel in the base of an ulcer that is visible during endoscopy in a patient who has bled or is bleeding from an ulcer in the upper gastrointestinal tract. These vessels vary in size, shape and location and have the dimensions of length, width and height. Their clinical significance is great in that they are predictive of recurrent or further bleeding and as such are associated with higher mortality rates.

Endoscopy has provided clinicians ready access to ulcers with visible vessels and with active bleeding. To treat these lesions required only the development of techniques to be applied through endoscopes. Technology responded. Although the new era of therapeutic endoscopy is in its infancy, several therapeutic endoscopic modalities, including laser photocoagulation, electrocoagulation, heater probes and injection techniques, are evolving in the treatment of visible vessels. These advances are reducing the incidence of recurrent bleeding, the need for transfusions, the need for emergency surgery and the mortality of patients with such lesions. This chapter deals specifically with the use of lasers in the treatment of bleeding ulcers and visible vessels.

NATURAL HISTORY OF UPPER GASTROINTESTINAL TRACT HEMORRHAGE

To ultimately reduce the mortality of upper gastrointestinal tract hemorrhage requires a knowledge of the natural history and outcome of patients with this problem. The extensive survey by the American Society for Gastrointestinal Endoscopy (1) and other studies (2–6) have defined the outcome and have identified patients at high risk for morbidity and mortality. It is for such patients that therapeutic endoscopy holds the greatest promise for reducing mortality.

Endoscopy has provided a methodology that allows an accurate diagnosis of upper gastrointestinal tract hemorrhage in approximately 90% of cases (1,2). Fortunately in some 80% of cases, bleeding stops spontaneously before admission or before endoscopy is performed (1,6,7). As has been pointed out by numerous investigators, however, the overall mortality rate for patients with upper gastrointestinal tract bleeding remains 8-10%. Factors increasing the risk of death have been identified and generally relate to the severity of bleeding, significant co-existing medical illnesses, age above 60 years, need for surgery and continued or recurrent bleeding (1–7).

An important endoscopic observation in patients with upper gastrointestinal hemorrhage has been the recognition of ulcers with "stigmata of recent hemorrhage" (SRH) (8–10). This term refers to those patients with current or recent ulcer bleeding in whom endoscopy reveals an ulcer with active bleeding, a

TABLE 1. Etiology of Upper Gastrointestinal Tract Hemorrhage (1)*

Peptic ulcers	
Duodenal	24%
Gastric	21%
Stomal	2%
Gastric erosions	23%
Varices	10%
Mallory-Weiss tears	7%
Esophagitis	6%
Duodenitis, erosive	6%
Tumors	3%
Esophageal Ulcers	2%
O-W-R Telangiectasia	0.5%
Other lesions	6%

*Total greater than 100% as several patients had more than one lesion.

visible vessel or a fresh clot. Although rebleeding has occured in up to 42% of patients with stigmata of recent hemorrhage (9), it appears that the risk of recurrent hemorrhage is greatest in those found to be actively bleeding (85% rebleed) (11) or who are found to have true visible vessels (50% to 56% rebleed) (10,11) at endoscopy. The importance of rebleeding, and hence of these lesions, is emphasized by the fact that rebleeding in hospitalized patients is associated with a 22% mortality compared to a 2% mortality for those who do not rebleed (7). Thus, a category of high-risk patients and lesions amenable to laser photocoagulation therapy has been identified.

Endoscopy has improved our ability to diagnose and access bleeding peptic ulcers and has provided a technique to identify high risk lesions and patients. Technological advances, such as laser photocoagulation, will allow therapeutic endoscopy in the treatment of upper gastrointestinal hemorrhage to make further progress in reducing the morbidity and mortality, as well as the treatment cost, of this life threatening problem.

HISTORY OF LASER TREATMENT OF UPPER GASTROINTESTINAL HEMORRHAGE

In 1975 Dwyer and colleagues (12–14) reported the sucessful application of the argon laser for the control of bleeding in humans. In Germany Frühmorgen et al. (15–17) reported in 1976 their success in coagulating bleeding lesions with the argon laser. In the following year Kiefhaber and associates (18), also in Germany, reported the use of the Nd:YAG laser for the control of massive upper gastrointestinal hemorrhage. Kiefhaber subsequently reported on his extensive experience with the Nd:YAG laser (19) with successful results in 94% of 692 unselected patients with various causes of upper gastrointestinal bleeding. Other studies to be discussed subsequently have reported on controlled trials with the argon and Nd:YAG lasers for the control of hemorrhage from peptic ulcers.

EXPERIMENTAL STUDIES IN LABORATORY ANIMALS

Stimulated by the initial reports on the use of laser therapy in animals and humans, a number of investigators have conducted extensive animal model research on the use of lasers for the control of ulcer hemorrhage. Utilizing the standard ulcer maker, essentially a modified intestinal biopsy tube (20), acute ulcers measuring 1 cm in diameter and 0.15 cm deep can be created in heparinized dogs which are then studied to evaluate the effectiveness of lasers in treatment of bleeding. Although certainly not comparable to the bleeding peptic ulcer seen clinically, the ulcer maker does provide a reliable model to be studied.

Animal studies (for a concise summary of laser studies in laboratory animals see Silverstein and colleagues [21]) with the argon laser have shown that high power settings (5 to 7 watts) are necessary to effectively coagulate bleeding lesions. Because blood absorbs argon laser energy, a coaxial carbon dioxide gas jet system (22) was incorporated into the laser probe emitting the gas jet coaxially to the laser beam clearing blood from the field. The proper rate of gas flow for clearing blood was studied by Johnston et al. (23). Over distention and consequent thinning of the stomach wall also was found to correlate with greater laser-induced full-thickness injury to the gastric wall.

Animal studies with the Nd:YAG laser have shown greater tissue injury correlating with higher power settings and longer times of application (24). Johnston et al. (25) found that high power settings and close proximity of the laser probe tip to the lesion produced more frequent full-thickness injury to the gastric wall. In such circumstances an erosive effect was occasionally seen which actually resulted in increased bleeding or rebleeding, an important clinical consideration that will be dealt with later. Bown et al. (26) suggested that the total energy delivered to the gastric mucosa also correlated with full-thickness injury. In dogs full-thickness injury and perforation appear to be well tolerated. Because peritonitis does not develop, extrapolation of results in animals to humans is somewhat difficult (27,28). A more recent study by Kelly et al. (29) demonstrated that the extent of damage and the rate of healing depended on the amount of laser energy used. As commonly used in humans, 75 watts with 0.4 second applications achieved hemostasis with total energy concentrations that neither produced full-thickness tissue damage nor altered the healing rate from that observed in untreated ulcers. It was found that thermal contraction was the primary hemostatic mechanism, with thrombosis occurring only as a secondary effect. The Nd:YAG laser effectively stops bleeding in the experimental setting (30).

Comparisons between the argon and the Nd:YAG lasers have been performed by several groups (24–26). Findings indicate that both lasers effectively coagulate bleeding lesions, with the Nd:YAG laser producing more rapid results. The Nd:YAG laser creates more frequent full-thickness injury in the dog gastric wall, but the significance of this information in the human is uncertain. Recent clinical studies have not reported perforation as a complication of Nd:YAG laser treatment. The experimental work by Kelly et. al. (29) confirms the relative safety of the Nd:YAG laser.

The following aspects of laser photocoagulation therapy have been studied: time required for therapeutic effect, the need for a gas jet to clear the field of blood, cessation of bleeding, depth of tissue injury, and the occurrence of perforation. According to observations made in animal models, power (watts) settings and time (duration) of laser application have been suggested as variables. However, the information gleaned from laboratory investigations is only partially transferable to the clinical setting. Organ movement from respiratory or peristaltic motion, organ distention from insufflation that thins the organ wall, presence of fluid or secretions, and variable distances from the bleeding lesion are simultaneously occurring factors in the clinical setting that are difficult to recreate in the laboratory. These variables represent critical elements in laser therapy which greatly influence the use and effectiveness of lasers in human beings.

CLINICAL STUDIES OF LASER CONTROL OF UPPER GASTROINTESTINAL HEMORRHAGE

Clinical studies of laser photocoagulation of upper gastrointestinal hemorrhage are difficult to compare. Most lesions stop bleeding spontaneously. Patient selection has varied considerably from one center to another, and details of techniques used differ. Classification of bleeding lesions is not standardized and has produced some confusion; however a number of prospective controlled studies are published. Some of these studies are ongoing and appear to show more favorable results as the series expand.

Nd:YAG STUDIES

Rutgeerts and colleagues (31) were able to control spurting arterial bleeding in 87% of 23 patients, but the recurrence of bleeding was high (55%). The incidence of surgery was less in this group (61%) compared to their historical rate (95%). In 86 patients with active, non-spurting bleeding, the Nd:YAG laser was significantly more effective ($p < 0.001$) than conservative treatment in stopping the bleeding. The rate of recurrence of bleeding and the need for surgery were lower, although statistical significance was not found ($p < 0.1$). In their patients with stigmata of recent hemorrhage, a numerical reduction in the rate of rebleeding and in the operative indications occurred, but again statistical significance was not achieved. In a subsequent report Rutgeerts et al. (32) found pretreatment with injection of adrenalin around arterial spurters or visible vessels in patients with transfusion needs of greater than 5 units significantly reduced further bleeding ($p < 0.005$), the operative rate ($p < 0.005$), and mortality ($p < 0.01$).

Swain et al.(33), in a randomized study involving 82 patients, found that Nd:YAG laser therapy significantly reduced the incidence of rebleeding ($p < 0.001$) and the need for emergency surgery ($p < 0.01$). In patients with visible vessels undergoing laser treatment only 3 of 22 rebled, as compared to

16 of the 27 control patients ($p < 0.005$). In patients with other stigmata of recent hemorrhage, rebleeding was found to be uncommon in treatment or control groups. Swain et. al. suggested that the Nd:YAG laser significantly reduced the rebleeding rate and the need for emergency surgery in patients with peptic ulcers and stigmata of recent hemorrhage that are accessible to laser therapy.

In 1981 Ihre and associates (34) reported on 135 patients with active or inactive bleeding of all types including varices. After selection and entry into the study, 23 patients were assigned to the laser group. Eight patients could not be treated for technical reasons. Fourteen of the 15 patients who underwent laser treatment stopped bleeding, but 7 rebled. There was no significant difference with regard to continued or recurrent bleeding, the need for emergency surgery or mortality between the treatment and the control groups.

In the same year Escourrou et al. (35) reported no difference in control or treated groups in permanent hemostasis, need for surgery, or mortality between patients who received Nd:YAG laser therapy and those who did not. Eight of the 42 randomly assigned to laser therapy were excluded because endoscopic therapy was not possible.

MacLeod and colleagues (36,37) studied 45 patients and found that bleeding from ulcers without spots stopped irrespective of the treatment allocated. Twenty patients were bleeding from arteries. Eight were allocated to placebo treatment and all later underwent emergency surgery for management of further hemorrhage. Twelve were allocated to receive Nd:YAG laser treatment and only one of eight who actually received laser therapy required surgery ($p < 0.002$). Four were not treated because of clinical or technical reasons and all of them required emergency surgery.

ARGON LASER STUDIES

In 1981, Vallon and colleagues (11) reported on 28 patients with actively bleeding ulcers, 35 patients with nonbleeding visible vessels, and 73 patients with nonbleeding ulcers without visible vessels but with a "central spot." They found no statistically significant difference in regard to prevention of bleeding or the need for emergency surgery.

Swain et al. (38) studied patients with active and inactive bleeding with visible vessels (Groups 1 and 2), patients with other stigmata of recent hemorrhage (Groups 3 and 4) and patients with overlying clots (Groups 5 and 6). Argon laser therapy in Groups 1 and 2 significantly reduced rebleeding or continued bleeding as well as mortality. There was no difference between patients who received argon laser therapy and those who did not in the other groups. On two occasions the laser was fired at visible but non-bleeding vessels and caused arterial hemorrhage which could not be stopped by further application of the laser. This complication will be discussed at a later point in this chapter.

Jensen et al. (39) also reported greater permanent hemostasis and less frequent need for emergency surgery in a small series of patients treated with the argon laser.

NEODYMIUM:YAG AND ARGON LASER CHARACTERISTICS

Considerable debate has occurred between advocates for each type of GI laser, each proclaiming the virtues and effectiveness of either the argon or the Nd:YAG laser in the treatment of upper gastrointestinal hemorrhage from peptic ulcers. The argon laser has the theoretical advantage of safety as the tissue penetration is shallow, usually stated to be 1 mm. In contrast the Nd:YAG laser penetrates tissue to a depth of 4 mm. In practice, perforation with either laser is practically non-existant when used by a competent, skilled endoscopist. The argon laser energy is absorbed by blood and therefore requires a high flow of carbon dioxide or air to clear the blood from the bleeding site in order for the laser energy to be applied effectively. The Nd:YAG laser energy is essentially not absorbed by blood and will therefore produce at least some tissue coagulation in spite of the presence of blood, thus making air flow a less critical element for this laser. However, in the case of a significantly bleeding lesion, gas flow to clear the field is necessary to allow proper visualization and laser application. Greater application time of laser energy is required for the argon laser as compared to the Nd:YAG laser, providing a theoretical, if not practical, advantage for the Nd:YAG laser. The argon laser aiming beam is visible, whereas the Nd:YAG laser beam is not. The Nd:YAG therefore requires an additional xenon or helium-neon aiming beam which represents a practical disadvantage for this laser. The Nd:YAG laser holds greater risk of potential damage to the eye of the examiner, observer or patient. However the argon laser can also injure the eye and the use of protective goggles (or an endoscope viewing lens cover) is recommended with both lasers.

Fleischer (40) has reported that the Nd:YAG laser represents the majority of GI lasers in use. Whether this represents theoretical, practical or marketing advantages over the argon laser is uncertain. What is certain is that successful laser use is dependent upon the dedication of the endoscopist in stopping upper gastrointestinal hemorrhage through precise, exacting and sometimes gruelling efforts. Tissue effects of edema, thermal contraction and thrombosis are essential, and both the argon and the Nd:YAG lasers will produce these results if properly used. It appears, however, that most endoscopists favor the Nd:YAG laser for the control of upper gastrointestinal hemorrhage.

INDICATIONS AND CONTRAINDICATIONS

Indications and contraindications for laser photocoagulation are generally similar to those for endoscopy in patients with upper gastrointestinal hemorrhage.

If endoscopy is indicated and feasable, laser therapy can be considered. For patients with torrential bleeding which can not be adequately cleared for visualization, emergency surgery is indicated in most situations. With lesser degrees of bleeding, attempts at laser therapy are possible. Patients with stigmata of recent hemorrhage including active bleeding, a visible vessel or a fresh clot are ideal candidates for laser photocoagulation. As discussed later, the visible gastroduodenal artery should be approached with great caution, if at all. The greatest contraindication is any one or a combination of: (1) the untrained endoscopist, (2) the unprepared assistant or (3) the inadequate facility.

PREPARATION PRIOR TO LASER PHOTOCOAGULATION

Several authors have described the techniques and requirements for dealing with bleeding peptic ulcers and visible vessels (13,28,41). Beyond the development of an adequate facility (42), it is of paramount importance that the endoscopist be trained and experienced in the use of endoscopy in upper gastrointestinal hemorrhage and that a competent team of endoscopic assistants be available.

EQUIPMENT AND DRUGS

Preparation prior to laser use is essential as laser therapy for upper gastrointestinal hemorrhage is exacting work. One must anticipate and prepare for the

TABLE 2. Laser Preparation: Equipment and Drugs

Large-bore irrigation tube
Vasopressin
Two-channel endoscope (white tip)
Snare
Water Pik or syringe irrigator
Blood pump
Cardiac monitor
Pulse and blood pressure monitor
Oxygen
Crash cart
Nasogastric tube taped onto endoscope (optional)
Williams "overtube" (optional)
Photography and television camera equipment (optional)

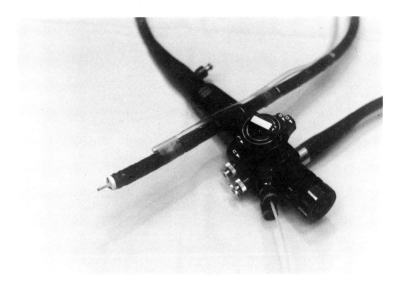

Fig. 1. A two-channel endoscope (white tipped). The laser probe is exiting one channel.

most difficult situation—the massive bleeder, and for the worst complication—laser induced massive arterial bleeding. Equipment and drugs must be available for immediate use.

A Monoject® or large-bore tube is used for thorough lavage of the stomach. Vasopressin must be available for intravenous use if uncontrollable bleeding occurs, to hopefully reduce the bleeding rate. A two-channel endoscope (Fig. 1) is preferred, although a large bore single channel instrument is acceptable. A white instrument tip is available from one manufacturer and can be used to reduce heating and damage to the instrument tip. A nasogastric tube can be taped alongside the instrument for recycling of air or gas allowing one channel to remain free for other uses. A snare should be available for transecting or removing large adherent clots, particularly those in the fundus. The Williams tube, which is used in sclerotherapy, is useful when inserted to serve as a splint to allow frequent, rapid and safe removal of the endoscope and clots. The tube also protects the patient's airway. The device is inserted over a Maloney number 44 dilator passed through the Williams tube; the dilator is removed and the tube is left in place as a splint. The side window is covered with tape to prevent mucosa from protruding into the lumen of the tube. If a large hiatal hernia or esophageal stricture is present this technique must be performed with caution. A quick endoscopic survey of the esophagus and stomach is advisable as a first step prior to introduction of the splint.

A Water Pik or syringe irrigator is needed to remove clots. A blood pump is also necessary to allow rapid blood infusion when needed. The availability of

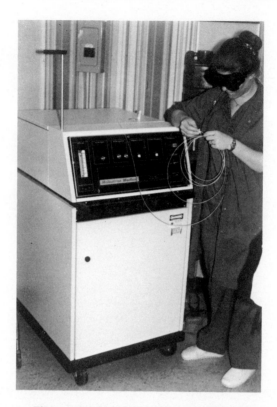

Fig. 2. An Nd:YAG laser. The flexible laser probe is exiting from the unit, and the tip is being cleaned.

cardiac, pulse and blood pressure monitors are advisable to assist in patient monitoring. Routine use of oxygen is advised as patients are often critically ill and in shock. A crash cart is essential in the event the need for it arises. Photographic and television equipment are helpful for purposes of documentation.

PERSONNEL

Competent endoscopic assistants are essential to a successful laser treatment facility. A minimum of two trained assistants should be available, with one being on call at all times. With such personnel, errors can be minimized. These assistants should be carefully trained and prepared for laser work. Team work is essential and rehearsal is necessary prior to beginning laser work and at periodic intervals if time between laser usage is excessive. The assistants should be capable of setting up for and participating in laser use as well as monitoring the patient. Their responsibilities should also entail alerting the operating suite of potential emergency surgery for treatment of massive upper gastrointestinal hemorrhage.

PHYSICIAN

Gastroenterologists using lasers in the treatment of massive upper gastrointestinal hemorrhage should always ensure that a surgeon is immediately available. The endoscopist should be prepared to expend 1½ to 3 hours or more on patients with active bleeding. Considerable scheduling flexibility is required. Treatment of visible vessels or spots may require less time, but to "sandwich" a laser case into a busy schedule without allowing adequate time is to invite disaster. Training and other requirements for physicians performing laser work have been discussed previously in this text.

THE LASER

Preparation of laser equipment should be automatic and should be checked by both the assistant and the physician (Fig. 2). The physician must be thoroughly familiar with the equipment. Signs should be posted on outside doors when the laser is in use. Protective goggles are necessary for assistants and observers. Endoscopists may use the goggles, or may rely on the protective ocular lens cover once the laser is inserted. The water cooling system must be in operation. The power emission from the laser probe should be checked. Firing the laser once on normal gastric mucosa to ascertain the "in vivo" tissue effect is another way to check adequate energy emission before treatment of a bleeding site is begun.

TECHNIQUE AND PROCEDURE

The physician should anticipate the need for laser therapy and be prepared for its use. Thorough irrigation of the stomach is necessary and a diagnostic EGD should be performed. An exact diagnosis is absolutely essential as laser application must be precise. The endoscopic suite should be cleared as the endoscopist must be able to give total and absolute concentration to the patient at all times. Observers and assistants likewise should be giving equal attention to the patient. Unnecessary talking and other distractions should not be tolerated.

The standard recommendations for use of the Nd:YAG laser are 80 watts energy over 0.5 second pulses from a distance of 1 centimeter. These are general guidelines only. In treating a deformed bulb with a visible artery, for example, one may be able to obtain only a distance of 0.5 cm and therefore 80 watts over 0.5 seconds may be too high a setting over too long an application time, requiring lower and shorter settings.

The quartz cable tip may become covered with coagulated blood and may need to be cleaned or exchanged for a second quartz cable. Air flow, both continuous and burst, may be reduced if the lesion is not actively bleeding in order to prevent possible over distention of the stomach. It is recommended, however, that gas flow be at least at a rate of 10cm^3 per second to prevent

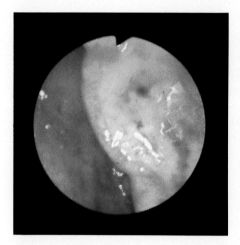

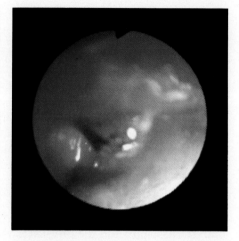

Fig. 3. A large visible artery at the periphery of a duodenal ulcer.

Fig. 4. An unearthed artery in the duodenal bulb without associated ulceration ("exulceratio simplex"; see text).

material from collecting on the laser tip and subsequently interfering with laser treatment, causing a burn, and destruction of the laser tip when fired. If the endoscopist cannot see the aiming light, the tip may be covered with debris and should be removed and cleaned prior to use. If a "flash-back" of light occurs along the laser quartz cable during use, it is probable that the tip has been damaged and should be removed for cleaning or replacement.

In discussing the actual technique of laser application, it behooves one to address the most difficult situation first, i.e. the gastroduodenal artery (Fig. 3). Principles of laser application discussed for this lesion also apply to the laser photocoagulation of all bleeding lesions or visible vessels. If located elsewhere, particularly in the stomach, access and therapy are easier but the basic principles of treatment remain the same. The gastroduodenal and infraduodenal arteries are arterial vessels measuring 1–4 millimeters in size and can be compared in size with the radial artery palpated at the wrist. Originating from the common hepatic artery, the gastroduodenal artery courses immediately posterior to and contiguous with the posterior surface of the duodenal bulb. As such, a penetrating duodenal ulcer will erode, in some instances, directly onto the gastroduodenal and infraduodenal arteries. For unexplained reasons these arteries occasionally will appear to penetrate mucosa without associated ulceration, similar to the lesion "exulceration simplex" (Fig. 4) (43–45). If eroded and massively bleeding, the gastroduodenal artery is a most difficult lesion to treat, even surgically. Due to the inability to clear the blood and to the urgency of the situation, such bleeding is generally untreatable endoscopically.

An oozing gastroduodenal artery, or one that has stopped bleeding is amenable to endoscopic therapy. Any treatment modality (injection, heater probe, monopolar or bipolar probe, laser, etc.) must be undertaken with extreme care, and absolute attention to preparatory steps outlined above is essential. Once

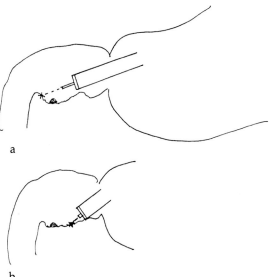

a

b

Fig. 5. Laser treatment of a visible vessel in a duodenal ulcer. The portion of the ulcer that can be readily approached is treated first (a). Treatment is completed by deflecting the folds by means of the tip (b).

preparation has been undertaken, treatment may, in certain situations be appropriate.

The base of an ulcer is covered with necrotic debris and edematous tissue. For this reason, the visible portion of the artery represents only a partial segment. Non-visible segments course underneath these tissues and may be covered only by necrotic debris for several millimeters from the visible portion of the artery. These segments are, in effect, exposed rather than enclosed by "normal" tissue. To laser the non-visible segment of the gastroduodenal artery (or any large artery) covered only by necrotic debris is similar to applying laser energy directly to an exposed artery, with resulting massive hemorrhage being a distinct possibility (38,46). An essential principle is therefore to begin laser therapy at least 2 to 3 mm away from the visible arterial segment.

Precise control of the instrument tip and precise eye-hand-foot coordination are also essential. Respiratory movement will change the position of the laser tip necessitating instantaneous reaction by the endoscopist when applying laser energy.

Edematous folds often prevent total visualization of the ulcer and make circumferential laser treatment around the visible artery extremely difficult. In such situations, first treat portions of the ulcer which can be readily approached. The fold should next be flattened with the instrument tip and laser energy should be applied to the remaining area when possible (Fig. 5). The endoscopist must visualize the site where the laser is being fired and, if the

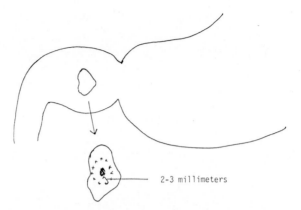

2-3 millimeters

Fig. 6. Laser treatment of a visible vessel. An attempt is made to rim the vessel from a distance of 2 to 3 mm. The x's denote sites of application of laser energy.

desired field is not visible, the laser should not be used. One should not risk hitting the visible gastroduodenal artery early in laser treatment, if at all. For small arteries or visible vessels, particularly those in the stomach, direct application of laser energy to the vessel can be considered once the lesion has been "rimmed" with laser energy, as will be described later. Glucagon can be administered intravenously to reduce duodenal spasm and thereby improve visualization. Laser settings should be reduced (e.g. time to 0.2 or 0.3 seconds; watts to 50 to 60 for the Nd:YAG laser) if duodenal spasm and deformity necessitate close proximity of the instrument and laser tip to the vessel.

An attempt should be made to rim the visible artery with laser energy applied 2 to 3 mm distant (Fig. 6). If orientation is possible, the initial treatment should be directed toward the superior portion of the artery as it courses from superior to inferior as in the case of the gastroduodenal artery (Fig. 7). Application of laser energy inferiorly may produce back pressure and exaccerbate bleeding. The endoscopist should work rapidly and attempt to apply a rim of laser therapy within 2 to 3 minutes, as heat induced edema occurs rapidly and will further impair visualization. Bleeding often occurs during such treatment and if a rim of laser treatment has first been created, the resulting edema may compress the bleeding vessel thus offering some protection against massive hemorrhage. Recent reports suggest that injecting adrenalin (0.1 ml, 1:10,000) (32) or 0.1 ml. absolute alcohol (47,48) in three or four sites immediately adjacent to the bleeding vessel, may help reduce bleeding.

A two channel endoscope is the preferred instrument, as one of the channels can be used to suction blood and secretions more effectively. In spite of the fact that a single channel instrument offers better visualization due to its smaller size, the larger channel scope is still preferable as more efficient aspiration becomes possible.

If active bleeding is not occurring, air or gas flow can be reduced during treatment to prevent overdistention. It should be remembered, however, that

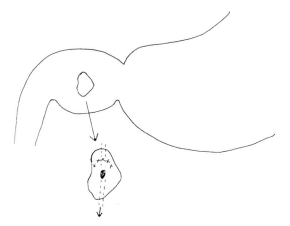

Fig. 7. Laser treatment of a visible vessel. If orientation in the duodenal bulb is possible, laser treatment should be begun at the superior portion of the artery as it courses from superior to inferior. The x's denote sites of application of laser energy.

gas flow at a rate of 10cc per second prevents material from collecting on the laser tip and subsequently interfering with laser treatment or causing a burn and destruction of the laser tip. If active bleeding occurs, air flow should be immediately increased to assist in clearing the field. If massive bleeding occurs during laser treatment, the endoscopist has only 1 minute, perhaps several minutes, to affect further treatment as the volume of blood rapidly obscures visualization. As has been mentioned, intravenous vasopressin can be used in patients without coronary artery disease to slow the bleeding rate. Some endoscopists start intravenous vasopressin therapy prior to laser application in these situations. A surgeon should be available and should be called immediately if massive bleeding occurs.

The precise techniques in the laser treatment of the exposed gastroduodenal artery are still evolving. The majority of such patients will need surgical intervention. At this time, because of the great risk of inducing massive bleeding, I recommend consideration of laser treatment of the visible gastroduodenal artery in limited clinical situations only:

• Chronically ill, poor surgical risk patients with documented and continued bleeding.

• Good surgical risk patients with documented recurrent bleeding (second episode).

Small visible vessels and other bleeding ulcers can be approached more aggressively provided the principles of therapy outlined above are considered.

After use of the laser, monitoring the patient remains an essential part of treatment. A nasogastric tube connected to dependent drainage and irrigated very gently will allow early detection of recurrent bleeding. Oozing of blood for a brief period may be anticipated, but fresh blood through the tube generally means active bleeding and suggests the need for repeated laser treatment.

COMPLICATIONS

Perforation and exaccerbation of massive hemorrhage are complications which do occur but at an acceptably low incidence. Johnston (46) has provided an excellent review of laser photocoagulation complications. Kiefhaber (19) reported 11 perforations in his 667 patients (incidence, 1.6%) with all types of GI bleeding. The combined experience of Kiefhaber (19), Dwyer (49) and Johnston (43) in practice settings, finds an incidence of laser induced perforation in 1 to 2% of Nd:YAG laser cases. Most perforations reported were delayed, being recognized 2 to 5 days after laser therapy. It should be pointed out that the controlled studies (31–37) for the Nd:YAG laser discussed earlier in this chapter resulted in no instance of perforation. For the argon laser, Brunetaud (50) reported no instance of perforation. As the endoscopist becomes more experienced in use of lasers, it would seem that perforation will occur infrequently.

Minor increases in bleeding during laser therapy are relatively common. Laser-induced massive arterial bleeding has occurred (31,38,43) and may require emergency surgical intervention. One death from exsanguination has occurred in a non-operable patient following inadvertent disruption of a large bleeding gastroduodenal artery. Attention to proper techniques of laser therapy and a thorough understanding of the limitations and risks of laser photocoagulation should be considered before using the laser on large bleeding arteries.

SUMMARY

The goal of laser treatment of the visible vessel or bleeding ulcer is to stop the bleeding to allow healing of the ulcer base. Adjuvant techniques, including the use of vasoconstrictive agents, tissue adhesives and tissue injection, hold future promise in further assisting laser therapy toward its goal. While still evolving, laser photocoagulation does appear to be an effective method of treatment. As experience increases and as new technology and techniques are applied, the development of still more effective treatment appears promising.

REFERENCES

1. Silverstein FE, Gilbert DA, Tedesco FJ, et al: The national ASGE survey on upper gastrointestinal bleeding. Parts 1–3. *Gastrointest Endosc* 27:73, 1981.
2. Cotton PB, Rosenberg MT, Waldram RPL, et al: Early endoscopy of the oesophagus, stomach and duodenal bulb in patients with haematemesis and melaena. *Br Med J* 2:505, 1973.

3. Allan R, Dykes P: A study of the factors influencing mortality rates from gastrointestinal hemorrhage. *Q J Med* [NS] 180:533, 1976.

4. Kang JY, Piper DW: Improvement in mortality rates in bleeding peptic ulcer disease. *Med J Aust* 1:213, 1980.

5. Schiller KFR, Cotton PB: Acute upper gastrointestinal haemorrhage. *Clin Gastroenterol* 7:595, 1978.

6. Schiller KFR, Truelove SC, Williams DG: Haematemesis and melaena, with special reference to factors influencing the outcome. *Br Med J* 2:7, 1970.

7. Avery-Jones F: Hemeatemesis and melaena with special reference to causation and to factors influencing the mortality from bleeding peptic ulcers. *Gastroenterology* 30:166, 1956.

8. Griffiths WJ, Neumann DA, Welsh JD: The visible vessel as an indicator of uncontrolled or recurrent gastrointestinal hemorrhage. *N Engl J Med* 300:1411, 1979.

9. Foster DN, Miloszewski KJA, Losowsky MS: Stigmata of recent hemorrhage in diagnosis and prognosis of upper gastrointestinal bleeding. *Br Med J* 1:1173, 1978.

10. Storey DW, Bown SG, Swain CP, et al: Endoscopic prediction of recurrent bleeding in peptic ulcers. *N Engl J Med* 305:915, 1981.

11. Vallon AG, Cotton PB, Laurence BH, et al: Randomized trial of endoscopic argon laser photocoagulation in bleeding peptic ulcers. *Gut* 22:228, 1981.

12. Dwyer RM, Yellin AE, Cherlow J, et al: Laser induced hemostasis in the upper gastrointestinal tract using a flexible fiberoptic endoscope. *Gastroenterology* 68:888, 1975.

13. Dwyer RM: The technique of gastrointestinal laser endoscopy, in Goldman L (ed): *The Biomedical Laser: Technology and Clinical Applications*. New York, Springer-Verlag, 1981, pp 253–269.

14. Dwyer RM, Yellin AE, Craig J, et al: Gastric hemostasis by laser phototherapy in man. *J Am Med Ass* 236:1383, 1976.

15. Frühmorgen P, Boden F, Reidenbach HD, et al: The first endoscopic laser coagulation in the human GI tract. *Endoscopy* 7:156, 1975.

16. Frühmorgen P, Boden F, Reidenbach HD, et al: The first successful endoscopic laser coagulations of bleeding and potential bleeding lesions in the human gastrointestinal tract. (abstract) *Gastrointest Endosc* 22:224, 1976.

17. Frühmorgen P, Boden F, Reidenbach HD, et al: Endoscopic laser coagulation of bleeding gastrointestinal lesions with report of the first therapeutic application in man. *Gastrointest Endosc* 23:75, 1976.

18. Kiefhaber P, Nath G, Moritz K: Endoscopic control of massive gastrointestinal hemorrhage by irradiation with a high power neodymium YAG laser. *Prog Surg* 15:140, 1977.

19. Kiefhaber P: Endoscopic applications of Nd:YAG laser radiation in the gastrointestinal tract, in Joffe SN (ed): *Neodymium-YAG Laser in Medicine and Surgery*. New York, Elsevier, 1983, pp 6–14.

20. Protell RL, Silverstein FE, Piercey J, et al: A reproducible animal model of acute bleeding ulcer—The "ulcer maker." *Gastroenterology* 71:961, 1976.

21. Silverstein FE, Gilbert DA, Feld AD, et al: Laser photocoagulation: Experimental and clinical studies, in Papp JP (ed): *Endoscopic Control of Gastrointestinal Hemorrhage*. Boca Raton, Florida CRC Press, 1981, pp 87–101.

22. Silverstein FE, Protell RL, Gulacsik D, et al: Endoscopic laser treatment. III: The development and testing of a gas-jet assisted argon laser waveguide in control of bleeding experimental ulcers. *Gastroenterology* 74:232, 1978.

23. Johnston JH, Jensen DM, Mautner W: Limitations of endoscopic argon laser with coaxial CO_2. (abstract) *Gastroenterology* 76:1161, 1979.

24. Silverstein FE, Protell RL, Gilbert DA, et al: Argon vs. neodymium-YAG laser photocoagulation of experimental canine gastric ulcers. *Gastroenterology* 77:491, 1979.

25. Johnston JH, Jensen DM, Mautner W: Is argon laser safe at close treatment distance or high powers? (abstract) *Gastroenterology* 76:1161, 1980.

26. Bown SG, Salmon PR, Kelly DF, et al: Argon laser photo-coagulation in the dog stomach. *Gut* 20:680, 1979.

27. Dixon JA, Berenson MM, McCloskey DW: Neodymium-YAG laser treatment of experimental canine gastric bleeding, acute and chronic studies of photocoagulation, penetration and perforation. *Gastroenterology* 77:647, 1979.

28. Dixon JA: General surgical and endoscopic applications of lasers, in *Surgical Application of Lasers*. Chicago, Year Book Medical Publishers, 1983, pp 72–99.

29. Kelly DF, Bown SG, Calder BM, et al: Histological changes following Nd:YAG laser photocoagulation of canine gastric mucosa. *Gut* 24:914, 1983.

30. Escourrou J, Frexinos J, Balos D, et al: Comparison of a new method of electrocoagulation and YAG laser photocoagulation in the treatment of bleeding canine gastric ulcers. (abstract) *Gastroenterology* 76:1128, 1979.

31. Rutgeerts P, Vantrappen G, Broecbaert L, et al: Controlled trial of YAG laser treatment of upper digestive hemorrhage. *Gastroenterology* 83:410, 1982.

32. Rutgeerts P, Vantrappen G, Coremans G, et al: Pretreatment of bleeding ulcers with adrenaline injections renders YAG laser photocoagulation highly efficacious. (abstract) *Gastroenterology* 84:1291, 1983.

33. Swain CP, Bown SG, Salmon PR, et al: Controlled trial of Nd:YAG laser photocoagulation in bleeding peptic ulcers. (abstract) *Gastroenterology* 84:1327, 1983.

34. Ihre T, Johansson C, Seligsson U, et al: Endoscopic YAG laser treatment in massive UGI bleeding. *Scand J Gastroenterol* 16:633, 1981.

35. Escourrou J, Frexinos J, Bommelaer G, et al: Prospective randomized study of YAG photocoagulation in gastrointestinal bleeding, in Atsumi K, Nimsakul N (eds): *Proceedings of Laser —Tokyo '81*. Tokyo, Intergroup, 1981.

36. MacLeod I, Mills PR, Mackenzie JF, et al: Neodymium yttrium aluminum garnet laser photocoagulation for major haemorrhage from peptic ulcers and single vessels: A single blind controlled study. *Br Med J* 286:345, 1983.

37. MacLeod I, Mills PR, Mackenzie JF, et al: Neodymium-YAG laser photocoagulation for major acute upper gastrointestinal haemorrhage. (abstract) *Gut* 23:A905, 1982.

38. Swain CP, Bown SG, Storey DW, et al: Controlled trial of argon laser photocoagulation in bleeding peptic ulcers. *Lancet* 2:1313, 1981.

39. Jensen DM, Machicado GA, Tapia JF, et al: Endoscopic argon laser photocoagulation of patients with severe gastrointestinal bleeding. *Gastroenterology* 84:572, 1983.

40. Fleischer DE: The current status of gastrointestinal laser activity in the United States. *Gastrointest Endosc* 28:157, 1982.

41. Johnston J: Specific treatment techniques for massive upper gastrointestinal bleed-

ing, in Fleischer D, Jensen D, Bright-Asare P (eds): *Therapeutic Laser Endoscopy in Gastrointestinal Disease*. Boston, Martinus Nijhoff, 1983, p. 173.

42. Overholt, B: Use of lasers in community hospitals in the United States, in Fleischer D, Jensen D, Bright-Asare P (eds): *Therapeutic Laser Endoscopy in Gastrointestinal Disease*. Boston, Martinus Nijhoff, 1983, pp 187–192.

43. Dieulafoy G: L'exulceratio simple, in Delahoye A (ed): *Manuel de Pathologie Interne*, Vol 4. Paris, Masson et Cie, 1908, pp 178–305.

44. Broberg A, Ihre T, Pyk E, et al: Exulceratio simplex as conceivable cause of massive gastric hemorrhage. *Surg Gynecol Obstet* 154:186, 1982.

45. Goldman RL: Submucosal arterial malformation of the stomach with fatal hemorrhage. *Gastroenterology* 46:589, 1964.

46. Johnston J: YAG laser treatment of high risk patients with severe upper gastrointestinal bleeding. *Gastrointest Endosc* 27:135, 1981.

47. Asaki S: Tissue solidification in coping with digestive tract bleeding: Hemostatic effect of local injection of 99.5% ethanol. *Tohoku J Exp Med* 134:223, 1981.

48. Asaki S, Nizhimura T, Satoh A, et al: Endoscopic control of gastrointestinal hemorrhage by local injection of absolute ethanol: A basic assessment of the procedure. *Tohoku J Exp Med* 140:339, 1983.

49. Dwyer RW: Safe and effective laser phototherapy in man using the Nd:YAG laser. (abstract) *Gastroenterology* 76:1126, 1979.

50. Brunetaud JM, Enger A, Flament JB, et al: Utilization d'un laser a argon ionise en endoscopie digestive: Photocoagulation des lesions hemorrhagiques. *Rev Phys Appl* 14:385, 1979.

8

Endoscopic Gastric Polypectomy

Rollin W. Hughes, Jr.

As advances in fiberoptic instruments continue to be made, diagnostic as well as therapeutic endoscopy is having an increasingly important role in the management of gastrointestinal polyps. It is the intent of the author to explain the principles of investigation and management of gastric polyps.

A polyp is defined as a lesion that projects from the mucosal surface into the lumen, and the term is used with varying degrees of accuracy. Morgagni (1), in 1769, made the first postmortem diagnosis of gastric polyps, and Quain (2) is credited with the first clinical diagnosis.

In 1888, Ménétrier (3) called attention to the relationship between gastric polyps and carcinoma. There has been a dispute among authors over the premalignant potential of gastric polyps, but this issue has been resolved by combining various elements in the classification schemes proposed by Monaco and colleagues (4), Ming and Goldman (5), Morson and Dawson (6), Elster (7) and Kozuka and coworkers (8).

Many early efforts to determine whether polyps were malignant were made without the benefit of histologic studies, and attention was focused on the size, shape and number of polyps (9). Recognizing that malignant degeneration is a cellular event and that neither size nor number of polyps is a reliable indicator, it has been universally accepted that the question of whether a polyp is malignant must be answered on the basis of histologic evaluation. A consensus has evolved that polyps are separable into hyperplastic and adenomatous types. Further, biopsy specimens obtained by forceps are unreliable in determining the type of polyp that is present (10). Therefore, a gastric polyp should be removed by snare polypectomy if excision by this means is technically feasible.

The clinical implications of epithelial gastric polyps relate to their potential for becoming malignant. Adenomatous polyps have a premalignant potential, as has been noted by Ming and Goldman (5) and Elster (7). Adenomatous polyps are the only type that demonstrate cellular atypism and high mitotic frequency and that harbor carcinoma in situ.

170

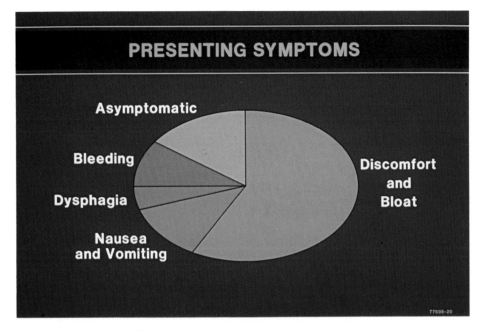

Fig. 1. The presenting symptoms of patients with gastric polyps.

The possibility that malignant degeneration will take place in a gastric polyp increases as the size of a polyp increases. The simultaneous development of carcinoma in a stomach that harbors a polyp has been well documented (5). A stomach that contains a polyp will likely show chronic gastritis and intestinal metaplasia. These pathologic states that are associated with gastric polyps also are seen in patients with gastric carcinoma. The mutual association of these phenomena supports the concept that a gastric mucosa that gives rise to a polyp is suitable soil for the development of a carcinoma.

Most hyperplastic, adenomatous and mesenchymal polypoid tumors are discovered serendipitously, either as an incidental finding at laparotomy or in the course of diagnostic x-ray or gastroscopic examination. Symptoms usually are the result of a complication, such as ulceration, which may give rise to hemorrhage, or intussusception through the pylorus, which causes obstruction. The clinical manifestations of gastric polypoid lesions depend on their location and size; the larger the polyp, the more likely the patient will experience symptoms and be anemic (Fig. 1) (11).

The histologic similarity between a stomach in which polyps are found and a stomach that harbors gastric carcinoma has been previously discussed. Achlorhydria has been reported in most patients with polyps (12), whereas pernicious anemia occurred in only 12.4% of the patients in one study (13). Yet, when Tatsuta and associates (14) employed Congo red staining at the time of endoscopy with gastrin augmentation, 20% of the polyps were seen in the acid-secreting area of the stomach, and half of them retained their acid-secreting activity. Chromoendoscopy and magnification endoscopy are evolving methods for studying gastric polyps that warrant further evaluation (15).

HISTOLOGIC FEATURES OF THE GASTRIC GLANDS

The arbitrary gross division of the stomach into the cardia, fundus, body and antrum may give a false impression that these areas correspond to the locations of the three types of gastric gland. An excellent study by Oi and colleagues (16) has demonstrated that there is a wide variation in the location of the junctional zone between the region that contains the pyloric glands and the region that harbors the fundic glands.

Polyps can originate from surface epithelium, the glandular neck region, gastric glands or combination of several types of epithelium. A clear under-standing of the pathologic alterations of the gastric mucosa requires familiarity with the various types of gastric glands. The cardiac glands are morphologically similar to the pyloric glands, yet they are restricted to a zone that measures only 1 to 1.5 cm at the cardiac end of the stomach.

The fundic and pyloric glands have the same type of mucous cell covering their surface and lining their foveolar, or pit, regions. These two types of glands have different configurations and cellular compositions. The fundic glands are straight tubules composed primarily of parietal cells in the superficial portion. Chief cells make up the deeper portion of the tubules. The pyloric glands are coiled and are composed almost exclusively of mucous cells; a few argentaffin cells also are present.

CLASSIFICATION

As has been previously stated, the term *polyp* is a gross descriptive classification, and the true nature of a polyp is determined by its histologic characteristics. Many inflammatory conditions may thicken the mucosa and submucosa to such a degree that a polypoidal mass will result. A polyp formed as a consequence of a local inflammatory reaction is rightly called an inflamma-tory or hyperplastic polyp. Such polyps have no premalignant potential and are secondary to the inflammatory condition that offends the gastric mucosa. Yet, it is known that many benign and malignant neoplasms may assume a polypoidal form and that benign and malignant polyps cannot be distin-guished solely on the basis of gross configuration.

The following classification scheme is proposed:

1. Epithelial polyps
   Hyperplastic polyp
   Adenomatous polyp
   Hamartomatous polyp (Peutz-Jeghers syndrome)
   Mucosal nodule or cyst
2. Mesenchymal neoplasms
   Leiomyoma
   Fibroma
   Neurogenic tumor
   Lipoma
   Vascular tumor
3. Miscellaneous tumors
   Aberrant or heterotopic pancreas
   Inflammatory pseudotumor

PATHOLOGIC CHARACTERISTICS OF GASTRIC POLYPS

Studies by Tomasulo (17) and by Ming and Goldman (5) have helped resolve the differences of opinion regarding the incidence of malignant degeneration of epithelial polyps. These authors recognize that all gastric polyps look alike on gross inspection. They can be divided into two distinct histologic types: hyperplastic and adenomatous polyps. Both types of polyp may coexist with gastric carcinoma, but only adenomatous polyps undergo malignant change.

HYPERPLASTIC POLYPS

Hyperplastic polyps outnumber adenomatous polyps by a factor of 8 to 1. They are randomly distributed throughout the stomach and usually are less than 2 cm in diameter. Most hyperplastic polyps are sessile or have a short pedicle and a smooth to slightly lobulated surface. Adherent mucus or superficial ulceration is frequently observed.

Under a microscope, hyperplastic polyps are found to consist of branching glands with cystic dilation by cells identical to those of the surface epithelium. Single layers of hyperplastic foveolar cells are seen sitting along a dilated cystic gland. The columnar cells have maintained their uniform configuration, al-

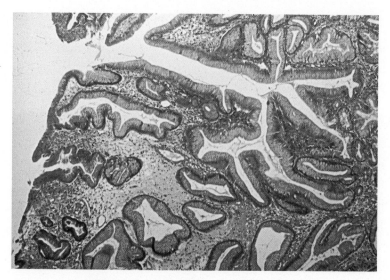

Fig. 2. A hyperplastic polyp shows branching cystic glands with mucous neck cells covering the tubules.

though their cytoplasm contains large amounts of mucus. The small nuclei are located basally and rarely exhibit mitoses. The lamina propria frequently has a moderate number of inflammatory cells; fibrotic and muscle cells are interspersed between the gastric glands (Fig. 2).

Intestinal metaplasia is absent and independent carcinoma is reported to coexist in less than 10% of stomachs that harbor a hyperplastic polyp.

ADENOMATOUS POLYPS

Adenomatous polyps are predominantly antral in location, and 80% of them are 2 cm or greater in diameter. A classic adenomatous polyp has a broad base and an irregular surface. Although the surface may be smooth, more often it is trabeculated with deep fissures or has a papillary configuration.

When an excised polyp is viewed under a microscope, a papillary or villous pattern is seen. The surface cells are poorly differentiated and pleomorphic. There is decreased secretory activity with a paucity of mucus-containing cells, and the nuclei of the surface cells are hyperchromatic and frequently show mitotic activity (Fig. 3).

A striking histologic distinction is found when adenomatous polyps are compared with hyperplastic polyps; in particular, the glandular compositions of the two types of polyps differ markedly. The glands of adenomatous polyps are composed of cells with elongated, hyperchromatic nuclei arranged in a picket-fence pattern. There is an abrupt transition between the epithelium of

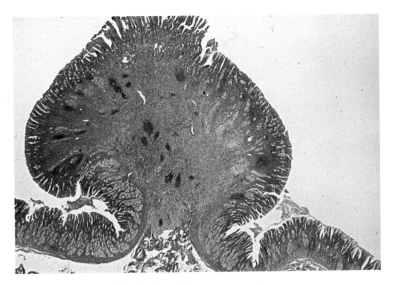

Fig. 3. An adenomatous polyp.

an adenomatous polyp and the adjacent "normal" epithelium of the gastric mucosa.

Inflammatory cells are infrequently seen in the submucosa of adenomatous polyps, and intestinal metaplasia may be present. Cellular dysplasia is frequently seen, and an independent carcinoma coexists in approximately 30% of stomachs that harbor an adenomatous polyp (Table 1).

TABLE 1. Comparison of Hyperplastic and Adenomatous Polyps

	Hyperplastic Polyps	Adenomatous Polyps
Larger than 2 cm	<10%	>80%
Configuration	Smooth or lobulated	Papillary
Pedicle present	<30%	>40%
Multiplicity	30%	0
Coexisting carcinoma	<10%	30%
Microscopic		
Malignant transformation	0	+ +
Anaplasia	Absent	Marked
Hyperplasia	Mild to moderate	Marked
Pyloric metaplasia	Marked	Absent to mild
Intestinal metaplasia	Absent to mild	Marked
Muscle tissue	Present	Absent
Cystic glands	Frequent	Infrequent
Inflammation	Prominent	Not prominent

INTESTINAL METAPLASIA

Intestinal metaplasia is frequently found in atrophic gastric mucosa or in loci associated with adenomatous epithelial polyps along with well-differentiated malignant gastric lesions. This observation supports the hypothesis that adenomatous polyps have a premalignant potential (Figs. 3 to 5). The metaplastic intestinal mucosa contains numerous goblet cells interposed by nonmucussecreting columnar cells that have striated luminal borders. A recent study by Winborn and Weser (18) with scanning electron microscopy vividly demonstrated the difference between the morphologic features of the gastric mucosa and those of areas of intestinal metaplasia.

The goblet cells alluded to above secrete an acid mucin that occupies the supranuclear portion of the cytoplasm, and this mucin stains brilliantly with mucicarmine, period acid Schiff or alcian blue at a pH of 2.5. These staining features have been the criteria used by pathologists in diagnosing intestinal metaplasia.

Kozuka and colleagues (8) used these staining qualities to classify polyps into metaplastic and gastric types. The latter type was subdivided into a true gastric form (without metaplasia) and a mixed form, which shows secondary metaplasia. If one adheres strictly to this classification scheme, the metaplastic type of polyp is found to show a clear correlation between size and degree of metapla-

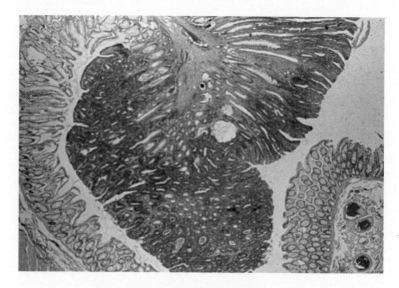

Fig. 4. An adenomatous polyp with a focus of carcinoma in the center. Note the abrupt transition from adenomatous to normal epithelium with marked intestinalization.

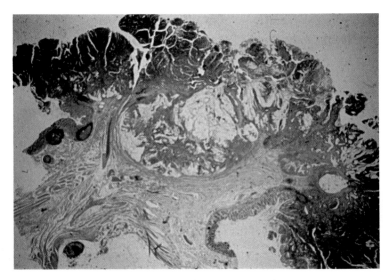

Fig. 5. A polyp with invasive carcinoma
in its stalk at the center of the section.

sia. As the histologic grade or degree of metaplasia increases, so does the
incidence of cancerous lesions.

MISCELLANEOUS POLYPOID
TUMORS

Additional polyps that have distinct histologic features require comment. Inflammatory fibroid polyps, or circumscribed eosinophilic granulomas, have an
oval, smooth surface that often is ulcerated. Under a microscope, such polyps
are found to be composed of a mixture of spindle fibroblasts, eosinophils,
plasma cells and lymphocytes. True granulomas are seldom seen, although
nests of histiocytes may be visualized. Salmon and Paulley (19) reviewed 122
patients who had eosinophilic gastroenteritis, 53 of whom had gastic involvement. In 17 of these 53 patients, the gastric lesions were polypoid (Figs. 6
and 7).

Recent studies have made investigators aware of the extracolonic occurrence
of polypoid lesions in patients with Gardner's syndrome (20). Fifty-five percent
of such patients have a number of polypoid lesions in the gastric fundus and
body. Studies with microscopy have demonstrated that the lesions are cysts of
the gastric glands or polyps of the fundic glands, as has been noted by
Watanabe and coworkers (21). The disordered glands show toruosity and bud-
ding of their structures, although the lining cells are normal and consist of

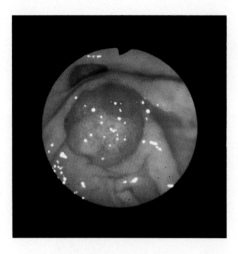

Fig. 6. An inflammatory fibroid antral polyp. The pylorus is seen in the background.

parietal, chief and mucus-secreting cells. Adenomatous polyps have been observed in the antrum, although 73% of such patients are found to have polyps in the duodenum, as shown by endoscopy. The duodenal polyps are adenomatous, as are the colonic polyps, and microadenomatous tissue is observed when biopsy specimens of normal-appearing mucosa are examined.

Bartholomew and associates (22) described the occurrence of hamartomatous gastric polyps in Peutz-Jeghers syndrome. Of 182 patients studied by these authors, 96% had small intestinal polyps, 29% colonic polyps, 30% rectal polyps and 24% gastric polyps.

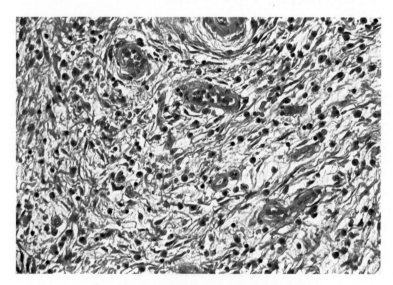

Fig. 7. An inflammatory fibroid polyp composed of spindle fibroblasts, plasma cells, lymphocytes and eosinophils.

In juvenile polyposis coli, hyperplastic gastric polyps rarely are seen. Regenerative polypoid folds are found in patients who have Canada-Cronkhite syndrome. Heterotopic pancreas presents as a nipple-like protrusion from the mucosal surface. In most instances, heterotopic pancreas is intramural and antral in location. Adenomas of Brunner's glands are more likely to be seen in the duodenal bulb, although they can occur in the antrum. Such adenomas consist of normal-appearing Brunner's glands separated by bands of smooth muscle fibers.

MESENCHYMAL TUMORS

Mesenchymal neoplasms comprise approximately one-eighth of all benign gastric tumors. Leiomyoma is by far the most common benign mesenchymal tumor. Gastric mesenchymal tumors usually are solitary, well-circumscribed, spheroidal masses that are located submucosally. The overlying mucosa can be ulcerated, and frank bleeding may be an ensuing consequence. Gross inspection by endoscopists and surgeons does not allow differentiation between leiomyoma and leiomyosarcoma. The leiomyoma or benign smooth muscle tumors are less than six cm in diameter, and at high magnification microscopy, it showed fewer than five mitoses per 50 fields. By contrast, more than five mitoses per 50 microscopic fields are seen in leiomyosarcomas, to label such tumors as sarcomas. There is an indeterminant group of tumors that are greater than 6 cm in diameter that show fewer than five mitoses per 50 high powered microscopic fields. On occasion, these large, smooth muscle tumors may metastasize but they lack the histologic features of malignant degeneration (Figs. 8 and 9) (23, 24). In the stomach, approximately 20% of smooth muscle tumors are malignant, and Carney (25) has recognized an association between

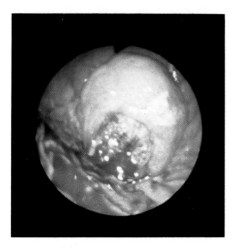

Fig. 8. A pedunculated leiomyoma with ulceration at its tip.

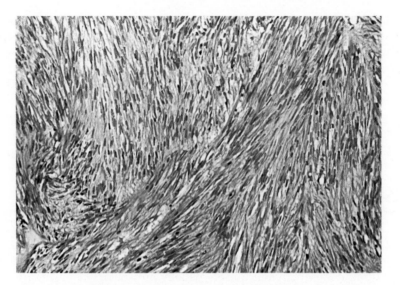

Fig. 9. A leiomyoma composed of a monotonous array of spindle-shaped cells showing absence of nuclear mitosis.

epithelioid leiomyosarcoma and functioning extraadrenal paraganglioma and pulmonary chondroma.

Leiomyoblastoma resembles leiomyoma on gross examination. However, microscopy reveals a bizarre histologic appearance, with large, round polygonal cells often having a perinuclear clear zone. The biologic activity of leiomyoblastoma appears to be intermediate between that of leiomyoma and that of leiomyosarcoma.

GOALS OF THERAPY

Questions that must be answered by endoscopists and pathologists are: 1) Is there a malignant lesion? 2) Is there a potential for malignant degeneration? 3) Is there an independent carcinoma? To determine whether there is a possibility of malignant change, a thorough histologic examination of a polypoid lesion is essential. It usually is necessary to subject an entire polyp to histologic examination. Gastroscopic polypectomy should be performed when a pedunculated polyp is encountered, and surgical excision is indicated if the polyp is sessile or has a broad base. An intramural polypoid lesion, such as a leiomyoma, should be removed surgically.

TECHNIQUE

The first gastroscopic polypectomy was performed in 1969 by Tsuneoko and Uchida (26), and the first excision by means of diathermy current was performed in 1971 by Classen and Demling (27), who used a snare developed by Deyhle. This method of removal carries a complication rate of 1% to 2% and can be performed with reasonable safety by use of various snares and grasping devices (Fig. 10) (28–34).

Once a polypoid lesion has been recognized, the patient's coagulation status must be normal and his or her general health must be suitable before endoscopic polypectomy can be considered. Endoscopic polypectomy should be deferred in patients who have external cardiac pacemakers. Patients are prepared for examination in an otherwise routine fashion, and an end-viewing fiberoptic endoscope is used. A single-channel endoscope usually suffices, although an end-viewing, double-channel endoscope is necessary in some patients, particularly those with broad-based, pedunculated polyps that must be lifted before they can be encircled with a loop. Glucagon is administered intravenously before polypectomy is begun. Glucagon inhibits gastric and duodenal peristalsis and thus facilitates retrieval of polyps.

After a polyp has been snared by means of a wire loop, electrocoagulation current alone is used if the polyp is attached by a thin pedicle. A blend of cutting and coagulation current usually is applied to a thick-based polyp.

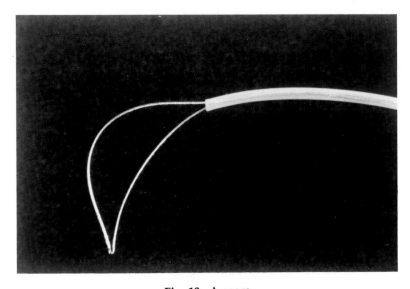

Fig. 10. A snare.

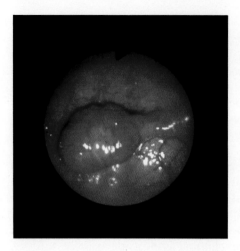

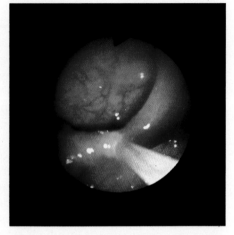

Fig. 11. An antral polyp with a long pedicle.

Fig. 12. An antral polyp with a snare placed on the middle of its stalk at the beginning of electrocoagulation.

Polyps are transected by use of a high-frequency current with coagulation and cutting effects that is produced by a generator attached to the sheathed snare. The current is applied for brief pulses until the pedicle is transected. It is important to position the snare so that it is not in contact with the gastric wall (Figs. 11 and 12).

Asaki and colleagues (35) used a double-snare technique for gastroscopic polypectomy when the pedicle was thick. Double strangulation affords control if a polyp bleeds. The distal loop is initially used for removal, and if bleeding occurs, the proximal snare is drawn tight and additional coagulation current is applied. These authors also have injected alcohol into the coagulated base to arrest bleeding when the double-loop technique cannot be used.

After polypectomy has been completed, the patient is kept at rest and fasted for 12 hours. If the patient is comfortable and without evidence of bleeding, he or she is initially fed clear liquids. The patient is placed on a normal diet within 24 hours. Once the polyp has been removed and retrieved, it is submitted for pathologic examination, and the patient is not discharged until the final report is available. For further details regarding the technique for polypectomy, the reader is referred to chapter 12.

Because such patients have had thermal, necrotic ulcers, a histamine 2 blocking agent is prescribed on an empiric basis, and they are instructed to take the medication for 1 month. It is recognized that many patients with gastric polyps are achlorhydric and do not need such medication. In most cases, however, secretory capacity has not been established before polypectomy, so the author routinely prescribes an agent that suppresses parietal cell activity.

COMPLICATIONS

Complications encountered during gastroscopic polypectomy are related mainly to endoscopy, adverse reactions to sedation and instrument-induced injury. Other complications may result from the use of high-frequency current that has coagulation and cutting effects. Such complications include bleeding, perforation, electric shock, high-frequency burns and residual thermal ulcers. The high-frequency current develops its cutting and coagulation effects through the accumulation of heat. The total heat produced is directly related to the square of the amperes multiplied by the tissue resistance.

Electric shock results from the leakage of low-frequency current, and application of high-frequency current can cause burns. To guard against electrical hazards, a ground system must be established, be it an isolated or a reference ground. Most burns caused by high-frequency current result from the discharge of a spark from the system or from a polyp in an undesired direction, producing a contralateral burn. It is necessary to position a polyp away from the gastric wall before activating the instrument so that the current does not make contact with any portion of the gastric wall and cause a contralateral burn.

To guard against electrical injury to the patient or operator, a wide-area ground plate should be in contact with the patient and an appropriately low power setting (less than 80 watts) should be used. Electrocardiographic monitoring instruments should be isolated or momentarily detached during application of current. It should be remembered that needles and metal points concentrate electrical energy and result in burns. It is for this reason that patients with external pacemakers are at high risk for injury when high-frequency current is used.

The endoscope should be attached by means of an "S" wire to the ground if a reference ground system is used. It is unclear whether the endoscope should be attached to the ground if an isolated ground system is being used. The author's practice is not to attach the endoscope to a ground system in this situation.

RECOMMENDED MANAGEMENT SCHEME

If a gastric polyp is found on x-ray study, endoscopy is recommended for the purposes of verification and biopsy. Further, it should be evaluated for suitability for snare removal. Large, broad-based polypoid lesions should be managed surgically. Polyps with a stalk may be safely removed by means of endoscopic snare polypectomy. If a biopsy specimen shows invasive carcinoma, gastric

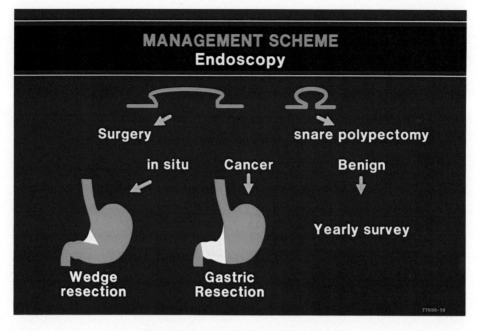

Fig. 13. A scheme for management.

resection should be performed. Carcinoma in situ may be managed by means of wedge resection if the patient's general health is suitable for this procedure. If conservative management is selected, the patient should undergo examination periodically because of the association of malignant change and the recognized recurrence of adenomatous polyps (Fig. 13).

SUMMARY

When a gastric polyp is found on x-ray examination it should be evaluated endoscopically and removed by means of snare polypectomy and/or by biopsy. The latter technique is the preferred method to allow pathologic examination, which can then determine its histologic composition. A pathologist can best determine if there is coexisting malignant degeneration when an entire polyp has been removed. If a polyp cannot be removed at gastroscopy and is large, it should be excised surgically. If the excised polyp is hyperplastic, no surveillance is necessary. Patients with adenomatous polyps should undergo endoscopy periodically, probably every 1 to 2 years.

REFERENCES

1. Morgagni JB: *Seats and Causes of Disease Investigated by Anatomy*. London, A. Miller and T. Cadell, 1769.

2. Quain R: Causes of polyps ejected from stomach. *J Pathol Soc London* 8:219, 1857.

3. Ménétrier P: Des polyadenomas gastriques de leur rapports avec le cancer de l'estomoc *Arch Phys Norm Pathol Paris* 1:32, 236, 1888.

4. Monaco AP, Roth SI, Castleman B, et al: Adenomatous polyps of the stomach: A clinical and pathological study of 153 cases. *Cancer* 15:456, 1962.

5. Ming SG, Goldman H: Gastric polyps: A histogenetic classification and the relation to carcinoma. *Cancer* 18:721, 1965.

6. Morson BC, Dawson IMP: *Gastrointestinal Pathology*. Oxford, Blackwell, 1972, pp 128–131, 161–171.

7. Elster K: A new approach to the classification of gastric polyps. *Endoscopy* 6:44, 1974.

8. Kozuka S, Masamoto K, Suzuki S, et al: Histogenetic types and size of polypoid lesions in the stomach with special reference to cancerous changes. *Gann* 68:267, 1977.

9. Yamada T, Ichikawa H: X-ray diagnosis of elevated lesions of the stomach. *Radiology* 110:79, 1974.

10. Seifert E, Elster K: Gastric polypectomy. *Am J Gastroenterol* 63:451, 1975.

11. Lanza FL, Graham DY, Nelson RS, et al: Endoscopic upper gastrointestinal polypectomy. Report of 73 polypectomies in 63 patients. *Am J Gastroenterol* 75:345, 1981.

12. Hitchcock CR, Sullivan WA, Wagensteen OH: The value of achlorhydria as a screening test for gastric cancer: A ten-year report. *Gastroenterology* 29:621, 1955.

13. Elsborg L, Mosbech J: Pernicious anemia as a risk factor in gastric cancer. *Acta Med Scand* 206:315, 1979.

14. Tatsuta M, Okuda S, Tamura H, et al: Polyps in the acid-secreting area of the stomach. *Gastrointest Endosc* 16:145, 1981.

15. Okuda T, Nishizawa M: Magnified observation of elevated borderline lesion (adenoma) of the stomach based on dissecting microscopy and magnifying fiberoptic endoscopy. *Endoscopy* 13:234, 1981.

16. Oi M, Oshida K, Sugimura S: The location of gastric ulcer. *Gastroenterology* 36:45, 1959.

17. Tomasulo J: Gastric polyp. Histologic types and their relationship to gastric carcinoma. *Cancer* 27:1346, 1971.

18. Winborn WB, Weser E: Scanning electron microscopy of intestinal metaplasia of the human stomach. *Gastrointest Endosc* 29:201, 1983.

19. Salmon PR, Paulley JW: Eosinophilic granuloma of the gastrointestinal tract. *Gut* 8:8, 1967.

20. Burt RW, Berenson MM, Lee RG, et al: Upper gastrointestinal polyps in Gardner's syndrome. *Gastroenterology* 86:295, 1984.

21. Watanabe H, Enjooji M, Yao T, et al: Gastric lesion in familial adenomatosis coli: Their incidence and histologic analysis. *Hum Pathol* 9:269, 1978.

22. Bartholomew LG, Moore CE, Dahlin DC, et al: Intestinal polyposis associated with mucocutaneous pigmentation. *Surg Gynecol Obstet* 115:1, 1962.

23. Appelman HD, Helwig EB: Gastric epithelioid leiomyoma and leiomyosarcoma. *Cancer* 3:708, 1976.

24. Ellis PSJ, Whitehead R: Mitosis counting: A need for reappraisal. *Hum Pathol* 12:3, 1981.

25. Carney JA: The triad of gastric epithelioid leiomyosarcoma, functioning extra-adrenal paraganglioma and pulmonary chondroma. *Cancer* 43:374, 1979.

26. Tsuneoko K, Uchida T: Endoscopic polypectomy of the stomach. *Gastrointest Endosc* 11:171, 1970.

27. Classen M, Demling L: Operative Gastroskopie: Fiberendoskopische Polypenatrogung in Magen. *Dtsch Med Wochenschr* 96:1466, 1971.

28. Sivak M, Sullivan BH: Gastroscopic polypectomy. *Cleveland Clin Q* 40:153, 1973.

29. Hargrove RL, Overholt BF: Polypectomy via the fiberoptic gastroscope. *J Am Med Ass* 224:904, 1973.

30. Gaisford W: Gastrointestinal polypectomy via the fiberendoscope. *Arch Surg (Chicago)* 106:458, 1973.

31. Appel MF: Endoscopic removal of gastric and duodenal polyps. *South Med J* 69:593, 1976.

32. Papp JP: Electrosurgical advances in upper gastrointestinal endoscopy. *Am J Gastroenterol* 66:248, 1976.

33. Jacobs WH; Endoscopic electrosurgical polypectomies of the upper gastrointestinal tract. *Am J Gastroenterol* 68:241, 1977.

34. ReMine SG, Hughes RW, Weiland LH: Endoscopic gastric polypectomy. *Mayo Clin Proc* 56:371, 1981.

35. Asaki S, Nishimura T, Sato M, et al: Endoscopic polypectomy using high frequency current: Double-snare method of polypectomy for prevention of incidental bleeding and perforation. *Tohoku J Exp Med* 136:215, 1982.

9

Topical Agents in the Management of Gastrointestinal Bleeding

Richard I. Breuer
Robert M. Craig

It is reasonable to believe that by 1980 at the latest the endoscopist will have available for routine use a safe, effective treatment for acute gastrointestinal hemorrhage (1).

Estimates suggest that each year, more than 300,000 patients enter U.S. hospitals with upper gastrointestinal tract bleeding (2). Endoscopy continues to be a remarkably accurate diagnostic tool, pinpointing bleeding lesions in more than 90% of patients (3–6). However, mortality has remained high at 8% to 9% (2–4,7–10). Since the advent of endoscopy, there have not been shorter hospital stays or a reduction of transfusion requirements (11,12). Patients who continue to bleed or who rebleed in the hospital setting have an especially poor prognosis (10). Emergency surgical intervention for bleeding from one common lesion, peptic ulcer, is much more risky than is elective surgical intervention for the same condition (13,14). Thus, a transendoscopic technique for stopping gastrointestinal bleeding, or at least for decreasing the rate of bleeding so that operations can be safer, is urgently needed. This chapter discusses the experience with, and prospects of, topical agents that can be applied through an endoscope to accomplish these goals.

DIFFICULTIES IN THE EVALUATION OF ENDOSCOPIC THERAPY FOR UPPER GASTROINTESTINAL TRACT BLEEDING

Between 75% and 90% of all patients admitted to hospitals stop bleeding with supportive care, antacids and/or histamine-blocker therapy (2,6,9,10). Thus, to detect even a 3% decrease in the mortality of patients who continue to bleed, at least 1300 patients would have to be assigned randomly to control and treatment groups (15). To prove that a proposed treatment reduced the rate of continuing hemorrhage due to esophagitis, gastritis and duodenal and gastric ulcers would also be difficult. Two hundred and fifty patients with bleeding from each type of lesion would have to be studied to enable detection of a decrease from 25% to 10% in the incidence of continuing hemorrhage with acceptable statistical confidence (16). Because not all patients initially screened would qualify, a reasonable estimate might be 1500 patients necessary for such a trial! No one medical center encounters such a large population of patients with such lesions. Further, the logistic and financial difficulties involved in completing such a study could be prohibitive. These issues and others inherent in prospective trials (17) make it difficult to show that any endoscopic therapy is effective by modern statistical standards.

Animal models have been used properly to provide an initial measure of the safety and efficacy of treatment. Such studies cost much less than do those conducted with human patients; however, the results may not be reliably extrapolated to the clinical setting. In most experiments, efficacy is defined as the ability to stop bleeding from standard-sized, acute ulcers induced with a large biopsy capsule in heparinized animals. Such ulcers are not comparable to those seen in clinical practice because they lack an inflammatory reaction; also, in animal models, bleeding occurs from several vessels, rather than from one or two, as occurs in most patients with ulcers. Bleeding rates may not be severe enough to simulate massive arterial bleeding in human beings, and there may be other species-specific differences (18). Moreover, appreciable slowing of bleeding, which in human patients would permit elective rather than emergency surgical intervention, usually is not measured in short-term animal studies (19). Thus, although efficacy can be measured on a standard scale and methods can be compared in a standard model, there are great limitations to the usefulness of even the best of the animal models.

In current surgical practice, there are several topical hemostatic agents that can control serious hemorrhage when they are applied under ideal conditions. For example, a standard-sized splenic laceration killed 100% of laboratory animals by exsanguination. Oxidized, regenerated cellulose (Surgicel), an absorbable gelatin sponge (Gelfoam), microcrystalline collagen (Avitene) and a bovine collagen (Collastat) each reduced that mortality to less than 25% (20). Even simpler methods, including the application of cold or heat, pressor agents and clotting factors, have been used with some success to manage various wounds.

Adaptation of these or other hemostatic agents for use through an endoscope is a great challenge. Distance from the mucosa is at times hard to judge and keep constant, and small endoscope channels may limit delivery rates. Further, safe pressure systems that would achieve initial hemostasis and that would allow fixation of material to bleeding sites have not been developed.

IDEAL TOPICAL THERAPY

An ideal topical endoscopic therapy should control hemorrhage from local and diffuse lesions, be relatively easy to apply through standard instruments and produce no local tissue destruction or systemic toxicity. Several agents have been tried; however, none has yet been shown convincingly to be effective in the endoscopic control of hemorrhage from the gastrointestinal tract in human beings. A survey of the methods used should highlight the problems and potential for success.

COLD, HEAT AND PRESSORS

The potential usefulness of topical instillation of cold substances into the stomach is supported by an experimental model in which rabbit stomachs were studied in vivo during gastric cooling (21). When the animals were not in shock, there was some protection of the gastric mucosa with regional cooling. However, when cooling was applied to the animals when they were in shock, there were more mucosal erosions, presumably due to further diminution of gastric blood flow. In dogs, gastric lavage with iced saline or water is a safe procedure that does not result in serious disruption of normal physiologic processes (22). Instillation of cold saline or water by means of a nasogastric tube is a time-honored ritual for immediate control of upper gastrointestinal tract hemorrhage in human beings despite the absence of controlled studies supporting its efficacy (23).

Ponsky and colleagues (24) showed that canine gastric pouches cooled to $-24°C$ had a marked decrease in gastric secretion. In the 1950s and 1960s, clinical trials of gastric freezing in the management of duodenal ulcer disease and in massive hematemesis were performed (25–28). These anecdotal reports indicated efficacy. Subsequently, the clinical effectiveness of gastric freezing was refuted by a well-controlled study of its use in duodenal ulcer disease. This trial failed to demonstrate relief of pain, suppression of secretion or a decrease in the rate of recurrence (29).

There also is a theoretical basis for the application of heat to arrest gastrointestinal hemorrhage. Sigel and Hatke (30) showed that the strength of the bond produced between the severed ends of a blood vessel during electrocoagulation varied with the amount of energy applied or the amount of heat generated. This principle has been extended to the use of a heater probe for upper gastrointestinal tract hemorrhage (31–33). The inner heating coil can be passed through a flexible endoscope, which is protected by a Teflon coating outside the probe. In the heparinized dog ulcer model, both the 6.4 mm and the 3.2 mm diameter probe promoted cessation of bleeding with no gross perforation. However, full-thickness injury was seen histologically 20% of the time, more frequently with the larger-diameter probe. The depth of injury seemed to be related to the pressure applied to the bleeding site. The smaller probe can be passed through an endoscope, but an average of 12 applications was necessary to promote cessation of bleeding. Despite these difficulties, clinical studies with a heater probe may be warranted because of its relative simplicity and low cost.

Direct instillation of pressors or other pharmacologic substances into a bleeding stomach is an attractive technique because of ease of administration. Kiselow and Wagner (34) treated 12 patients with massive bleeding from upper gastrointestinal tract lesions other than varices. Eight milligrams of norepinephrine in 100 ml of saline was instilled through a nasogastric tube, which was then clamped for 30 minutes. This procedure was repeated every hour for 4 to 6 hours. Bleeding ceased from seven of 13 lesions. There was no morbidity or mortality from the procedure. LeVeen and coworkers (35) also reported a series in which norepinephrine was administered intraperitoneally or intragastrically in bleeding patients. Bleeding ceased in 12 of the 18 patients. In addition, with a canine model of gastrointestinal hemorrhage reported by the same investigators, mortality was reduced by intraperitoneal administration of norepinephrine (35). Intraperitoneal use of pressors seems too unwieldy for clinical application, but pressors introduced into the stomach through a nasogastric tube or directed through an endoscope might be effective.

Although endoscopic injection techniques have been used primarily to control bleeding from esophageal varices, bleeding from other lesions has been managed in the same manner (36). Ulcers were injected with 5 to 10 ml of a dilute solution of epinephrine, and hemostasis was effected in 75% of cases. This technique also seemed useful for controlling bleeding from Mallory-Weiss tears. No complication was reported. However, the study was done in an uncontrolled manner, and the method of patient selection was not clearly specified.

There are few data on the topical administration of other pressors or such agents as vasopressin or prostaglandins. However, topical administration of 16,16-N,N-dimethyl prostaglandin E_2 has been shown to increase the production of alkaline secretions in the stomach, and this technique may be useful in promoting cessation of gastric bleeding (37).

CLOTTING FACTORS

Linsheer and Fazio (38) have demonstrated that direct endoscopic application of clotting factors on bleeding sites is feasible. Their preliminary data are encouraging. These investigators used a relatively simple four-channel tube that fit through a standard biopsy channel to deliver in sequence: saline to wash a lesion, carbon dioxide to dry it and then, simultaneously, two parts of cryoprecipitate and one part of thrombin to induce hemostasis (Fig. 1). Cryoprecipitate was used instead of fibrinogen to reduce the potential risk for hepatitis because the former is prepared from 1 unit of plasma rather than from many units of pooled human plasma. The cryoprecipitate/thrombin spray produced hemostasis in all ulcers that were treated. The authors considered the method most useful for arresting persistent, low-grade bleeding and postulated that it might be ineffective for "an arterial gusher or massive bleeding from a large, ruptured esophageal varix." The spray also was applied in a nonrandomized manner in 12 patients who were considered poor risks for surgical intervention and who suffered from persistent upper gastrointestinal tract bleeding. The cryoprecipitate/thrombin spray seemed effective and without untoward side effects. This technique appears to be safe, and the spray is simple to deliver with an appropriate system. However, the clotting factors are expensive, and there is a minor risk for hepatitis, depending on the amount of spray that is administered. The real issue, nonetheless, is efficacy. Even though they used

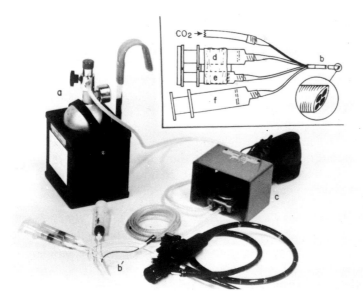

Fig. 1. The spraying device used by Linscheer and Fazio. Reprinted from Linscheer WG, Fazio TL: Control of upper gastrointestinal hemorrhage by endoscopic spraying of clotting factors. *Gastroenterology* 77:642, 1979, with permission. (a) Carbon dioxide pressure tank with pressure reducer; (b) four-lumen catheter, 2 mm in diameter and 250 cm in length; (c) foot pedal; (d) twin syringes [10 ml, cryoprecipitate; (e) 5 ml, thrombin]; (f) saline syringe (30 ml).

almost identical spraying equipment and the same animal model, Jensen and colleagues (39) failed to confirm the results of Linsheer and Fazio. Inspection of the data fails to reveal an obvious explanation for the discrepancy between the results of the two studies. However, less than ideal adherence of the clotting factors to the bleeding sites may well explain the difference.

A novel approach with this technique was reported by Smith and associates (40), who used a ferromagnetic/thrombin mixture in the heparinized dog ulcer model. A strong magnetic field kept the mixture in the ulcer and promoted cessation of bleeding. Another group (41) used the same principle, placing the ferromagnetic/thrombin mixture through an endoscope in the same canine model. However, in this study, only 48% of the ulcers stopped bleeding. No studies with this technique have been performed in human patients. Thus, because of the conflicting results in the canine model, only controlled clinical trials may demonstrate whether endoscopic application of clotting factors is helpful in controlling gastrointestinal hemorrhage.

CYANOACRYLATE TISSUE GLUES

Cyanoacrylate polymers, which have the unique property of bonding mammalian tissues, have been investigated to determine their hemostatic properties (42,43). One compound, trifluoro-isopropyl-α cyanoacrylate MBR 4197, polymerized uniformly in less than 10 seconds and showed minimal animal toxicity (43,44). Moreover, good hemostasis could be achieved when the material was applied by a freon aerosol propellant, making it an ideal candidate for endoscopic application. Its apparent mechanism of action is mechanical tamponade of a bleeding lesion. The Minneapolis group (45) showed that ulcers created experimentally by the lift and cut technique in dogs bled less when they were treated with MBR 4197 than when the propellant was used alone. Neither the compound nor the propellant caused tissue damage, and ulcer healing proceeded normally. However, Protell and associates (46) used the same delivery system and found no hemostatic advantage for MBR 4197 in the heparinized dog ulcer model. Because of the different techniques of ulcer induction, these studies are difficult to compare. In an uncontrolled clinical study, endoscopic application of MBR 4197 seemed to control relatively severe bleeding from a variety of lesions in the upper gastrointestinal tract in five of six critically ill patients who had been considered poor surgical risks (47).

A prospective, randomized, controlled multicenter trial with the polymer was terminated after 52 patients had been studied. Only patients who had "active bleeding" from, or a "fresh clot" in a gastric or duodenal ulcer that was accessible for application of the polymer had been included in this study. There appeared to be no benefit for patients treated with MBR 4197 as compared with patients who received conventional treatment. Neither blood transfusion requirements nor frequency of emergency surgical intervention differed between the two groups. One factor in this negative study was that despite the selection of only patients with active bleeding or adherent clots, conventional treatment was successful in 86% of patients. Thus to prove that MBR 4197 is indeed an effective agent, it would require hundreds of patients, carefully selected to be among those at highest risk for continued bleeding or rebleeding.

Moreover, several studies have shown that gentle pressure seems to enhance the effectiveness of the polymer (42). Animal studies also have shown that MBR 4197 works best on a clean, dry surface (42). Despite washing with saline and drying with carbon dioxide through a special irrigation pump, these conditions cannot always be satisfied in the clinical setting. The catheter system sometimes becomes clogged with prematurely dried polymer. The authors emphasized the need for a more reliable delivery system and for a polymer that could be applied under less than ideal conditions (48).

TOPICAL COLLAGEN HEMOSTATS

Collagen hemostats have been used in general, vascular, plastic and oral surgery since the 1970s (49–52). Microcrystalline collagen hemostat was initially described in 1967 as a novel child of polymer chemistry (53). It is a water-insoluble acid salt of bovine collagen that is prepared by a process that conserves the normal helical configuration of collagen molecules and most of the bonding forces between them. It is a dry, tangled, fibrous substance that is easily compressible. In a remarkable series of experiments, Abbott and Austen (54) showed that microcrystalline collagen hemostat promotes hemostasis when a large, reproducible defect is induced experimentally in the carotid arteries of mongrel dogs. Cessation of bleeding occurred in 93% of such major arterial lesions, as compared to a success rate of only 4% in arteries wrapped at similar pressure with surgical gauze alone. Microcrystalline collagen hemostat also was superior to oxidized cellulose cloth in producing hemostasis in this model (92% vs. 42% efficacy, $p < 0.01$). Further, the hemostat maintained most of its effectiveness when animals had previously been heparinized (76%), after salicylate-induced inhibition of platelet function (85%) and even after induction of profound thrombocytopenia (71%). It also substantially decreases capillary bleeding in the skin graft donor site model in human beings (55). In these studies, 40% to 50% reductions of the frequency of bleeding were reported. Interestingly enough, application of gentle pressure had a tendency to improve the performance of the hemostat. Recently, this substance and Collastat, a native collagen from bovine corium, were found to be effective in slowing bleeding from splenic lacerations (20). Therefore, topical collagen compounds have the potential to staunch major arterial bleeding as well as to control oozing from denuded surfaces—the two clinical conditions found in upper gatrointestinal tract bleeding in human patients. Studies in laboratory animals and human beings have shown that microcrystalline collagen hemostat is minimally antigenic and safe, being without danger of sensitization or anaphylactic reactions or other toxicity (56). With this proven effectiveness and safety, the potential for endoscopic application had to be explored.

Klein and associates (19) used the heparinized dog ulcer model. Microcrystalline collagen hemostat was applied as 100 mg of the dry powder and, to simulate endoscopic conditions, as a slurry of 1 g in 10 cm^3 of water. Ulcers treated with the slurry as well as the powder bled much less than did ulcers that were not treated. Many hemostat-treated ulcers, but no control ulcers, stopped bleeding completely. However, in an abstract, Feld and coworkers (57) reported that a smaller amount of slurry at the same concentration did not seem effective in the same animal model.

In a limited, uncontrolled clinical feasibility study, microcrystalline collagen hemostat was used at a concentration of 1 g in 15 ml of water instilled through a washing catheter inserted through the biopsy channel of a standard endoscope. Bleeding stopped in eight of nine patients who had shown continuing hemorrhage from various mucosal lesions despite histamine 2 blocking agent and antacid therapy for at least 72 hours before application of the hemostat (Fig. 2, a to c) (19). A prospective, controlled clinical study that was being conducted by the author and his colleagues to evaluate the efficacy of the slurry was stopped when it was realized that clinical resources were inadequate for providing the necessary 250 patients bleeding from each of four sites to show a diminution of continued bleeding from 25% to 10% with proper α and β errors (16). The author remains convinced, however, that, when applied as a slurry, microcrystalline collagen hemostat is effective in patients in whom there is continued oozing from diffuse lesions and that the hemostat prevents rebleeding in some patients in whom bleeding has stopped temporarily after major arterial hemorrhage. If a delivery system were developed that allows delivery

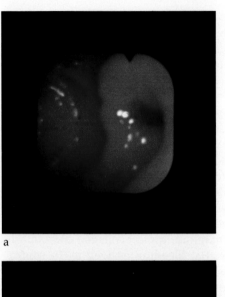
a

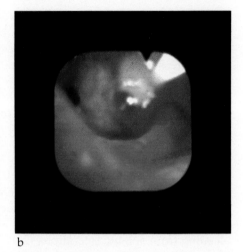
b

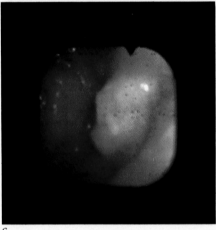
c

Fig. 2. Application of MCH (microcrystalline collagen hemostat) to a bleeding gastric lesion. (a) The gastric ulcer is hemorrhaging rapidly. (b) An endoscopic catheter is inserted through the 2.2-mm biopsy channel of a standard 9-mm gastroduodenal panendoscope, washing is completed and slurry is being applied. (c) MCH slurry covers the ulcer site immediately after application, and bleeding has stopped. The slurry was made by mixing MCH powder with 20 cm^3 of saline and was forced through a washing catheter by applying hand pressure to a 10-cm^3 syringe.

in powder form or application of gentle pressure, microcrystalline collagen hemostat could be a highly effective agent for endoscopic management of most cases of gastrointestinal bleeding.

Thus, topical agents that are safe and that can control bleeding are available today. Some such agents have been administered through endoscopes with partial success. However, stumbling blocks remain to the conclusive demonstration that endoscopic application of any agent consistently stops gastrointestinal hemorrhage in human beings. Major issues include the lack of an animal model that accurately reflects the situation in patients with hemorrhage, the large-scale clinical trials that must be conducted to prove efficacy and the less than ideal endoscopic delivery systems that are currently available. Some of these problems are potentially solvable, and much progress already has been made. Perhaps, as was suggested in 1976, with the ". . . close cooperation of the gastroenterologist, surgeon, pathologist, pharmacologist, chemical and electrical engineer . . ." (1), the goal may soon be achieved.

REFERENCES

1. Katon RW: Experimental control of gastrointestinal hemorrhage via the endoscope: A new era dawns. *Gastroenterology* 70:272–277, 1976.

2. Cutler JA, Mendeleff AI: Upper gastrointestinal bleeding: Nature and magnitude of problem in the United Sates. *Dig Dis Sci* 26:90S–96S, 1981.

3. Silverstein FE, Gilbert DA, Tedesco FJ, et al: The national ASGE survey on upper gastrointestinal bleeding. Parts I–III. *Gastrointest Endosc* 27:73–102, 1981.

4. Cotton PB, Rosenberg MT, Waldram RPL, et al: Early endoscopy of oesophagus, stomach, and duodenal bulb in patients with haematemesis and melaena. *Br Med J* 2:505–509, 1973.

5. Sugawa C, Werner MH, Hayes DF, et al: Early endoscopy. A guide to therapy in the acute hemorrhage of the upper gastrointestinal tract. *Arch Surg (Chicago)*, 107:133–137, 1973.

6. Palmer ED: The vigorous diagnostic approach to upper gastrointestinal hemorhage. *J Am Med Ass* 207:1477–1480, 1969.

7. Ihre T, Johansson C, Seligsson V, et al: Endoscopic YAG-laser treatment in massive upper gastrointestinal bleeding. *Scand J Gastroenterol* 16:633–640, 1981.

8. Hunt PS, Hansky J, Korman MG: Mortality in patients with haematemesis and melaena: A prospective study. *Br Med J* 1:1238–1240, 1979.

9. Morgan AG, Mac Adam WAF, Walmsley GL, et al: Clinical findings, early endoscopy, and multivariate analysis in patients bleeding from the upper gastrointestinal tract. *Br Med J* 2:237–240, 1977.

10. Fleischer D: Etiology and prevalence of severe persistent upper gastrointestinal bleeding. *Gastroenterology* 84:538–543, 1983.

11. Peterson WL, Barnett CC, Smith HJ, et al: Routine early endoscopy in upper gastrointestinal tract bleeding. *N Engl J Med* 304:925–929, 1981.

12. Sandlow LJ, Becker GH, Spellberg MA, et al: A prospective randomized study of the management of upper gastrointestinal hemorrhage. *Am J Gastroenterol* 61:282–289, 1974.

13. Brooks JR: Factors affecting the mortality from peptic ulcer. The bleeding ulcer and ulcer in the aged. *N Engl J Med* 271:803, 1974.

14. Dorsey JM, Burkhead HC, Bonus RL, et al: Five-year study on gastrointestinal bleeding. *Surg Gynecol Obstet* 120:784, 1965.

15. Erickson RA, Glick ME: Can early diagnostic esophagogastroduodenoscopy (EGD) decrease the mortality associated with upper gastrointestinal bleeding (UGIB)? (abstract) *Gastroenterology* 84:1146, 1983.

16. Dunn JK: Personal communication, 1981.

17. Feinstein AR: An additional basic science for clinical medicine: ii. The limitations of randomized trials. *Ann Intern Med* 99:544–550, 1983.

18. Jensen DM: Topics in endoscopy. Part A. Upper gastrointestinal bleeding, in Gitnick GL (ed): *Current Gastroenterology & Hepatology*. New York, Wiley, 1979, pp 64–78.

19. Klein FA, Drueck C, Breuer RI, et al: Control of upper gastrointestinal bleeding with a microcrystalline collagen hemostat. *Dig Dis Sci* 27:981–985, 1982.

20. Coln D, Horton J, Ogden M, et al: Evaluation of hemostatic agents in experimental splenic locations. *Am J Surg* 145:256–259, 1983.

21. Menguy R, Masters YF: Influence of cold on stress ulceration and on gastric mucosal blood flow and energy metabolism. *Ann Surg* 194:29–34, 1981.

22. Larson DA, Farnell MB: Upper gastrointestinal hemorrhage. *Mayo Clin Proc* 58:371–387, 1983.

23. Bryant LR, Mobin-Uddin K, Dillon ML, et al: Comparison of ice water with iced saline for gastric lavage in gastroduodenal hemorrhage. *Am J Surg* 124:570–572, 1972.

24. Ponsky JL, Hoffman M, Swayngrin DS: Saline irrigation in gastric hemorrhage: The effect of temperature. *J Surg Res* 28:204–205, 1980.

25. Wangensteen OH, Peter ET, Bernstein EF, et al: Can physiologic gastrectomy be achieved by gastric freezing? *Ann Surg* 156:579–591, 1962.

26. Wangensteen OH, Root HD, Jenson CB, et al: Depression of gastric secretion and digestion by gastric hypothermia: Its clinical use in massive hematemesis. *Surgery* 44:265–274, 1958.

27. Salmon PA: Local gastric hypothermia induced by direct perfusion of the gastric lumen. *Can Med Ass J* 97:944–949, 1967.

28. Rogers JB, Older TM, Stabler EV: Gastric hypothermia: A critical evaluation of its use in massive upper gastrointestinal bleeding. *Ann Surg* 163:367–372, 1966.

29. Ruffin JM, Grizzle JE, Hightower NC, et al: A co-operative double-blind evaluation of gastric freezing in the treatment of duodenal ulcer. *N Engl J Med* 281:16–19, 1969.

30. Sigel B, Hatke FL: Physical factors in electrocoagulation of blood vessels. *Arch Surg (Chicago)* 95:54–58, 1967.

31. Rubin C, Auth D, Silverstein F, et al: Preliminary study of a Teflon-coated heater for endoscopic control of upper gastrointestinal bleeding in a standard ulcer model. (abstract) *Gastrointest Endosc* 22:235, 1976.

32. Protell RL, Rubin CE, Auth DC, et al: The heater probe: A new endoscopic method for stopping massive gastrointestinal bleeding. *Gastroenterology* 74:257–262, 1978.

33. Protell RL, Lawrence DM, Peoples JE, et al: A new endoscopic thermal cautery which stops experimental bleeding safely. (abstract) *Gastroenterology* 78:1239, 1980.

34. Kiselow MC, Wagner M: Intragastric instillation of levarterenol. *Arch Surg (Chicago)* 107:387–389, 1973.

35. LeVeen H, Diaz C, Falk G, et al: A proposed method to interrupt gastrointestinal bleeding: Preliminary report. *Ann Surg* 175:459–469, 1972.

36. Soehendra N, Kempeneers I, de Heer K: Endoskopische Injektionsmethode zur Blutstillung im Verdanungstrakt. *Deutsche Med Wochenschr* 107:1474–1476, 1982.

37. Kauffman GL, Grossman MI: Gastric alkaline secretion: Effect of topical and intravenous 16-16 dimethyl prostaglandin E_2. (abstract) *Gastroenterology* 76:1165, 1979.

38. Linsheer WG, Fazio TL: Control of upper gastrointestinal hemorrhage by endoscopic spraying of clotting factors. *Gastroenterology* 77:642–646, 1979.

39. Jensen DM, Machicado G, Tapia J, et al: Clotting factors fail to control bleeding from standard ulcers or gastric erosions. *Gastroenterology* 78:1187, 1980.

40. Smith FW, Heinonen LA, Peterson EC, et al: The use of a strong magnetic field in the control of gastrointestinal bleeding. (abstract) *Gastroenterology* 78:1264, 1980.

41. Carlson D, Jensen DM, Machicado G, et al: Treatment of experimental bleeding gastric ulcers and erosions with ferromagnetic tamponade. *Gastroenterology* 78:1147, 1980.

42. Matsumoto T, Hardaway RM, Heisterkamp CA, et al: Cyanoacrylate adhesive and hemostasis. *Arch Surg (Chicago)* 94:858–860, 1967.

43. Nelson RA, Banitt EH, Kvam DC, et al: A new fluoroalkyl cyanoacrylate surgical adhesive. *Arch Surg (Chicago)* 100:295–298, 1970.

44. Ousterhout DK, Larsen HW, Margetis PM, et al: Effect of ingested n-butyl alpha-cyanoacrylate on the growth of weaning rats. *Oral Surg Oral Med Oral Pathol* 27:275–280, 1969.

45. Martin TR, Silvis SE: The endoscopic control of GI blood loss with a tissue adhesive (MBR 4197). (abstract) *Gastroenterology* 72:1098, 1977.

46. Protell RL, Silverstein FE, Gulacsik C, et al: Failure of cyanoacrylate tissue glue (flucrylate, MBR 4197) to stop bleeding from experimental canine gastric ulcers. *Dig Dis Sci* 23:903–908, 1978.

47. Martin TR, Onstad GR, Silvis SE: Endoscopic control of massive upper gastrointestinal bleeding with a tissue adhesive (MBR 4197). *Gastrointest Endosc* 24:74–76, 1977.

48. Peura DA, Johnson LF, Burkhalter EL, et al: Use of trifluoroisopropyl cyanoacrylate polymer (MBR 4197) in patients with bleeding peptic ulcers of the stomach and duodenum: A randomized controlled study. *J Clin Gastroenterol* 4:325–328, 1982.

49. Hait MR, Robb CA, Baxter CR, et al: comparative evaluation of Avitene microcrystalline collagen hemostat in experimental animal wounds. *Am J Surg* 125:284–287, 1973.

50. Abbott WM, Austen WG: Microcrystalline collagen as a topical hemostatic agent for vascular surgery. *Surgery* 75(6):925–933, 1974.

51. Vistnes LM, Goodwin DA, Tenery JG, et al: Control of capillary bleeding by topical application of microcrystalline collagen. *Surgery* 76:291–294, 1974.

52. Hunt LM, Benoit PW: Evaluation of a microcrystalline collagen preparation in extraction wounds. *J Oral Surg* 34:407–414, 1976.

53. Battista OA, Erdi NZ, Ferraro CF, et al: Novel microcrystals of polymers. *J Appl Polym Sci* 11:481–498, 1967.

54. Abbott WM, Austen WG: The effectiveness and mechanism of collagen-induced topical hemostasis. *Surgery* 78:723–729, 1975.

55. Wilkinson TS, Tenery J, Zufi D: The skin graft donor site as a model for evaluation of hemostatic agents. *Plast Reconstr Surg* 55:541–544, 1973.

56. Tenery J, Clemmons RG: Technical Report Code No. 072-3310-005, Alcon Laboratories, October 9, 1972.

57. Feld AD, Silverstein FE, Keegan MD: Failure of microfibrillar collagen hemostat (MCH Avitene®) to stop bleeding from experimental canine ulcers. (abstract) *Gastrointest Endosc* 27:132, 1981.

10

Endoscopic Retrograde Sphincterotomy

Stephen E. Silvis
Jack A. Vennes

In the 1950s, sphincterotomy was occasionally performed to manage obstruction of the common bile duct following surgical duodenotomy. In many cases, the sphincterotomy became strictured, so the technique for sphincteroplasty was developed. The mucosa of the common bile duct was sutured to the duodenal mucosa, and stenosis was a much less frequent occurrence after such surgical repair (1–5).

More than a decade ago, Koch and colleagues (6,7) performed endoscopic retrograde sphincterotomy (ERS) in dogs by passing an exposed wire attached to a cannula up the bile duct and applying high-frequency current to cut the sphincter. The sphincterotomies stayed open. Koch and colleagues and other investigators (8–13) then performed sphincterotomy in patients to remove stones from the common bile duct. Because of lingering concern about the possibility of eventual stricturing, use of the procedure developed slowly, particularly in the United States. However, it has become apparent that stricturing is an uncommon occurrence, and over the past five years use of ERS has increased rapidly (14–18). A survey conducted in 1983 reported on more than 5000 patients treated by 75 physicians in the United States (19). Large series of patients have also been reported from around the world (14–18). Endoscopic retrograde sphincterotomy is now clearly the procedure of choice for the management of recurrent common duct stones after cholecystectomy (20–36).

REVIEW OF THE ANATOMY OF THE BILIARY AND PANCREATIC DUCTS

A basic understanding of the normal anatomy of the pancreaticobiliary system is of utmost importance when ERS is being contemplated.

The gallbladder, intrahepatic and extrahepatic bile ducts, liver, pancreas and pancreatic duct are derived from diverticula that originate in the foregut. At

198

two weeks of gestation, diverticula develop in this region. The dorsal diverticulum eventually becomes the body and tail of the pancreas. The more distal ventral diverticulum develops into the bile duct system, gallbladder and head of the pancreas. During the development of the ventral pancreas and distal bile duct, posterior rotation behind the duodenum results in fusion of the dorsal and ventral pancreatic anlagen, which forms the mature pancreas. The ducts within the dorsal and ventral pancreatic buds usually fuse in a predictable fashion. The main duct (duct of Wirsung) results from fusion of the ventral and dorsal pancreatic ducts. It enters the duodenum along with the distal common bile duct at the major papilla (papilla of Vater). A minor pancreatic duct (duct of Santorini) also may be present and results from persistence of the remnant of the dorsal pancreatic duct. If the duct of Santorini is present and patent, it drains into the duodenum via the minor papilla, which is located a few centimeters proximal to the major papilla.

Many anomalies in the biliary and pancreatic duct systems have been reported; however, such anatomic variations are rarely clinically important (37). One of the most frequent anomalies is pancreas divisum (Fig. 1, a and b). This

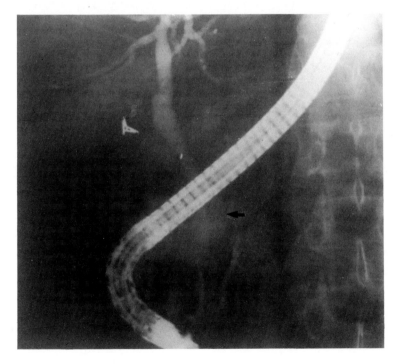

Fig. 1a. This cholangiopancreatogram shows a small ventral pancreas, which reflects nonfusion of the ventral and dorsal pancreatic anlagen. This patient had recurrent pancreatitis. The pancreatic duct is not obstructed because there are fine terminal branches coming off the duct that fill from the papilla of Vater (short arrow). The apparent stenosis of the common duct is a streaming artifact that filled out with further injection of contrast material. It was necessary to opacify the major component of the pancreatic duct from the papilla of Santorini.

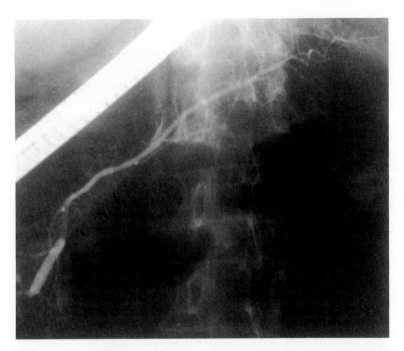

Fig. 1b. This pancreatogram was obtained with a tapered cannula from the papilla of Santorini and is entirely normal. The small area of the pancreas that is fed by the ventral duct is outlined by the arrows. It remains controversial whether pancreas divisum is the etiologic basis of acute recurrent pancreatitis, as seen in this patient.

anomaly is seen in approximately 5% of patients and is due to failure of fusion of the dorsal and ventral pancreatic ducts (38). In this situation, a variable portion of the pancreatic head is drained into the major papilla through a small ventral pancreatic duct. The remainder of the head, the body and the tail of the pancreas drain via the persistent duct of Santorini, the minor papilla. Controversy exists over whether this embryologic defect is a cause of acute recurrent pancreatitis (39–44).

In the parenchyma of the liver, the interlobular ducts eventually fuse to form the right and left hepatic ducts, which join at the porta hepatis to form the common hepatic duct. Usually, within 4 to 5 cm of the porta hepatis, the cystic duct can be seen joining the common hepatic duct. There is marked variation in the point of union of the cystic and common hepatic ducts to form the common bile duct. The common bile duct courses posteriorly through the head of the pancreas and then turns laterally to enter the second portion of the duodenum. The distal common bile duct and pancreatic duct frequently join to form a common channel in the ampulla of Vater. Autopsy studies reveal that a common channel occurs in approximately 85% of cases (Fig. 2). In the remaining 15% of cases, the pancreatic and bile ducts open separately in the duodenum

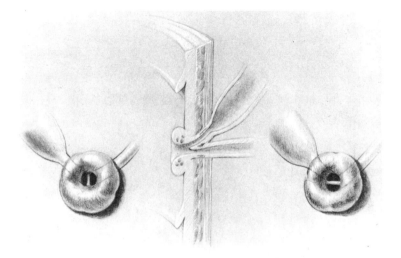

Fig. 2. This drawing of the papilla of Vater illustrates a number of points. Obviously, the orifice is never seen this clearly because it is filled with frondlike mucosa. Major points of illustration are that the common duct, when viewed *en face*, swings at a moderate angle to the left, and the pancreatic duct swings slightly to the right. There frequently is a short common channel with a very narrow septum between the two ducts. Although the septum can be orientated in all angles, in this illustration, it is shown facing directly horizontally and vertically. Its angle of orientation varies among patients, creating problems in locating the desired duct. The cross-sectional view shows that the pancreatic duct tends to run directly through the duodenal wall, where the common bile duct runs tangentially and in a cephalad direction. The length of this tangential segment in the duodenal wall is, of course, the area that is incised for sphincterotomy. In many cases, the length of the tangential segment is far longer than is shown, and the angle may be much sharper. It is of critical importance both in ERCP and sphincterotomy to be aware of these anatomic relationships and the variations that occur.

on the major papilla. The incidence of separate orifices is probably lower than has been reported in autopsy series because the common channel frequently is only a few millimeters in length during life; with fixation of specimens, the opening of the common channel appears to be composed of two separate orifices. The distal common bile duct enters the duodenal wall obliquely and courses within the wall for approximately 5 to 30 mm before opening into the papilla (45,46). It is this portion of the duct that is divided at the time of ERS (Fig. 3).

It should be noted that the head of the pancreas lies slightly to the right of the spine and that the body of the gland crosses the spine at approximately the second lumbar vertebra. The body of the pancreas is the most anterior portion of the pancreas, crossing over the vena cava and aorta. The tail of the pancreas

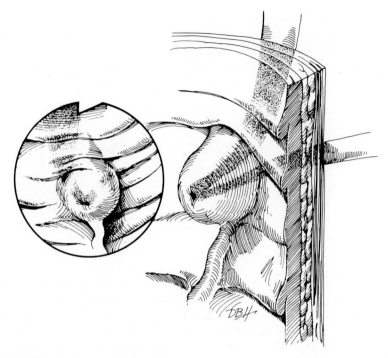

Fig. 3. This drawing is an artist's conception of the papilla of Vater viewed *en face*. The dotted arrangement of the pancreatic and common bile ducts is shown. There is marked variation in the first few millimeters of the ducts in the papilla. There are sphincters around the common channel, the common bile duct and the pancreatic duct. Variation in the microanatomic structure of the papilla is one factor that makes ERCP and sphincterotomy difficult. On the other hand, the tangential angle of the common bile duct in the duodenal wall makes ERS possible and reasonably safe.

then courses posteriorly; thus, if a patient lies prone on an x-ray table, the portion of the pancreatic duct in the body of the gland is actually uphill from the portion in the head of the gland.

The region where the duodenal wall is penetrated by the biliary and pancreatic ducts has been termed the choledochoduodenal junction (Fig. 3). During their passage through the duodenal wall, the common bile duct, pancreatic duct and ampulla of Vater are surrounded by a complex arrangement of smooth muscles, which has been designated the sphincter of Oddi. The most detailed dissections of this area in human beings were performed by Boyden (45,46), who divided the sphincter of Oddi into four sections: a sheath of circular muscle that surrounds the common bile duct from its entrance into the duodenal wall to the junction with the pancreatic duct, a group of longitudinally arranged muscle fibers that occupy the space between the biliary and pancreatic ducts, a network of muscle fibers that encircles the ampulla of Vater and the common channel and a circular muscle fiber that surrounds the pancreatic duct until the point where it unites with the common bile duct.

In human beings, the common bile duct contains only sparse longitudinal muscle fibers that do not influence the flow of bile (47). The duct acts mainly as a passive conduit for the approximately 1000 ml of bile that are produced daily by the liver. The rate of flow of bile through this system is quite variable, being as low as 0.4 ml per minute during fasting to as high as 2 to 3 ml per minute after gallbladder contraction. By contrast, pressure within the common bile duct remains fairly constant, usually about 12 mm of mercury above the pressure within the duodenum. Recent pressure studies in human beings indicate that the sphincter of Oddi is approximately 6 mm long (48). These studies were performed in patients without pancreatic or biliary disease and revealed that the average pressure of the basal sphincter was about 4 mm of mercury above the pressure within the bile duct. In addition, superimposed on the resting pressures are distinct phasic pressure waves, which have been demonstrated throughout the length of the sphincter segment. These phasic contractions occur at a rate of about four per minute and have an average amplitude of 100 ± 50 mm of mercury above duodenal pressure (48–50). Such phasic waves are not recorded from the common bile duct and do not correlate with any phase of duodenal motor activity. Further studies have shown that approximately 60% of the phasic waves progress toward the duodenum, 25% are simultaneous and approximately 15% move in a retrograde fashion. Control mechanisms that regulate the contractions of the sphincter of Oddi are not well understood (48–54). Current thinking is that hormones are the primary mediators of sphincter pressure and that gastrointestinal peptides function as modulators; however, the possibility of neurogenic control still exists.

ENDOSCOPIC RETROGRADE CHOLANGIOPANCREATOGRAPHY

It is obvious that an operator must have skill and experience with endoscopic retrograde cholangiopancreatography (ERCP) before considering ERS. The latter procedure is considerably more difficult than ERCP; therefore, an operator must have a high level of expertise with ERCP before contemplating therapeutic endoscopic procedures on the common duct. The technique of ERCP is beyond the scope of this chapter and has been described previously in detail (55). However, a brief discussion of prerequisites for success may be beneficial. The patient must have optimal preparation to achieve sedation and relaxation of smooth muscle tone. Duodenal atony must be induced by use of atropine, glucagon or the two agents in combination (56). Control over motility facilitates location and cannulation of the papilla of Vater.

An endoscopist who performs ERCP should be able to cannulate the common bile duct selectively and freely. This maneuver is best accomplished with the patient in the prone position, which also permits much clearer interpretation of resulting x-ray films. After the papilla of vater has been located, it frequently is necessary to straighten out the loop in the stomach to obtain a better closeup position for cannulation. Attempting to cannulate from far away is a major cause of failure.

It is important to view the papilla of Vater closely to identify its orifice(s). These details should be memorized because in the event the papilla is difficult to cannulate, each cannula mark will appear as an orifice or obscure landmarks. Small moves are necessary to achieve precise orientation of the cannula into the axis of the common bile duct. It is necessary to practice hand and eye coordination, particularly the coordinated movement of the cannula upward with the lever while it is being advanced forward with the right hand. The endoscopist must not become impatient. The axis of the cannula and duct needs to be aligned properly, a maneuver that is accomplished by means of combinations of lateral or vertical flexion or rotation of the endoscope. Failure to make these small moves to align the axis properly is a cause of problems in selective cannulation.

It is important to be able to deal with problems when they arise by modifying aspects of the procedure; for example, the patient can be changed from the prone to an oblique position, a tapered cannula can be subsituted or the procedure can be attempted again in 1 to 3 days. Certain problems predict trouble in ERCP. An example is distortion of the normal anatomic structure as a result of previous duodenal or gastric surgery. Billroth II gastrectomy also makes the procedure difficult to perform (57–60). On the other hand, Billroth I gastrectomy usually causes only minor difficulty. Previous biliary surgery with common duct exploration and/or choledochoduodenostomy occasionally causes problems because of fixation and nonrotation of the duodenal loop.

The papilla of Santorini may be large and can be confused with the major papilla. However, it usually is firm and resists cannulation (61). If the papilla of Santorini is resistant to cannulation, the operator should look downward and rotate slightly to the left in the visual field to locate the papilla of Vater. Diverticula are extremely common in older patients and usually occur in a juxta-ampullary position (62). The papilla of Vater usually sits on the rim of a diverticulum and is rarely located in a diverticulum, a location that would prohibit cannulation. Therefore, a careful search around the rim of the diverticulum is warranted. The reader may wish to review details of the technique of ERCP in other publications (55).

ENDOSCOPIC RETROGRADE SPHINCTEROTOMY

INDICATIONS

The usual indication for endoscopic sphincterotomy is recurrent or residual common duct stones. Cholelithiasis is a common problem in the United States. It has been estimated that each year, 600,000 cholecystectomies are performed in this country. In 1% to 10% of cases, the common duct becomes obstructed by

TABLE 1. Indications for and Complications of
Endoscopic Retrograde Sphincterotomy, Survey of
75 U.S. Physicians (19)

	Attempts	Complications
Common bile duct stones	4815	312 (6.5%)
Biliary pancreatitis	218	8 (3.7%)
Papillary stenosis	669	61 (9.1%)
Malignant lesions	88	12 (13.6%)
Total	5790	393 (6.7%)

gallstones some time after cholecystectomy (63–68). The procedure has been shown to be satisfactory for the management of gallstone pancreatitis and acute suppurative cholangitis (69–81). Important considerations in the performance of ERS are that biliary pancreatitis must be documented and that open drainage must be obtained after sphincterotomy. In addition, ERS has been used for the management of papillary stenosis (82–92) and malignant lesions of the distal common bile duct (93–95).

A survey of 75 physicians in the United States (19) revealed that, as in other reports (96–101), common duct stones were the indication for ERS in 83% of 5790 procedures (Table 1). Extremely large stones are probably a contraindication to the procedure. Stones with diameters greater than 2.5 cm often cannot be removed by means of ERS. The survey noted that if a Billroth II operation has been done, it represents a major problem for the performance of ERS. In the same survey, 84 ERSs were attempted in patients who had previously undergone a Billroth II gastrectomy. The success rate in such patients was only 60%, as compared to 87% in all patients in whom ERS had been performed.

Before making a final decision to proceed with ERS, a high-quality cholangiogram must be obtained (102–109). The sizes of the common duct stones in relation to the length of the apparent intraduodenal segment of the common bile duct and the surgical risk factors for a patient influence the decision to proceed with ERS. It is desirable to perform ERS after ERCP has been completed; therefore, advance preparation must be made for ERS. Surgical consultation should be obtained before ERCP is done, and a surgeon should be available before ERS is performed. Clotting factor studies should have been obtained, and blood must be available in the event that transfusion becomes necessary.

Figures 4a and 4b are cholangiograms that show numerous small stones. There is a relatively long intraduodenal segment of the common duct. This situation is excellent for endoscopic removal of stones. Figure 5 shows stones of a moderate size in the gallbladder and common duct. Indications for the procedure in this situation would depend on a patient's immediate medical condition and the risks for surgical intervention. Endoscopic retrograde sphincterotomy should be performed if the patient has gallstone pancreatitis or suppurative cholangitis or if the patient is at high risk for surgical intervention.

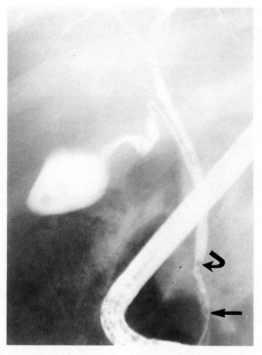

Fig. 4a. This cholangiogram shows a number of radiolucent stones in the gallbladder. The arrow indicates a small stone in the common bile duct. This patient was admitted with pancreatitis. Because of the very small diameter of the stone in the common bile duct, only a short sphincterotomy was required, even though the cannula in the common bile duct reveals a long segment of duct in the wall between the two arrows. Endoscopic retrograde sphincterotomy was performed to remove the small calculi, and the pancreatitis resolved.

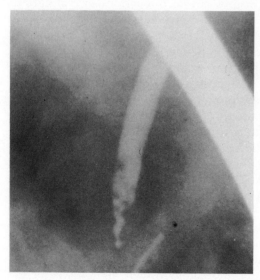

Fig. 4b. This cholangiogram shows a magnified view of only the distal portion of the common bile duct. The numerous small irregularities, which represent stones, can easily be overlooked on contrast studies. It is necessary to use fluoroscopy and to obtain spot films before the contrast material becomes dense and/or to use dilute contrast material. The sphincterotomy for these very small stones does not need to be of great length.

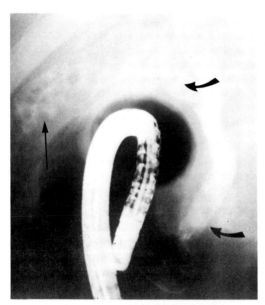

Fig. 5. These stones in the gallbladder (small arrow), cystic duct and common bile duct (large arrow) are easily seen. When measured in comparison to the dimensions of the endoscope, they are found to be approximately 2 to 5 mm in diameters. Stones of this size are readily removed by ERS. In this picture, the papillotome is seen just entering the distal portion of the common bile duct. Because of other medical conditions, this elderly, ill man was treated with ERS. It remains unclear which patients should undergo ERS with their gallbladders in situ.

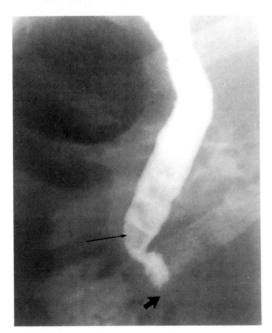

Fig. 6. This cholangiogram shows a magnified view of the distal portion of the common bile duct in which there are stones with diameters of 1 to 1.5 cm. It illustrates a number of points. The short arrow shows the entrance of the papilla. A long horizontal portion of the papilla must be excised before the dilated segment of the common duct is entered. At the long arrow, the duct turns sharply away from the duodenum. The operator should not extend the sphincterotomy into this area, which may be outside the duodenal wall. Stones of this size with this anatomic configuration of the duct may be successfully managed by ERS.

For patients with intact gallbladders who are at standard risk for surgical intervention, the question of whether ERS is indicated remains unanswered. Figure 6 shows common duct stones having diameters of 1 to 1.5 cm. There is a long intraduodenal segment of the common bile duct. Endoscopic retrograde sphincterotomy was performed successfully in this patient. By contrast, some patients have a short intraduodenal segment that will permit creation of a sphincterotomy of only modest length (Fig. 7). Figure 8 shows common duct stones having diameters greater than 2 cm. Several treatment options can be considered for patients with such large stones. Surgical removal should be strongly considered if such a patient is a standard risk for surgical intervention. Endoscopic retrograde sphincterotomy is feasible only if the intraduodenal segment is prominent and long, so that a generous cut can be safely made. After a cut has been made, the stones will likely remain in the duct, and a nasobiliary tube may be positioned in the duct and left clamped; the tube remains available as a decompression device should the stones reobstruct the duct. The operator may then wait 5 to 7 days for edema and inflammation to subside; when the tissue shrinks, large calculi may pass. Another final option is to drip monooctanoate via the nasobiliary tube. This agent dissolves cholesterol-containing calculi in approximately 50% of cases or may soften large calculi so that they can be extracted a few days later as "mud." These alternatives are discussed to demonstrate that the decision to perform ERS can be made only after a high-quality cholangiogram has been obtained.

USE OF RADIOFREQUENCY CURRENT

An endoscopist must have a basic knowledge of electrosurgery before contemplating ERS. By 1900, it was known that radiofrequency currents pass through the human body without causing adverse effects. Initially, high frequencies were used to coagulate skin tissue or internal tissue during surgical procedures. An excellent review of early electrosurgery has been published by McLean (110,111). Today, there are a number of small electrosurgical generators that are effective and usually safe (112). Such generators produce alternating current in the range of 400,000 to 1,000,000 cycles per second. Although high-frequency current has long been used for therapeutic purposes, the precise details of the interactions between tissue and electric current are not well known (113–117). It is important to bear in mind that electrosurgical generators not only have variable power output (watts) but that they also produce mark-

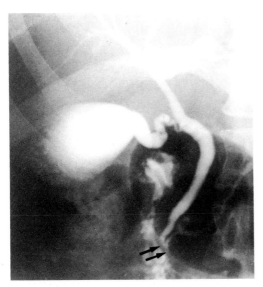

Fig. 7. This cholangiopancreatogram shows an anatomic arrangement in which the pancreatic and bile ducts are in the duodenal wall for only a very short segment. The entrance of the papilla is indicated by an arrow, and its exit from the duodenum, only a few millimeters away, is indicated by a second arrow. Patients with this anatomic configuration can tolerate only a very short sphincterotomy. In some patients, this anatomic configuration constitutes a contraindication to ERS.

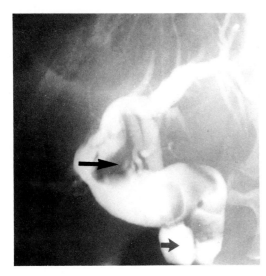

Fig. 8. This elderly patient had massive dilatation of the common bile duct with huge radiolucent stones. These findings on a cholangiogram should prompt a reevaluation of the decision to perform ERS. The short arrow indicates a periampullary diverticulum filled with contrast material. Whether sphincterotomy could or should be performed in this patient would depend on the length of the intraduodenal segment as visualized endoscopically and on x-ray study. In addition, the overall condition of the patient must be considered. If sphincterotomy is performed in this patient, the operator is likely to have difficulty removing the stones. Removal of stones may require a second procedure or infusion of monooctanoate to dissolve them. If this patient represented a reasonably standard surgical risk, it would be prudent to remove the stones by surgical exploration of the common bile duct. In this case, sphincterotomy was done because the patient was elderly. The large stone indicated by the long arrow was actually a cluster of stones that broke up during the second manipulation, after the sphincterotomy had been extended.

edly different waveforms of current. Both the power output and type of current produced vary widely from one manufacturer's generator to another.

Figures 9 and 10 show different waveforms of current that have cutting and coagulation effects. Coagulation currents usually are composed of short, repetitive cycles interspersed by periods when the current is off. Cutting currents are composed of continuous sinusoidal waves or bursts that are active most of the time (Fig. 10). Although these modulations are in thousands of cycles per second, the tissue effects are strikingly different.

It is useful to review some of the basic principles of the effect of radiofrequency current on tissue. Because alternating current is being used, the term *impedance* is more precise than *resistance*. Tissue impedance is the mathematic combination of resistance and capacitance. Tissue capacitance is the result of the presence of capacitors in the radiofrequency circuit. Capacitors measure a tissue's ability to store energy. Tissue resistance dissipates the energy as heat. Current density is quantified as the amount of current in a given cross-sectional area of an electrode or a sphincterotome wire. The heat generated is proportional to the square of the current density. This relationship is an extremely important concept to keep in mind during ERS. If a power setting is kept constant, the current density depends on the area of the wire electrode that is in contact with tissue. Contact varies constantly during ERS and frequently is not under the precise control of the operator.

The primary difference between cutting and coagulation currents relates to the percentage of time that the current is active, that is the duty cycle (Fig. 11). Currents that have a cutting effect produce intense heat at the point of contact, probably vaporizing and exploding cells. An arc, as visible sparking, can be seen forming and reforming in the same area, and this arc gradually advances. The exploding cells probably cut with a steam wedge effect. Currents that have a coagulation effect are composed of short, repetitive cycles, usually at a frequency of about 20,000 cycles per second (Fig. 10). These dampened bursts have a significantly lower duty cycle. It is important to be aware that high power coagulation current can produce cutting, while low power cutting current will produce tissue coagulation.

Radiofrequency generators offer many benefits but also pose a number of real and potential problems. It should be remembered that current flows along the path of least impedance (resistance); if the current density is high, a burn

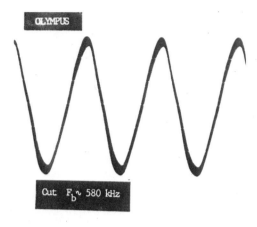

Fig. 9. The waveform of a current that has a cutting effect is shown in the top of this frame. It is a simple sinusoidal current, which is active all the time. The lower panel shows the waveform of a current with a coagulation effect from the same unit. The time when the current is active is markedly reduced. The percentage of time that the current is active is referred to as the "duty cycle," and it represents the basic difference between the waveforms of currents that have a cutting effect and those that have a coagulation effect.

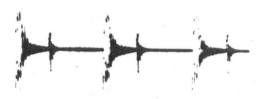

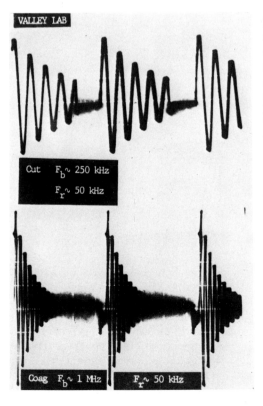

Fig. 10. The top of this frame shows a different waveform of a current that has a cutting effect; these are bursts with very short off periods. A current that has a coagulation effect, in which the current declines most of the time, is shown in the lower panel. F_b denotes frequency of the basic current; the frequency of the current with a coagulation effect is 1 megahertz (MHz; megacycles per second), and F_r is the frequency of the repetitions at 50 kilohertz (kHz). Although the upper waveform is labeled as a current with a cutting effect, it is very similar to blended currents in many electrosurgical units.

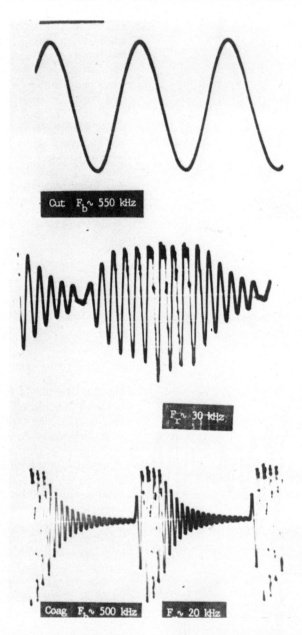

Fig. 11. The upper panel of this frame shows a current with a cutting effect that has a basic frequency of 550 kHz in a sinusoidal pattern. The middle panel shows a blended current in which a 30,000-hertz oscillation occurs with a very short off period in the duty cycle. In the lower panel, the coagulation mode has the current off approximately half of the time to allow cooling; it coagulates rather than cuts. Most endoscopists who perform sphincterotomy use units or settings that give blended currents similar to that shown in the center of this frame, or the cutting current of the generator (Fig. 10, *top*) produces a similar current. It is undesirable to use a simple sine-wave current that has a cutting effect.

will result. For this reason, the ground plate must be large enough to prevent the production of heat as current returns through this electrode. If the gelled pad becomes partially detached with only a small area of contact, a high enough current density can be produced to cause burning. Prevention of burns is the primary advantage of capacitively coupled plates (disposable grounds). As such plates become detached, their impedance rises, thus reducing the flow of current before a substantial increase in temperature occurs. On the other hand, gelled pads conduct almost the entire current through a narrow area of contact, and burns at the return electrode are possible. The possibility of burns is a problem in confused, unconscious or heavily sedated patients, who may not respond quickly to discomfort, as is the experience with many patients undergoing ERS.

An appreciable percentage of the radiofrequency current produced by electrosurgical generators is transmitted. This is well demonstrated by the interference produced on monitors such as x-ray, television or electrocardiography. Most modern pacemakers are adequately shielded from radiofrequency currents.

Radiofrequency current can flow without apparent connection by means of capacitive coupling. A capacitor is a plate of electrical material that conducts electric current separated by a layer of insulation to which is attached another layer of conducting material. Figure 12 shows an endoscope acting as a conductor with a sphincterotome acting as another conductor. The Teflon sheath acts as an insulator. This setup functions as a capacitor. The operator can sustain burns as a result of capacitive coupling with an endoscope that has no electric circuit fault. Burns can occur when a small area of the operator's skin is in contact with the ground, as would occur if an elbow were rested against a grounded x-ray table.

Nerves, and therefore muscles, can be stimulated at frequencies below 3000 cycles per second. Currents below this frequency apparently are produced by tissue because they are not produced by electrosurgical generators that are connected to a purely resistive circuit. All electrosurgical generators have low-frequency current blocking condensers to eliminate such unwanted current frequencies. Typically, approximately 0.01 to 0.5 milliampere of low-frequency current flows during a normal operation. Such low-frequency currents are probably harmless, except if they are introduced directly into the heart by a

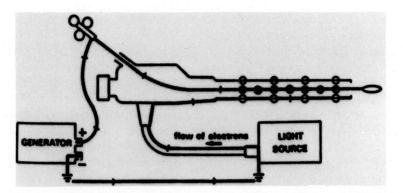

Fig. 12. This drawing illustrates the principle of escape, or secondary currents. The wire of the sphincterotome acts as one plate and the metal of the endoscope acts as the other, with the Teflon sheath producing insulation. The plate and metal of the endoscope function as a capacitor, allowing coupling of the high-frequency current to the endoscope. High-frequency current that is produced will not cause shocks to the operator, patient or other personnel; however, if a small area of contact is present, heat will be generated. This heat probably is the cause of most of the "shocks" reported during endoscopic procedures. If a small area of contact between the operator and ground is present, sudden heating will occur and give the impression of electric shock.

catheter, for example, by a transvenous cardiac pacemaker. If the blocking condensers fail in the closed position, dangerous low-frequency currents, in the range of 2 to 5 milliampers, can be produced (117). If failure occurs, the patient will experience nerve stimulation with each activation of the electrosurgical generator. Failure of the blocking condensers may be responsible for rare cases of ventricular fibrillation associated with electrosurgery (118). Obviously, if stimulation occurs with each activation of the electrosurgical generator, a different generator should be used to complete the procedure.

The use of electrosurgery in ERS involves a number of considerations. The ultimate goal of producing a smooth cut through the papillary muscle into the intraduodenal segment of the common bile duct should be constantly remembered. The cut should be made in such a manner that minimal bleeding and necrosis result. It is necessary to bear in mind that the length of wire that is in contact with the papilla varies continually during the cutting. When cutting is initiated, it may be necessary to reduce the amount of current that is delivered by shortening the bursts or by lowering the power setting.

A number of electrosurgical generators that produce blended current have been satisfactorily used in the performance of ERS. It is desirable not to vary the unit being used. Changes in the power setting do not result in equal changes in generator output from unit to unit, even among units from the same manufacturer. With good understanding of the electrosurgical generator and the results that are desired, the endoscopist should be able to apply electrosurgical current for ERS with few complications. Probably the best single reference on the basic principles of electrosurgery is that of Barlow (119).

TECHNIQUE (5,7,17,120–125)

The goal of ERS is to sever the sphincter fibers from the distal common bile duct as well as any soft tissue that impedes the passage of bile and/or common duct stones. The length of the sphincterotomy should be tailored to the size of the common duct stones. The apparent length of the intraduodenal segment of the common bile duct and the length of the narrow portion of the duct until the point where the duct becomes dilated are of great importance. Obviously, a sphincterotomy must be extended to the dilated portion of the duct, but it must also remain within the intraduodenal segment of the duct. Patients with long strictures of a distal common duct that extends outside the duodenal wall or patients with failure of the distal segment of the preampullary duct to dilate are not good candidates for this endoscopic procedure (Fig. 13)

A wide variety of instruments for sphincterotomy are available from a number of manufacturers (Figs. 14 to 17). Most of them are modifications of the original Erlangen design in which the cannula is fitted with a wire that exits and reenters the end of the cannula, leaving an exposed length of wire. In various designs, the length of exposed wire ranges from 20 to 40 mm. The proximal handle of the papillotome controls the tension of the wire and the flexion of the cannula, so that during cutting, the wire is held against the roof of the papilla. The wire must be directed toward the duodenal lumen.

Figures 18a and 18b show the schematic orientation of a sphincterotome in the common bile duct. In this view, the artist illustrates the idealized position of the sphincterotome. The endoscopic view that should be seen immediately

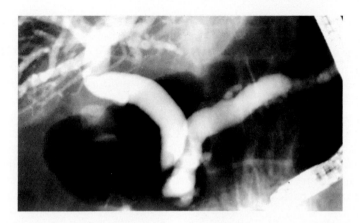

Fig. 13. This cholangiopancreatogram shows marked enlargement of the pancreatic duct with dilatation and beading of the side branches of the duct, indicating chronic pancreatitis. In addition, there is a narrow stricture of the common bile duct (between the two arrows). The bile duct was slightly enlarged (14 to 16 mm). There is some dilatation of the intrahepatic ducts. Patients with strictures of the distal portion of the common bile duct usually are not good candidates for ERS because there is concern about malignant degeneration in the bile duct and because the stricturing may be be-yond the duodenal wall. This patient had undergone six operations in the upper abdominal area, including cholecystectomy, exploration of the common bile duct, drainage of a pancreatic abscess, vagotomy, pyloroplasty and drainage of two pseudocysts. Because of these previous surgical procedures and the patient's poor medical condition, a decision was made to attempt sphincterotomy through the area of stricture on the assumption that it probably was encased in extensive scar tissue. The patient tolerated the procedure without difficulty and has had no further cholangitis.

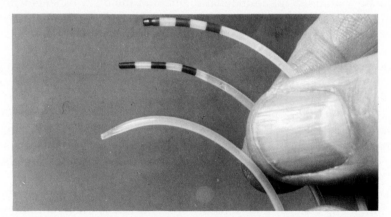

Fig. 14. The upper cannula is a standard ERCP cannula. The middle cannula is a slightly tapered, marked cannula, and the lower cannula is a homemade, markedly tapered cannula. Tapered cannulas are useful in the papilla of Santorini and are occasionally used in very tight papil-las of Vater. They should not be used routinely in that they have a marked tendency to produce artifactual marks on the papilla, making it more difficult to perform a second cannulation or to introduce a sphincterotome.

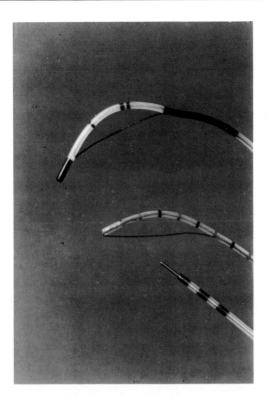

Fig. 15. The sphincterotome on the top is a standard instrument with 30 mm of exposed wire and marked tip. This instrument can be flexed by means of its proximal handle to varying degrees; the authors prefer to cut with the degree of flexion shown here. It is desirable to have a number of sphincterotomes available because each sphincterotome assumes a different position in the papilla of Vater. Designs are available with longer and shorter exposed wires; however, a 30-mm wire is adequate for most patients. The papillotome in the middle is a "precut" instrument. The primary difference with this type of papillotome is that the exposed wire runs all the way to the tip of the instrument. It is designed for use in cutting when a standard papillotome will not slide further than the duct and, obviously, a papillotome should cut at its tip. The desired result is to allow the endoscopist to cut into the duct. The instrument on the bottom is a needle electrode for cutting through the duodenal wall into the common bile duct. Cutting should be done only when there is a marked bulge of the bile duct into the duodenum and when the operator is absolutely certain of the position of the bile duct in relation to the duodenal wall. After the common bile duct has been entered, a catheter can be passed up the duct to confirm the position of the duct, and then a standard papillotome can be introduced to perform the sphincterotomy. The authors believe that precut papillotomes and needle electrodes should be used only under special circumstances and only in patients at high risk for abdominal surgery. After these instruments have been used, marked edema occasionally develops, and the operator will have great difficulty introducing a standard papillotome.

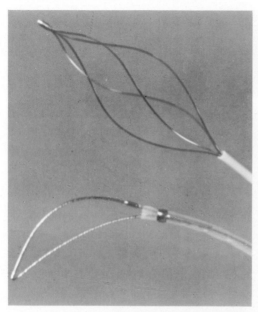

Fig. 16. The instrument at the top is a standard spiraling wire basket. This type of basket is more difficult to introduce into the common bile duct than is a balloon or papillotome. On occasion, the operator has difficulty entrapping stones in a basket, and there have been reports of impaction of baskets with entrapped stones in the distal portion of the common bile duct. Some patients have required surgical intervention for removal of impacted baskets with entrapped stones. The instrument at the bottom is a modified papillotome, similar to a polypectomy snare, in which the stone can be hooked in the wire loop and extracted. The authors more frequently use balloons, as shown in Figure 17.

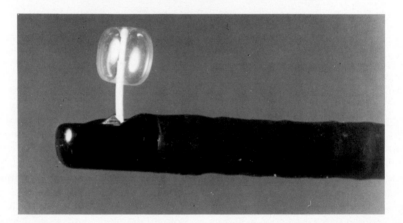

Fig. 17. This balloon is a modified Swan-Ganz catheter that can be inflated and deflated with an external syringe. There is a lumen for injecting contrast material into the duct. When fully inflated, the balloon is approximately 1 cm in diameter. Usually, however, it cannot be inflated to less than 0.75 cm. It is useful for passing up beyond stones to pull down and drag them through a sphincterotomy incision, for determining the size of the incision, for determining the presence of and removing gravel and for performing cholangiography after sphincterotomy or choledochoduodenostomy. In these instances, it usually is necessary to occlude the stoma to obtain adequate visualization of the bile duct. As shown in Figure 22, considerable traction often is required for pulling a stone through a sphincterotomy incision. Balloons break readily when they snap through incisions, probably by striking the elevator. The cannula elevator lever can be seen alongside the balloon catheter.

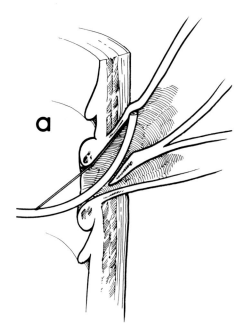

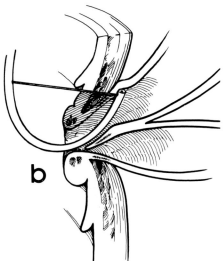

Fig. 18a. This drawing shows a cross-sectional view through the area of the papilla of Vater. A sphincterotome is in position, and there is moderate flexion on the wire. The sphincterotome is in the longitudinal axis of the common bile duct and is directed toward the duodenal wall.

Fig. 18b. This drawing shows the sphincterotomy near completion. As can be seen, a longitudinal incision has been made in the duodenal wall of the common bile duct. The sphincter fibers of the papilla of Vater have been severed. The bowing of the sphincterotome has been increased and is somewhat greater than is normally used. This figure illustrates primarily the ideal component of the sphincterotomy incision through the sphincter fibers and into the common duct wall.

before sphincterotomy is shown in Figures 19 and 20a. The wire will be withdrawn from the papilla and directed toward the duodenum. Figures 20b to 20f show gradual cutting of the sphincter by the wire. We advise a staged cutting approach in which only a few millimeters of the sphincter are cut at a time: we stop briefly to reexamine the area of the cut and reconfirm its proper orientation and the need for additional cutting. Figure 21 shows sizing of a sphincterotomy with a flexed papillotome, and Figures 22a and 22b depict sizing of the sphincterotomy with a 10-mm balloon catheter. Figure 23 shows a healed sphincterotomy.

We will now give a step-by-step description of ERS and will then discuss removal of common duct stones. After a high-quality cholangiogram has been obtained, the first step is to insert a papillotome freely into the common bile duct. Insertion of a papillotome may be more difficult than insertion of a

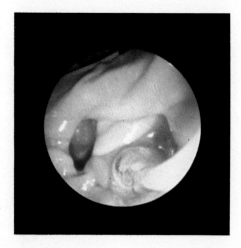

Fig. 19. In this endoscopic photograph, a papillotome is shown inserted into the common bile duct. There is a small periampullary diverticulum to the right of the papilla of Vater and a large periampullary diverticulum on the left side. The papillotome is clearly visualized following the course of the common bile duct in the ridge between the two diverticula. The operator can safely cut up between these two diverticula if the incision stays on the ridge. Obviously, the operator should not begin to cut until contrast has been injected to confirm the position of the common bile duct, and until the orientation of the wire has been confirmed by pulling it back into the duodenum. Close observation reveals just a few millimeters of wire coming out in the middle of the papilla directed toward the duodenal wall.

cannula for two reasons. The exposed wire forces the endoscopist to work at a greater distance from the papilla, and the sphincterotome is somewhat more rigid. It is important to identify carefully and remember the location of the orifice of the common bile duct and the angle at which the cannula entered the common duct. The operator must be certain that precise contact with the papilla has been made. After contact has been made, the papillotome is directed into the common bile duct at the previously determined angle. The papillotome can be directed at the appropriate angle by raising or lowering the cannula lever, by changing the angle of the endoscope by rotation, by changing the vertical or lateral flex or, occasionally, by adding some bow to the sphincterotome. Frequently, the sphincterotome hangs up in the papilla, sometimes for an extended period, after it has been advanced a few millimeters. In this situation, the best technique usually is to wiggle the sphincterotome by means of vertical and lateral flexes, adding in and out motions of the cannula with the right hand. If the operator is certain that contact was made precisely, the wiggling motions should be extended for a few minutes, particularly if the sphincterotome has been advanced slowly up the common bile duct. In some patients, pressure on the sphincterotome can be increased by moving the vertical flex of the endoscope or by withdrawing the instrument, which may allow it to pop into the common bile duct. In attempting to insert the sphincterotome into the common bile duct, the orientation of the wire is not important; however,

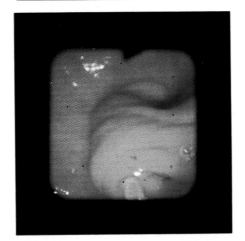

Fig. 20a. A sphincterotome is shown in the common bile duct. The endoscopist can identify the prominent longitudinal fold that distended on injection of contrast material, establishing that this structure is the segment of the common bile duct within the duodenal wall. From this position, the papillotome is withdrawn until 4 to 10 mm of wire are visible.

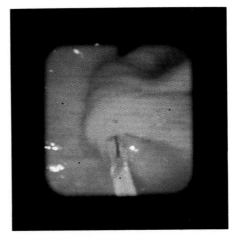

Fig. 20b. After the sphincterotome has been withdrawn, 4 to 5 mm of the wire can be seen protruding into the duodenum and directed toward its lumen. At this point, high-frequency current can be applied. Before the operator begins to cut, he or she should orientate the sphincterotome and determine how far up the duct the incision should be made. In this instance, an extensive sphincterotomy was needed, and a decision was made to extend the incision to the prominent crossing fold below the arrow.

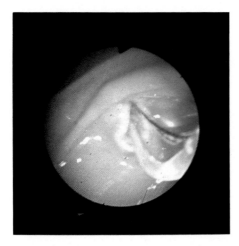

Fig. 20c. The sphincterotomy is now almost complete. In this instance, a decision was made to extend the incision up through the prominent crossing fold. This cutting usually is done with a partially flexed papillotome at a very low power setting or with very short bursts of current to carry the incision through the fold 1 mm at a time.

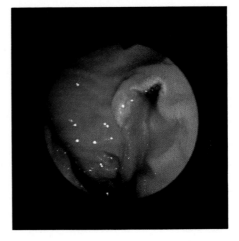

Fig. 20d. Completion of a sphincterotomy usually is signaled by a gush of bile containing some blood. The gush of bile signals that the sphincter fibers have been severed and usually indicates that the sphincterotomy is adequate.

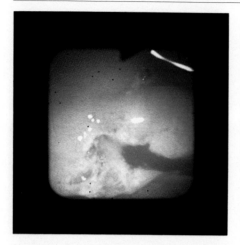

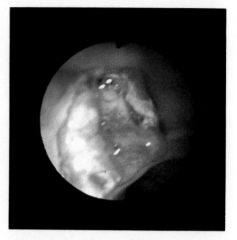

Fig. 20e. After contrast material and bile have stopped flowing from the common bile duct, the operator usually observes only a small trickle of blood. The initial gush of bile containing blood frequently is alarming; indeed, severe bleeding occurs in a small proportion of patients. The endoscopist should not attempt to assess the severity of bleeding in the first few seconds after completion of a sphincterotomy. The size of a sphincterotomy must be measured with a balloon, basket or papillotome.

Fig. 20f. A long sphincterotomy is shown immediately after completion. This is the same patient shown in Figure 20a. Note the prominent edema, which may occur within seconds after completion of the procedure. The edema sometimes makes extraction of stones a difficult maneuver to perform at the time the procedure is completed. Extraction probably would be easier at a later date.

orientation of the wire becomes a critical consideration before current is applied. The initial goal is to position the papillotome freely in the common bile duct.

After the sphincterotome has been passed freely into the common bile duct, it should be advanced only a short distance before contrast material is injected to identify the duct. If the sphincterotome has been inserted into the pancreatic duct, it must be removed. When the sphincterotome has been advancing slowly, it may be desirable to confirm fluoroscopically that it is directed toward the common bile duct. It is possible for an operator to be confident that he or she has advanced the sphincterotome at the same angle that the cannula entered the common bile duct, only to find that it has entered the pancreatic duct instead. This mistaken impression is probably related to the fact that cannulation is being done from a greater distance and with a stiffer instrument. Because of this possibility, contrast material must be injected after each insertion of the sphincterotome.

After the sphincterotome has been inserted, the next steps are to determine the orientation of the wire in relation to the common bile duct and duodenal

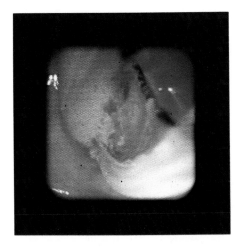

Fig. 21. A fully flexed papillotome is shown coming through a sphincterotomy incision with minimal resistance. Minimal resistance indicates that the opening into the duct is approximately 10 mm in diameter. The papillotome will stretch the incision in an anteroposterior direction; therefore, the sphincterotomy opening may not be as large as this maneuver would suggest.

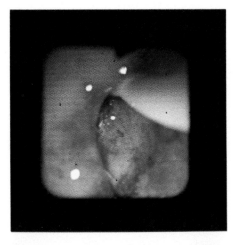

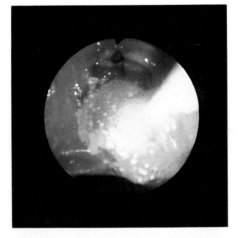

Fig. 22a. A balloon is shown bulging through a sphincterotomy incision. Sludge is seen below the balloon. Sludge frequently is found in common bile ducts that contain stones.

Fig. 22b. After the balloon has popped through into the duodenum, soft sludge, or mud, is seen adhering to the catheter. If the balloon has been fully inflated, this demonstrates that a 1-cm stone should pass through the opening. The authors sometimes make repeated passes through a sphincterotomy to remove mud and small stones.

wall and to determine the length of sphincterotomy that is desired. The operator knows the size of the calculus and, therefore, the approximate size of the ductal opening that is required. In addition, the operator must be sure that no cutting occurs beyond the duodenal wall. Because precise measurement is difficult, it is fortunate that the intraduodenal segment of the common bile duct is nearly always long enough to accomodate a standard cut, which is 10 to 12 mm. The operator may view endoscopically the impression on the duodenal wall of the common bile duct as it courses through the wall from the papilla. If this area of bulging distends when the duct is filled with contrast material, the operator can be certain of its course and that it represents the common bile duct. During the drainage phase of the cholangiogram, the intraduodenal portion of the bile duct may appear radiographically as a narrowed segment with a regular contour that fills and empties in a phasic manner with duodenal motility. It is neither necessary nor desirable to make a sphincterotomy longer than that which is required to allow passage of the largest common duct stones. The sphincterotome is then flexed to a one-quarter or one-half bow and is withdrawn slowly until the wire becomes visible (Fig. 24).

The operator should note the length of the wire that is in contact with tissue; therefore, if a short sphincterotomy is desired, a longer segment of wire needs

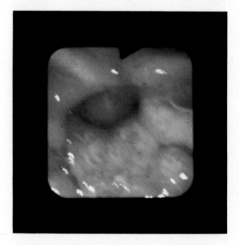

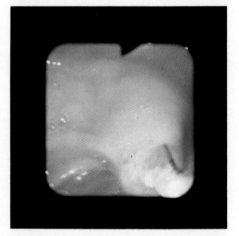

Fig. 23. A fully healed sphincterotomy is shown 6 weeks after the procedure. Such a gaping opening usually is not present, and a balloon is needed to measure the ductal orifice. (See Figure 22a, b.)

Fig. 24. This closeup view of a wire being pulled back into the duodenum shows the precise orientation of the wire toward the duodenal lumen. If electric current was applied at this point but cutting did not begin promptly, the papillotome would be withdrawn to shorten the length of wire in contact with the tissue.

to be made visible within the duodenum. The sphincterotomy wire should be oriented between the 11 and 2 o'clock positions, with the vertical axis of the duodenum being at 12 o'clock. Usually, 5 to 10 mm of the gently bowed 30-mm sphincterotome will lie within the duodenal lumen. The wire now lies firmly up against the roof of the papilla. It usually is not necessary or desirable to flex the tip fully as this may force the sphincterotome into the duodenum or up the common bile duct. The roof of the papilla and the intraduodenal segment of the common bile duct may be gently raised toward the lumen of the duodenum. When these structures are in the proper position, the operator may apply current. The sphincterotomy wire should be in close contact with the papillary orifice, thereby acting as a cutting edge along the longitudinal axis of the common bile duct. The wire usually acts as a cutting edge along the visible length of the intraduodenal segment of the duct. The whole procedure should be performed under direct visual guidance. At this point, it is advisable to be certain that all aspects of the procedure are under excellent control, that sedation is adequate and that control over motility is completely satisfactory. If there is any doubt about the position of the wire, it must be rechecked endoscopically and fluoroscopically. If the wire is not oriented properly, the first maneuver is to pass the sphincterotome back up the common bile duct. It should be flexed slightly more and withdrawn again to determine whether its position will rotate. If the sphincterotome still comes out in an unsatisfactory position, it should again be passed up the common bile duct and relaxed from its flexed state, and the endoscope should be rotated in an attempt to change the sphincterotome to the desired position. Occasionally, it is advisable to remove the instrument and select another sphincterotome before achieving proper positioning. For this and other reasons, a minimum of four sphincterotomes should be available.

The operator is ready to apply current at a predetermined power setting when he or she has broad knowledge of electrosurgical current and an understanding of the capabilities of the generator that is being used, confirmed the position of the sphincterotome in the common bile duct by injecting contrast material under fluoroscopic guidance and determined the length of the cut that has to be made. Current is delivered in the form of short bursts that are less than 1 second in duration. If the tissue does not begin to blanch within a few seconds, it is desirable to lengthen the duration of the bursts or to increase the power setting or retract some of the wire. After 3 to 5 mm of tissue has been cut, it is helpful to stop and briefly survey the direction of the cut and confirm that cutting is in the longitudinal axis of the common bile duct. Short, intermittent bursts of current are then applied to extend the sphincterotomy to the desired length. When the sphincterotomy is being extended in this manner, a gush of bile signals that the sphincteric fibers have been severed. After the sphincterotomy has been completed, the operator determines the size of the opening and patency to the bile duct. The size and patency may be determined by use of a flexed papillotome and then a balloon. If a 1-cm balloon does not come through, stones having diameters of 1 cm or greater usually will not pass, and the sphincterotomy will probably need to be extended. The sphincterotomy can be extended during the initial procedure, or the operator may decide to wait for the edema to subside and/or the stones to pass spontaneously. Sphincterotomies whose lengths are equal to the diameters of the stones usually allow passage of the stones. By contrast, sphincterotomies whose lengths are less than the diameters of the stones do not allow immediate passage of most stones.

A number of instruments have been designed to remove stones from the common bile duct. The various instruments are either baskets (Fig. 16) or balloons (Fig. 17). The authors prefer to use balloons because they can be deflated and removed if the stone(s) does not come through the sphincterotomy (Fig. 25). Balloons are relatively easy to position above stones in the common bile duct. It is desirable to attempt to remove the stones one at a time. Although vigorous traction is required to remove the stones, excessive pulling on the balloon may cause it to rupture. In addition, the balloon may snap through the sphincterotomy (Figs. 22a and 22b). Most breakage occurs when the balloon strikes the cannula elevator lever (Fig. 17).

Some operators prefer to use baskets to entrap stones and to extract the basket through the sphincterotomy. It is difficult to capture stones by use of baskets, and entrapment of baskets in sphincterotomies has been reported. In some such instances, surgical removal of the basket and stone has been necessary.

A number of special techniques have been described (126–136); however, evaluation of most such techniques is not possible because of insufficient experience. Recently, a mechanical lithotripsy device has been described in Germany (137–139). This device consists of a basket of high tensile strength wires with a Teflon sheath that can be removed and replaced by a coil spring sheath that allows application of firm traction on the stone; mechanical cutting through the stone is accomplished with the wires. Experience with this device is too sparse to allow a determination of its safety and efficacy, although it does appear to show promise. Electric spark pulsing lithotripsy, which has been useful for removing stones from the urinary tract, is now being studied to determine its effectiveness in the removal of gallstones. In addition, Orii and colleagues (140) have reported severing a gallstone with a YAG laser in two patients.

When stones cannot be removed after the sphincterotomy has been created, there are several options. The patient's problem should be reevaluated, and his or her risks for surgical intervention should be reconsidered. Radiographic and endoscopic studies should be done to determine whether there is an additional intramural segment of the common bile duct that will permit safe extension of

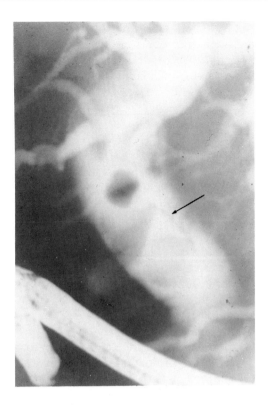

Fig. 25. A balloon catheter is shown in a greatly dilated common bile duct. The air-filled balloon and the air-filled catheter coming down from it (arrow) can be seen. This balloon has a diameter of 1 cm when fully inflated, which means that the stones in the duct have diameters of 2 to 4 cm. This patient required a very large the sphincterotomy. A major problem with extraction of stones from such a huge duct by means of a balloon catheter is that the stones tend to slip around the catheter. In this patient, the sphincterotomy was extended, and time was allowed for spontaneous passage of the stones.

the sphincterotomy. Radiographic studies should determine whether extension of the sphincterotomy will produce enlargement of the opening into the common bile duct. Extending the sphincterotomy beyond the dilated segment of the duct does not increase the diameter of the opening. If this ERS is the initial procedure, it usually is advisable to allow the stones to remain until the edema and reaction to the sphincterotomy have subsided. The patient is then reexamined in 5 to 14 days to determine whether the stones have passed. If the sphincterotomy is wide open and the patient has not had fever or shown an elevation of the white cell count, the authors' policy at this point is observation. If any of these factors is absent, a nasobiliary drain or a stent should be placed during the period of observation (141–144).

During the second examination, the operator may again consider extending the sphincterotomy and attempting extraction of the stones. If these maneuvers are unsuccessful, the operator should again reconsider the patient's risks for surgical intervention. In patients who are high surgical risks, it is probably appropriate to undertake a trial infusion of monooctanoate through a naso-biliary catheter, although the success rate with this procedure is probably less than 50% (145–148). Infusions of monooctanoate take 6 to 14 days, must be done on an inpatient basis and frequently cause epigastric distress and/or diarrhea.

SPECIAL PROBLEMS

There is an upper limit to the size of a stone that can be removed. The size limit varies with the anatomy of the patient, but for stones beyond 1½ cm in diameter, success rates begin to fall sharply. With current instrumentation, few stones having diameters greater than 2.5 cm can be safely removed by this technique. If methods for fragmenting stones become practical, this problem could be solved. It is the authors' belief that certain patients are not candidates for ERS. For example, the cholangiogram illustrated in Figure 7 shows the common bile duct passing almost directly through the duodenal wall. This intraduodenal segment would provide room for only a short sphincterotomy and would allow the removal of only small stones. Almost every experienced operator has seen certain patients whose anatomic structure was not amenable to the creation of a sphincterotomy of adequate length. It is possible that balloon dilators may be helpful in such patients for enlarging the sphincter to the point where the stones may be extracted. There is only preliminary experience with balloon dilatation of the sphincter (136). However, dilatation in dogs appears to have a permanent effect, with the ampulla remaining open for a number of weeks (149).

Periampullary diverticula (Fig. 19) were originally thought to represent a major hindrance to ERS. However, with increasing experience, it has been found that such diverticula often do not constitute a contraindication. However, in this situation, the papilla may be more difficult to locate and cannulate. Moreover, the sphincterotome must be oriented with greater care, and caution must be exercised to avoid inserting instruments into the tic. Concern had been expressed about the possibility of cutting through the wall of the common duct on the edge of a diverticulum but this complication has not been reported. Most patients with periampullary diverticula may be considered as candidates for ERS with the anticipation of a successful outcome.

The most common problems in ERS are failure to achieve free cannulation of the common bile duct and failure to insert the sphincterotome at the proper angle into the common bile duct. When the operator is having difficulty cannulating the common bile duct, the first step is to use a tapered cannula to outline a tract for the sphincterotome. Unsatisfactory orientation of the sphincterotome usually can be corrected by repositioning the instrument in the common bile duct or by using a different instrument. Only after prolonged efforts should the operator decide that precut or cutting into the common bile duct is indicated. In the authors' opinion, these procedures carry some risk for injury to the pancreatic duct and should be done only after the patient's risks for choledochoduodenostomy have been reevaluated.

Duodenotomy with or without sphincterotomy or choledochoduodenostomy makes ERS more difficult. The difficulty encountered in this situation probably is related to fibrosis, fixation and rotation of the duodenum as a result of mobilization of the duodenal loop during the exploratory procedure. The duodenotomy appears as a longitudinal fold that can easily be confused with the longitudinal fold of the papilla. Sutures may be seen that identify this fold as the duodenotomy. The papilla ordinarily is located on the opposite wall. Surgical sphincterotomy markedly alters anatomic structure. The orifice of the common bile duct is at the upper end, or at the apex of the sphincterotomy, and the pancreatic duct is at the lower end. Some patients with stenosis from previous sphincteroplasty present with evidence of obstruction. Since the surgical incision usually is carried to the cephalad end of the intramural segment, further extension by ERS usually is ill advised because no intramural portion of the duct remains uncut. The pancreatic duct sits on a flat surface of ductal mucosa near the previous papilla and may be difficult to locate.

Choledochoduodenostomy is performed by means of side-to-side anastomosis in the roof or just beyond the apex of the duodenal bulb. The area of the apex of the duodenal bulb is poorly visualized. In many instances, this procedure is better performed with an end-viewing gastroduodenoscope. The presence of air within the common bile duct after choledochoduodenostomy does not exclude the possibility of stones or stricturing. It may be necessary to occlude the stoma with a balloon to obtain a high-quality cholangiogram to rule out intraductal stones, particularly to exclude air as opposed to intraductal stones. The distal common bile duct is visualized by conventional cannulation of the papilla. There have been reports of patients with residual stones or debris in the distal limb of the choledochoduodenostomy, and in a few such patients, the stones or debris appeared to cause sepsis and cholangitis (sump syndrome) (150–155). Endoscopic retrograde sphincterotomy on the major papilla almost invariably relieves this symptom complex. Enlargement of the choledochoduodenostomy with a sphincterotome probably is dangerous because the area cannot be incised for a great distance without being outside the common duct. If the common duct is open to the papilla, it probably is more desirable to perform ERS on the normal papilla. Previous common duct exploration may rotate the duodenum up out of the right gutter. Simple cholecystectomy does not appreciably affect the anatomic structure of the duodenum.

Previous Billroth II anastomosis creates a major problem for the performance of ERCP and ERS. In patients who have a Billroth II anastomosis, the ampulla must be approached through the gastrojejunostomy from below. This approach reverses everything in the field of vision. The cannula and papillotome have a tendency to flex caudally, directing these instruments toward the duodenal wall. The operator is looking up at the papilla, which makes cannulation of the bile duct easier and the pancreatic duct more difficult to visualize. In such patients, the authors have found that a forward-viewing endoscope is useful for finding the papilla and cannulating the common bile duct. Occasionally, it is necessary to change to a side-viewing endoscope after the papilla has been identified. Reverse-cutting sphincterotomes that have been designed for use in such patients have not been useful in the authors' experience.

Surprisingly enough, ERS may be difficult to perform in patients with Billroth I gastrectomies. During this Billroth operation, most of the duodenal bulb usually is resected along with the antrum. There often is rotation between the duodenum and the stomach. In patients with this anastomosis, the papilla is located immediately beyond the stoma, which makes adequate positioning of an endoscope a difficult maneuver.

Abnormal clotting mechanisms also pose a problem. If administration of fresh-frozen plasma or specific clotting factors corrects the abnormal clotting mechanism, ERS probably can be done with only a slight increase in risk to the patient. The operator must remember that for several days, a raw area persists at the incision of the sphincterotomy, and abnormal clotting mechanisms should be corrected during this healing phase, which lasts 7 to 10 days.

RESULTS

Successful results are most often obtained when ERS is performed for removal of common duct stones. In this situation, the procedure is successful in 80% to 90% of patients (Table 2). Removal of stones at the initial procedure with a basket or balloon is accomplished in more than 50% of patients, and experience improves the success rate. In some patients, it is desirable to allow the stones to remain in the common duct in the hope that they will pass spontaneously. The common bile duct is free of stones in many patients when they return after 5 to 15 days for reexamination. If all the stones have not passed, extraction can be attempted with a basket or balloon, and the sphincterotomy may be extended.

A malignant lesion of the ampulla of Vater may be an indication for ERS. It should be noted that the complication rate is somewhat higher in patients with cancer; in the 1983 survey (19) noted previously, complications occurred in 12 of 88 patients with such lesions (Table 1). Endoscopic retrograde sphincterotomy is not a curative procedure, but it does relieve itching and pain. If the sphincterotomy is adequate, drainage may remain adequate for long periods.

In a survey of physicians who had performed ERS in the Unites States (19), 579 patients (slightly more than 10%) underwent the procedure because of papillary stenosis. This entity is difficult to define and is associated with a complication rate of 9%. If the condition is defined by the criteria of Geenen and colleagues (27,50,51), the diagnosis is probably accurate. However, if any of those criteria (i.e., biliary colic, recurrent cholestasis, dilatation of the bile

TABLE 2. Removal of Common Bile Duct Stones by
Endoscopic Retrograde Sphincterotomy, Survey of
75 U.S. Physicians (19)

	Number	Percent
Attempts	4815	
Successful	4426	90.0
Complications	312	6.5

TABLE 3. Complications of Endoscopic Retrograde Sphincterotomy

	Number of Patients	Complications	Mortality
Europe (Safrany) (101)	3618	7.0%	1.4% (1979)
United States (Geenen) (17)	1250	8.7%	1.4% (1980)
United Kingdom (Cotton) (29)	679	10.0%	1.2% (1980)
Total	5547	8.6%	1.4%

duct, delayed emptying of the common bile duct or elevated pressures) is eliminated, the diagnosis becomes increasingly less certain. In the authors' opinion, difficulty in cannulating the ampulla of Vater must not be considered evidence of papillary stenosis.

Table 3 shows the results of surveys that recorded complication rates ranging from 7% to 10%; definitions of complications may vary. Table 4 shows that the acute complication rate recorded in a recent U.S. survey was 6.7%. Reported complications included bleeding, panceatitis, perforation, cholangitis and entrapment of baskets. It should be noted that half of the fatalities were caused by bleeding. Common duct stones in patients with intact gallbladders represent a special problem. In 374 such patients, the complication rate was 8%; 75 (20%) of those patients underwent cholecystectomy. It is unclear in how many patients cholecystectomy was an elective procedure and in how many patients gallbladder disorders necessitated surgical intervention. Regardless of these uncertainties, only 20% of the 374 patients underwent gallbladder removal.

Late complications of ERS have not been completely defined, but such complications occur in approximately 1% of cases. A great concern of most investigators was that restenosis would be a common occurrence. In this series of 5790 patients, however, only 31 cases of restenosis were recorded. Stones can reform after adequate ERS, although this phenomenon is relatively rare. In this survey (19), stones reformed in only 31 patients in whom stricturing of the sphincterotomy had not occurred.

TABLE 4. Acute Complications of Endoscopic Retrograde Sphincterotomy (5790 cases in U.S. survey) (19)

	Number of Patients	Surgical Intervention	Death
Bleeding (nontransfused)	38	0	0
Bleeding (transfused)	85	18	11
Pancreatitis	122	5	6
Perforation	57	28	1
Cholangitis	78	26	2
Entrapped basket	13	9	2
Total	393 (6.7%)	86 (1.4%)	22 (0.4%)

TREATMENT OF COMPLICATIONS (156–165)

The bleeding that occurs after ERS usually can be managed by observation and/ or transfusion. Only 18 of the 122 patients with bleeding required surgical intervention; 11 of the 18 patients died. The surgical procedure that arrests such bleeding is difficult to perform. The bleeding site is difficult to locate, possibly being within the common bile duct or within the coagulated area of the sphincterotomy, which retains stitches poorly. A number of experienced European authors have recommended ligating the pancreaticoduodenal artery before undertaking a direct approach through a duodenotomy.

The pancreatitis that can develop after sphincterotomy is difficult to diagnose. Many patients with this complication have an elevated amylase level, and there may be abdominal pain from the gaseous distention that the procedure entails. If patients with pancreatitis have had cholangitis previously, they may have a residual elevation of the white cell count. A number of patients considered to have pancreatitis may have a confined perforation into the pancreatic bed. Most such patients can be adequately treated with antibiotics and conservative follow-up. If air is seen retroperitoneally, such patients probably should be observed and treated expectantly with nasogastric suction and antibiotics. Patients with free intraabdominal air probably should undergo an exploratory procedure. At the time of exploration, it usually is not advisable to make an extensive attempt to locate the perforation, which may be impossible to find. Drains should be placed around the duodenum and the lesser sac. Cholangitis is a complication that is becoming less frequent, and it can be prevented by placing a stent in the bile duct or by adding a nasobiliary catheter. When adequate sphincterotomy and drains are used, this complication should be a less common occurrence.

The complication of basket entrapment can be eliminated by using balloons to extract the stones or by being certain that the sphincterotomy is adequate to allow the passage of a basket with a trapped stone. If the recently developed lithotripsy device becomes practical, use of this device could eliminate the problem of large stones.

SUMMARY

In summary, endoscopic retrograde sphincterotomy is an evolving technique that shows promise for the nonoperative removal of common duct stones. It is a highly technical procedure with a low margin for error. However, when ERS is performed with great care, the complication rate remains at an acceptable level; mortality from ERS is considerably lower than it is with surgical removal of retained common duct stones. Two recent series (166,167) have shown a mortality of 3% to 4.5% with surgical removal of common duct stones. By contrast, the mortality reported with ERS is less than 1.5%. It would appear that ERS is the procedure of choice for removing common duct stones in patients in whom the gallbladder has previously been removed. It is an excellent form of management for acute suppurative cholangitis and gallstone pancreatitis. Its role in the management of malignant lesions of the ampulla of Vater and in common bile duct and papillary stenosis remains to be defined. The most effective therapy for patients with intact gallbladders is an issue that requires intense study. It appears that most patients do not have complications from the remaining cholelithiasis, and elective cholecystectomy may not be indicated.

REFERENCES

1. Doubilet M, Mulholland JH: Eight years study of pancreatitis and sphincterotomy. *J Am Med Ass* 160:521, 1956.

2. Bartlett MK, Nardi GL: Treatment of recurrent pancreatitis by transduodenal sphincterotomy and exploration of the pancreatic duct. *N Engl J Med* 262:643, 1960.

3. Moody FG, Berenson MM, McCloskey D: Transampullary septectomy for post-cholecystectomy pain. *Ann Surg* 186:415, 1977.

4. Nardi GL, Michelassi F, Zannini P: Transduodenal sphincteroplasty: 5-25 year follow-up of 89 patients. *Ann Surg* 198:453, 1983.

5. Siegel JH: Endoscopic papillotomy: Sphincterotomy or sphincteroplasty. *Am J Gastroenterol* 72:511, 1979.

6. Koch H, Classen M, Schaffner O, et al: Endoscopic papillotomy. Experimental studies and initial clinical experience. *Scand J Gastroenterol* 10:441, 1975.

7. Koch H, Rösch W, Schaffner O, et al: Endoscopic papillotomy. *Gastroenterology* 73:1393, 1977.

8. Kawai K, Akasaka Y, Murakami K, et al: Endoscopic sphincterotomy of the ampulla of Vater *Gastrointest Endosc* 20:148, 1974.

9. Seifert E, May B: Endoscopic papillotomy. *Acta Gastro-Enterol Belg* 40:31, 1977.

10. Cotton PB, Chapman M, Whiteside CG, et al: Duodenoscopic papillotomy and gallstone removal. *Br J Surg* 63:709, 1976.

11. Osnes M, Kahrs T: Endoscopic choledochoduodenostomy for choledocholithiasis through choledochoduodenal fistula. *Endoscopy* 9:162, 1977.

12. Rösch W, Koch H, Demling L: Manometry studies during ERCP and endoscopic papillotomy. *Endoscopy* 8:30, 1976.

13. Geenen JE, Hogan WJ, Shaffer RD, et al: Endoscopic electosurgical papillotomy and manometry in biliary tract disease. *J Am Med Ass* 237:2075, 1977.

14. Reiter JJ, Bayer HP, Mennicken L, et al: Results of endoscopic papillotomy: A collective experience from nine endoscopic centers in West Germany. *World J Surg* 2:505, 1978.

15. Classen M, Burmeister W, Hagenmüller F, et al: Long term examinations after endoscopic papillotomy (EPT). *Gastrointest Endosc* 25:37, 1979.

16. Cotton PB, Vallon AG: British experience with duodenoscopic sphincterotomy for removal of bile duct stones. *Br J Surg* 68:373, 1981.

17. Geenen JE, Vennes JA, Silvis SE: Resume of a seminar on endoscopic retrograde sphincterotomy (ERS). *Gastrointest Endosc* 27:31, 1981.

18. Nakajima M, Kizu M, Akasaka Y, et al: Five years experience of endoscopic sphincterotomy in Japan: A collective study from 25 centres. *Endoscopy* 11:138, 1979.

19. Vennes JA, Silvis SE: Survey of endoscopic retrograde sphincterotomy in the United States, in Classen M, Demling L. (eds): *Proceedings of the Tenth Anniversary of Sphincterotomy Conference*, Erlangen, West Germany (to be published).

20. Classen M, Safrany L: Endoscopic papillotomy and removal of gallstones. *Br Med J* 4:371, 1975.

21. Zimmon DS, Falkenstein DB, Kessler RE: Endoscopic papillotomy for choledocholithiasis. *N Engl J Med* 293:1181, 1975.

22. Seigert E: Endoscopic papillotomy and removal of gallstones. *Am J Gastroenterol* 69:154, 1978.

23. Safrany L: Duodenoscopic sphincterotomy and gallstone removal. *Gastroenterology* 72:338, 1977.

24. Siegel JH: Endoscopic papillotomy in the treatment of biliary tract disease: 258 procedures and results. *Dig Dis Sci* 26:1057, 1981.

25. Mee AS, Vallon AG, Croker JR, et al: Non-operative removal of bile duct stones by duodenoscopic sphincterotomy in the elderly. *Br Med J* 283:521, 1981.

26. Passi RB, Raval B: Endoscopic papillotomy. *Surgery* 92:581, 1982.

27. Geenen JE: New diagnostic and treatment modalities involving endoscopic retrograde cholangiopancreatography and esophagogastroduodenoscopy. *Scand J Gastroenterol Suppl* 77:93, 1982.

28. Siegel JH: Endoscopy and papillotomy in diseases of the biliary tract and pancreas. *J Clin Gastroenterol* 2:337, 1980.

29. Cotton PB: Nonoperative removal of bile duct stones by duodenoscopic sphincterotomy. *Br J Surg* 67:1, 1980.

30. Summerfield JA, Hunt RH, Lister AH, et al: Endoscopic sphincterotomy for bile duct stones. *Br J Radiol* 53:1041, 1980.

31. Rösch W, Riemann JR, Lux G, et al: Long-term follow-up after endoscopic sphincterotomy. *Endoscopy* 13:152, 1981.

32. Kozarek RA, Sanowski RA: Endoscopic papillotomy in the high-risk and aging patient with biliary tract disease. *J Clin Gastroenterol* 2:375, 1980.

33. Kozarek RA, Sanowski RA: Nonsurgical management of extrahepatic obstructive jaundice. *Ann Intern Med* 96:743, 1982.

34. Weitemeyer RA: Endoscopic sphincterotomy: A procedure of choice in the management of retained common bile duct stones and papillary stenosis. *Am J Surg* 143:536, 1982.

35. Safrany L, Cotton PB: Endoscopic management of choledocholithiasis. *Surg Clin North Am* 62:825, 1982.

36. Mazzeo RJ, Jordan FT, Strasius SR: Endoscopic papillotomy for recurrent common bile duct stones and papillary stenosis. A community hospital experience. *Arch Surg (Chicago)* 118:693, 1983.

37. Siegel JH, Yatto RP, Vender RJ: Anomalous pancreatic ducts causing "pseudo mass" of the pancreas. *J Clin Gastroenterol* 5:33, 1983.

38. Belber JP, Kazuko B: Fusion anomalies of the pancreatic ductal system: Differentiation from pathologic states. *Diagn Rad* 123:637, 1977.

39. Heiss FW, Shea JA: Association of pancreatitis and variant ductal anatomy. *Am J Gastroenterol* 70:158, 1978.

40. Rösch W, Koch H, Schaffner O, et al: The clinical significance of the pancreas divisum. *Gastrointest Endosc* 22:206, 1976.

41. Gregg JA: Pancreas divisum: Its association with pancreatitis. *Am J Surg* 134:539, 1977.

42. Cotton PB: Congenital anomaly of pancreas divisum as a cause of obstructive pain and pancreatitis. *Gut* 21:105, 1980.

43. Cremer M, Toussaint J, Dunhan F: Endoscopic management of chronic pancreatitis. *Gastrointest Endosc* 26:65, 1980.

44. Phillip J, Koch H, Classen M: Variations and anomalies of the papilla of Vater, the pancreas and the biliary duct system. *Endoscopy* 6:70, 1974.

45. Boyden EA: The sphincter of Oddi in man and certain representative mammals. *Surgery* 1:25, 1937.

46. Boyden EA: The anatomy of the choledochoduodenal junction in man. *Surg Gynecol Obstet* 104:641, 1957.

47. Ryan JP: Motility of the gallbladder and biliary tree, in Johnson LR (ed): *Physiology of the Gastrointestinal Tract*. New York, Raven Press, 1981, pp 473–494.

48. LoGiudice JA, Hogan WJ, Geenen JE, et al: Variations in propagation of phasic pressure waves in the human sphincter of Oddi. *Gastroenterology* 76:1187, 1979.

49. Riedel D, Geenen JE, Hogan WJ, et al: Endoscopic sphincterotomy: Follow-up evaluation of effects on sphincter of Oddi. *Gastrointest Endosc* 25:47, 1979.

50. Geenen JE, Hogan WJ, Dodds J, et al: Intraluminal pressure recording from the human sphincter of Oddi. *Gastroenterology* 78:317, 1980.

51. Bar-Meir S, Geenen JE, Hogan WJ, et al: Biliary and pancreatic duct pressures measured by ERCP manometry in patients with suspected papillary stenosis. *Dig Dis Sci* 24:209, 1979.

52. Carr-Locke DL, Gregg JA: Endoscopic manometry of pancreatic and biliary sphincter zones in man. *Dig Dis Sci* 26:7, 1981.

53. Scott GW, Smallwood RE, Rowlands S: Flow through the bile duct after cholecystectomy. *Surg Gynecol Obstet* 140:912, 1975.

54. Funch-Jensen P, Csendes A, Kruse A, et al: Common bile duct and Oddi sphincter pressure before and after endoscopic papillotomy in patients with common bile duct stones. *Ann Surg* 190:176, 1979.

55. Vennes JA: Technique of ERCP, in Stewart ET, Vennes JA, Geenen JE (eds): *Atlas of Endoscopic Retrograde Cholangiopancreatography*. St. Louis, Mosby, 1977, pp 4–18.

56. Silvis SE, Vennes JA: The role of glucagon in endoscopic pancreatography. *Gastrointest Endosc* 21:162, 1975.

57. Siegel JH, Yatto RP: ERCP and endoscopic papillotomy in patients with a Billroth II gastrectomy: Report of a method. *Gastrointest Endosc* 29:116, 1983.

58. Rosseland AR, Osnes M, Kruse A: Endoscopic sphincterotomy (EST) in patients with Billroth II gastrectomy. *Endoscopy* 13:19, 1981.

59. Safrany L, Neuhaus B, Portocarrero G, et al: Endoscopic sphincterotomy in patients with Billroth II gastrectomy. *Endoscopy* 12:16, 1980.

60. Urakami Y, Seki H, Kishi S: Endoscopic retrograde cholangiopancreatography after Billroth II operation and endoscopic sphincterotomy. *GEN* 30:251, 1976.

61. O'Connor KW, Lehman JA: Accessory papilla (AP) cannulation at ERP, aided by IV secretin and needle-tipped cannula. *Gastrointest Endosc* 29:172, 1983.

62. Urakami Y, Kishi S, Seifert E: Endoscopic papillotomy (EPT) in patients with juxtapapillary diverticula. *Gastrointest Endosc* 25:10, 1979.

63. Cattell RB, Warren KW: Surgery of the biliary tract. *N Engl J Med* 255:761, 1956.

64. Girard RM, Legros G: Retained and recurrent bile duct stones. Surgical or non-surgical removal? *Ann Surg* 193:150, 1981.

65. Riemann JF, Lux G, Rösch W, et al: Non-surgical biliary drainage: Technique, indications and results. *Endoscopy* 13:157, 1981.

66. Birkett DH, Williams LF Jr: Prevention and management of retained bile duct stones. *Surg Clin North Am* 61:939, 1981.

67. DenBesten L, Doty JE: Pathogenesis and management of choledocholithiasis. *Surg Clin North Am* 61:893, 1981.

68. Mazzariello RM: Residual biliary tract stones: Nonoperative treatment of 570 patients. *Surg Ann* 8:113, 1976.

69. Van Der Spuy S: Endoscopic sphincterotomy in the management of gallstone pancreatitis. *Endoscopy* 13:25, 1981.

70. Kelley TR, Swaney PE: Gallstone pancreatitis: The second time around. *Surgery* 92:571, 1982.

71. Thomas E, Reddy KR: Cholangitis and pancreatitis due to juxtapapillary duodenal diverticulum. Endoscopic sphincterotomy is the other alternative in selected cases. *Am J Gastroenterol* 77:303, 1982.

72. Jensen PB, Vallon AG: Hemobilia with jaundice: Treatment by endoscopic papillotomy. *Am J Gastroenterol* 77:162, 1982.

73. Safrany L, Cotton PB: A preliminary report: Urgent duodenoscopic sphincterotomy for acute gallstone pancreatitis. *Surgery* 89:424, 1981.

74. Tanker M, Sivak MV Jr: Endoscopic retrograde pancreatography (ERP) for acute recurrent pancreatitis (ARP). *Gastrointest Endosc* 28:154, 1982.

75. Hamilton I, Bradley P, Lintott DJ, et al: Endoscopic retrograde cholangio-pancreatography in the investigation and management of patients after acute pancreatitis. *Br J Surg* 69:504, 1982.

76. Zimmon DS, Falkenstein DB, Abrams RM, et al: ERCP in the diagnosis of pancreatic inflammatory disease. *Radiology* 113:287, 1974.

77. Urakami Y, Kitamura Y, Kishi S: Endoscopic papillotomy (EPT) for parapapillar choledochoduodenal fistula. *Gastrointest Endosc* 24:107, 1978.

78. Cotton PB, Beales JSM: Endoscopic pancreatography in management of relapsing acute pancreatitis. *Br Med J* 1:608, 1974.

79. Lam SK, Wong KP, Chan PKW, et al: Recurrent pyogenic cholangitis: A study of ERCP. Gastroenterology 74:1196, 1978.

80. Saharia PC, Cameron JC: Clinical management of acute cholangitis. *Surg Gynecol Obstet* 142:369, 1976.

81. Welch JP, Donaldson GA: The urgency of diagnosis and surgical treatment of acute suppurative cholangitis. *Am J Surg* 131:527, 1976.

82. Tanaka M, Ikeda S, Nakayama F: Nonoperative measurement of pancreatic and common bile duct pressures with a microtransducer catheter and effects of duodenoscopic sphincterotomy. *Dig Dis Sci* 26:245, 1981.

83. Grage TH, Lober P, Imamoglu K, et al: Stenosis of sphincter of Oddi: Clinicopathologic review of 50 cases. *Surgery* 48:304, 1960.

84. Siegel JH: Endoscopic management of choledocholithiasis and papillary stenosis. *Surg Gynecol Obstet* 148:747, 1979.

85. Csendes A, Kruse A, Funch-Jensen P, et al: Pressure measurements in the biliary and pancreatic duct systems in controls and in patients with gallstones, previous cholecystectomy, or common bile duct stones. *Gastroenterology* 77:1203, 1979.

86. Tanaka M, Ikeda S, Nakayama F: Continuous measurement of common bile duct pressure with an indwelling microtransducer catheter introduced by duodenoscopy: New diagnostic aid for postcholecystectomy dyskinesia. A preliminary report. *Gastrointest Endosc* 29:83, 1983.

87. Pace RF, Chamberlain MJ, Passi RB: Diagnosing papillary stenosis by technetium-99m HIDA scanning. *Can J Surg* 26:191, 1983.

88. Classen M: Endoscopic approach to papillary stenosis (PS). *Endoscopy* 13:154, 1981.

89. Guelrud M, Mendoza S, Vicent S, et al: Pressures in the sphincter of Oddi in patients with gallstones. *J Clin Gastroenterol* 5:37, 1983.

90. Toouli J, Geenen JE, Hogan WJ, et al: Sphincter of Oddi motor activity: A comparison between patients with common bile duct stones and controls. *Gastroenterology* 82:111, 1982.

91. Akasaka Y, Nakajima M, Kawai K: Electromyographic study of the postoperative function of duodenal papilla. Does the endoscopic sphincterotomy of the ampulla of Vater destroy the bile flow mechanism? *Am J Gastroenterol* 66:337, 1976.

92. Partington PF: Twenty-three years of experience with sphincterotomy and sphincteroplasty for stenosis of the sphincter of Oddi. *Surg Gynecol Obstet* 145:161, 1977.

93. Mirkin KR, Rosson R: Long-term palliation of ampullary carcinoma using endoscopic papillotomy. *Conn Med* 46:4, 1982.

94. Alderson D, Lavello M, Venaliles G: Endoscopic sphincterotomy before pancreatic duodenectomy for ampullary carcinoma. *Br Med J* 282:1109, 1981.

95. Rösch W: Endoscopic sphincterotomy in carcinoma of the ampulla of Vater. *Gastrointest Endosc* 28:203, 1982.

96. Mullens JE, Laufer I: Endoscopic retrograde cholangiopancreatography in the management of pancreatic and biliary disease. *Can J Surg* 19:405, 1976.

97. Soehendra N, Kempeneers I, Eichfuss HP, et al: Early post-operative endoscopy after biliary tract surgery. *Endoscopy* 13:113, 1981.

98. Meyhoff HH: Sphincterotomy treatment for biliary tract stones. A retrospective review. *Acta Chir Scand* 141:645, 1975.

99. Stout DJ, Sivak MV, Sullivan BH: Endoscopic sphincterotomy and removal of gallstones. *Surg Gynecol Obstet* 150:673, 1980.

100. Safrany L: Duodenoscopic sphincterotomy and gallstone removal. *Gastroenterology* 72:338, 1977.

101. Safrany L: Endoscopic treatment of biliary-tract diseases. An international study. *Lancet* 2:893, 1978.

102. Moss AA, Goldberg HI, Stewart ET: Radiographic technique, Stewart ET, Vennes JA, Geenen JE (eds): in *Atlas of Endoscopic Retrograde Cholangiopancreatography*. St. Louis, Mosby, 1977, pp 19–28.

103. Goldberg HI, Bilbao MK, Stewart ET, et al: Endoscopic retrograde cholangiopancreatography: Radiographic technique. *Am J Dig Dis* 21:270, 1976.

104. Varley TF, Rohrmann CA, Silvis SE, et al: The normal endoscopic pancreatogram. *Radiology* 118:295, 1976.

105. Rohrmann CA, Silvis SE, Vennes JA: The significance of pancreatic ductal obstruction in differential diagnosis of the abnormal endoscopic retrograde pancreatogram. *Radiology* 121:311, 1976.

106. Rohrmann CA, Ansel HJ, Ayoola EA, et al: Endoscopic retrograde intrahepatic cholangiogram: Radiographic findings in intrahepatic disease. *Am J Radiol* 128:45, 1977.

107. Lasser RB, Silvis SE, Vennes JA: The normal cholangiogram. *Am J Dig Dis* 23:586, 1978.

108. Cotton PB: The normal pancreatogram. *Endoscopy* 6:65, 1974.

109. Sivak MV, Sullivan BH: Endoscopic retrograde pancreatography. Analysis of the normal pancreatogram. *Am J Dig Dis* 21:203, 1976.

110. McLean AJ: The Bovie electrosurgical current generator. *Arch Surg (Chicago)* 18:1863, 1929.

111. McLean AJ: Characteristics of adequate electrosurgical current. *Am J Surg* 18:417, 1932.

112. Geddes LA, Silva LF, DeWitt DP, et al: What's new in electrosurgical instrumentation? *Med Instrum (Baltimore)* 11:355, 1977.

113. Editor, Electrosurgery, J. Operating Room Research Institute. vol I (4):10, vol I (5):30, vol I (6):21, August/September, October, November 1981.

114. Hudrlik TR, Silvis SE, Schmitt OH, et al: Further studies in the control of electrocoagulation (EC). *Gastrointest Endosc* 25:40, 1979.

115. Tucker RD, Hudrlik TR, Silvis SE, et al: Automated impedance: A case study in microprocessor programming. *Comput Biol Med* 11:153, 1981.

116. Tucker RD, Schmitt OH, Sievert CE, et al: Targets of convenience for computer automated measurements of electrical tissue impedance. *IEEE Spectrum* 82:1000, 1982.

117. Schmitt OH, Tucker RD, Sievert CE, et al: A miniature current probe for measuring electrosurgical currents. *Med Instrum (Baltimore)* 17:276, 1983.

118. Hungerbuhler RF, Swope JP, Reves JG: Ventricular fibrillation associated with use of electrocautery. *J Am Med Ass* 230:432, 1974.

119. Barlow DE: Endoscopic applications of electrosurgery: A view of basic principles. *Gastrointest Endosc* 28:73, 1982.

120. Geenen JE, Stewart ET: Endoscopic papillotomy, in Stewart ET, Vennes JA, Geneen JE (eds): *Atlas of Endoscopic Retrograde Cholangiopancreatography.* St. Louis, Mosby, 1977, pp 334–341.

121. Wurbs D: Endoscopic papillotomy. *Scand J Gastroenterol Suppl* 77:107, 1982.

122. Greenberg HM, Goldberg HI, Shapiro HA, et al: The importance of radiographic monitoring of endoscopic sphincterotomy. *Radiology* 141:295, 1981.

123. Safrany L, Neuhaus B: Intraduodenal manipulations of the common bile duct. *Surg Ann* 12:301, 1980.

124. Rosseland AR, Osnes M: Endoscopic papillotomy: Technique and experience with 204 patients. *Curr Surg* 37:152, 1980.

125. Siegel JH, Harding GT, Chateau F: Endoscopic incision of choledochal cysts (choledochocele). *Endoscopy* 13:200, 1981.

126. Siegel JH: Precut papillotomy: A method to improve success of ERCP and papillotomy. *Endoscopy* 12:130, 1980.

127. Wurbs D, Hagenmüller F, Classen M: Descending sphincterotomy of the papilla of Vater through a choledochoduodenostomy under endoscopic view. Another variant of endoscopic papillotomy (EPT). *Endoscopy* 12:38, 1980.

128. Weizel A, Stiehl, Raedsch R: Passage of a large bilirubin stone through a narrow papillotomy. *Endoscopy* 12:191, 1980.

129. Mason RR, Cotton PB: Combined duodenoscopic and transhepatic approach to stenosis of the papilla of Vater. *Br J Radiol* 54:678, 1981.

130. Mason RR, Cotton PB: Combined endoscopic and percutaneous transcystic approach to a retained common duct stone. *Br J Radiol* 53:38, 1980.

131. Wurbs D, Dammermann R, Ossenberg A, et al: Descending sphincterotomy of the papilla of Vater through the T-drain under endoscopic view. Variants of endoscopic papillotomy (EPT). *Endoscopy* 10:199, 1978.

132. Witzel L, Wolbergs E, Halter F: Removal of gallstones by a catheter loop after duodenoscopic sphincterotomy. *Lancet* 2:295, 1978.

133. Mason RR, Shorvon PJ, Cotton PB: Percutaneous descending biliary sphincterotomy with a choledochoscope passed through the cystic duct after cholecystostomy. *Br J Radiol* 55:595, 1982.

134. Siegel JH, Mayer LF: Percutaneous choledochoscopy and cholecystoscopy: Diagnostic and therapeutic uses. *Endoscopy* 13:124, 1981.

135. Thompson G, LeBrun PG, Fried L, et al: Radiologically assisted endoscopic papillotomy. *J Can Ass Radiol* 33:265, 1982.

136. Staritz M, Ewe K, Meyer zum Buschenfelde KH: Endoscopic papillary dilatation, a possible alternative to endoscopic papillotomy. *Lancet* 1:1306, 1982.

137. Riemann JF, Seuberth K, Demling L: Clinical application of a new mechanical lithotripter for smashing common bile duct stones. *Endoscopy* 14:226, 1982.

138. Koch H, Stolte M, Walz V: Endoscopic lithotripsy in the common bile duct. *Endoscopy* 9:95, 1977.

139. Koch H, Rösch W, Walz V: Endoscopic lithotripsy in the common bile duct. *Gastrointest Endosc* 26:16, 1980.

140. Orii K, Nakahara A, Takase Y, et al: Choledocholithotomy by YAG laser with a choledochofiberscope: Case reports of two patients. *Surgery* 90:120, 1981.

141. Wurbs D, Phillip J, Classen M: Experiences with the long standing nasobiliary tube in biliary diseases. *Endoscopy* 12:219, 1980.

142. Cotton PB, Burney PG, Mason RR: Transnasal bile duct catheterization after endoscopic sphincterotomy: Method for biliary drainage, perfusion, and sequential cholangiography. *Gut* 20:285, 1979.

143. Osnes M, Geiran O, Gronoeth K, et al: Nonoperative internal drainage of obstructive common bile ducts. *Arch Surg (Chicago)* 114:862, 1979.

144. Zimmon DS, Clemmet AR: Endoscopic stents and drains in the management of pancreatic and bile duct obstruction. *Surg Clin North Am* 62:87, 1982.

145. Witzel L, Wiederholt J, Wolbergs E: Dissolution of retained duct stones by perfusion with monoctanoin via a Teflon catheter introduced endoscopically. *Gastrointest Endosc* 27:63, 1981.

146. Venu RP, Geenen JE, Toouli J, et al: Gallstone dissolution using monooctanoin infusion through an endoscopically placed nasobiliary catheter. *Am J Gastroenterol* 77:227, 1982.

147. Gadacz TR: The effect of monooctanoin on retained common duct stones. *Surgery* 89:527, 1981.

148. Motson RW: Dissolution of common bile duct stones. *Br J Surg* 68:203, 1981.

149. Vennes JA, Silvis SE: Endoscopic retrograde balloon dilation. *Gastrointest Endosc* 28:149, 1982.

150. Barkin J, Silvis SE, Greenwald R: Endoscopic therapy of sump syndrome. *Dig Dis Sci* 25:597, 1980.

151. Siegel JH: Endoscopic management of the choledochocholecystoenterostomy sump syndrome. Definitive therapy for recurrent cholangitis. *Gastrointest Endosc* 26:77, 1980.

152. Siegel JH: Duodenoscopic sphincterotomy in the treatment of "sump" syndrome. *Dig Dis Sci* 26:922, 1981.

153. Siegel JH: Peroral choledochoscopy in the sump syndrome: Use of a thin caliber endoscope to negotiate a choledochoduodenostomy. *Gastrointest Endosc* 28:192, 1982.

154. Tanaka M, Ikeda S, Yoshimoto H: Endoscopic sphincterotomy for the treatment of biliary sump syndrome. *Surgery* 93:264, 1983.

155. Siegel JH: Biliary bezoar: The sump syndrome and choledochoenterostomy. *Endoscopy* 14:238, 1982.

156. Geenen JE: Endoscopic sphincterotomy: Indications and complications. *Postgrad Med* 70:235, 1981.

157. Neuhaus B, Safrany L: Complications of endoscopic sphincterotomy and their treatment. *Endoscopy* 13:197, 1981.

158. Sonnenshein M, Siegel JH, Rosenthal WS, et al: Recurrent choledocholithiasis following cholecystectomy, sphincterotomy and choledochoduodenostomy: Successful treatment with chenodeoxycholic acid. *Am J Med* 69:163, 1980.

159. Stout DJ, Sivak MV Jr, Sullivan BH Jr: Endoscopic sphincterotomy and removal of gallstones. *Surg Gynecol Obstet* 150:673, 1980.

160. Silvis SE, Nebel OT, Rogers G, et al: Endoscopic complications: Results of the 1974 American Society for Gastrointestinal Endoscopy survey. *J Am Med Ass* 235:928, 1976.

161. Vennes JA: Infectious complications of gastrointestinal endoscopy. *Dig Dis Sci* 26:60s, 1981.

162. Gerding D, Peterson L, Vennes JA: Cleaning and disinfection of fiberoptic endoscopes: Evaluation of glutaraldehyde exposure time and forced-air drying. *Gastroenterology* 83:613, 1982.

163. Meuwissen S, Maclaren DM: Disinfection of gastrointestinal fibre endoscopes. *Neth J Med* 26:23, 1983.

164. Friedman CJ, Leavell BS Jr, Adams K: A new complication of endoscopic papillotomy. *Gastrointest Endosc* 29:62, 1983.

165. Halter F, Bangerter U, Gigon JP, et al: Gallstones ileus after endoscopic sphincterotomy. *Endoscopy* 13:88, 1981.

166. Martin JK, Van Heerden JA: Surgery of the liver, biliary tract and pancreas. *Mayo Clin Proc* 55:333, 1980.

167. McSherry CK, Glenn F: The incidence and causes of death following sugery for non-malignant biliary tract disease. *Ann Surg* 191:271, 1980.

11

Endoscopic Decompression of the Biliary Tree

Jerome H. Siegel

Techniques for endoscopic decompression of the biliary tree were introduced a short time after endoscopic retrograde cholangiopancreatography (ERCP). This diagnostic technique became established as an integral modality in the management of diseases of the biliary tree and pancreas (1–8). The level of obstruction is identified by this endoscopic technique, and in many instances, the cause of jaundice may be partially eliminated through manipulative techniques during performance of the diagnostic procedure. The initial endoscopic technique for the management of stone disease was irrigation of the bile ducts, which was done in the hope that this procedure would wash out small stones and gravel (9). As experience with endoscopy increased, obstruction as a result of large stones, stenosis, inflammatory disease or tumor was successfully managed by use of the first therapeutic application of ERCP, sphincterotomy (papillotomy) (10–15).

The nomenclature for sphincterotomy has varied as efforts have been made to distinguish between surgical and endoscopic methods. To simplify this discussion, I will use the term *sphincterotomy* or *duodenoscopic sphincterotomy* to imply that the procedure is performed endoscopically.

Obstructive jaundice that results from stones in the common bile duct, with or without cholangitis and/or pancreatitis, is readily amenable to management with sphincterotomy (10–15). The first sphincterotomies, which were performed more than a decade ago, offered a nonsurgical alternative for the management of stones in the bile duct, stenosis and ampullary tumors. Reports presented at a recent symposium in Erlangen, West Germany have summarized worldwide experience with sphincterotomy. As of June 1983, there had been more than 20,000 attempts at duodenoscopic sphincterotomy (16). Complications associated with this procedure have occurred; however, as individual and cumulative experience has increased, the morbidity and mortality

241

associated with sphincterotomy have declined (15). In this discussion of endoscopic decompression of the bile duct to relieve obstruction, the role of duodenoscopic sphincterotomy will not be addressed. For the details of this technique as used in the management of specific obstructive diseases, the reader is referred to Chapter 10.

PERCUTANEOUS TECHNIQUES

Reports on decompression with percutaneous transhepatic cholangiography (PTC) appeared in the literature as early as 1978, providing an opportunity for radiologists and clinicians to participate for the first time in the management of obstruction due to malignant processes (17–21). This discussion will briefly describe decompression by means of PTC. Contraindications to PTC and decompression obviously include: lack of patient cooperation, sensitivity to iodinated contrast material, ascites and coagulopathy (8,17,20).

Percutaneous transhepatic cholangiography is performed as follows: The patient is positioned on an x-ray table that has fluoroscopic capabilities, anatomic landmarks are identified and marked for reference points, a "skinny" needle is inserted into the liver under fluoroscopic guidance and contrast material is injected as the needle is slowly withdrawn until the biliary tree has been opacified. The degree and level of obstruction are determined by this technique. After the biliary tree has been opacified, the skinny needle is removed. A larger needle (18 gauge, having a Teflon sheath) is then advanced into the liver and directed toward a large biliary radical. Once the needle has entered a large duct, it is removed; the catheter remains in place, providing access for passage of special guide wires that can be manipulated toward the obstruction. In most instances, the area of stricturing can be traversed by the guide wire, which can then enter the duodenum. An appropriate drainage catheter is advanced over the guide wire and placed into the duodenum. Occasionally, when the area of stricturing cannot be traversed, the catheter is left in place proximal to the obstruction to permit external drainage and decompression. If the narrowed area has been traversed and the distal end of the catheter is in the duodenum, the external connection of the catheter can be clamped to allow internal drainage and physiologic flow of bile. However, the external drain still protrudes from the lateral thoracic cage and may ultimately contribute to complications, including pneumothorax, infection, hemangioma or other vascular lesions of the liver (which have been responsible for bleeding episodes), peritoneal leaks and dislodgement of the drainage catheter (18–21). A permanent endoprosthesis, which lacks the external connection, has been developed and successfully placed (22,23). This endoprosthesis eliminates many complications attributed to the external drain but remains subject to occlusion by bile and sludge, which results in cholangitis and cholestasis. Access to the obstructed internal drain may be difficult, requiring a number of percutaneous punctures until the prosthesis can be irrigated or retrieved or irrigation or removal by means of an alternative endoscopic technique.

Success with immediate decompression and the results of long-term follow-up in patients treated in this manner have been good to excellent. Preoperative restoration of bile flow and/or replacement of needed electrolytes while obstruction is being relieved has been accomplished either in preparation for surgical intervention or in long-term palliation (18–21). In most reported series, long-term biliary tract decompression and drainage were provided for patients in whom surgical intervention had been contraindicated. The major shortcoming of this procedure is the placement of an external catheter, which requires care from the patient, the family or health personnel. The most common complaint of patients who have undergone the procedure is the extreme discomfort that is experienced during percutaneous manipulation and insertion of a drain. The persistent pain experienced by some patients after the procedure necessitates continuous management with analgesics.

There have been conflicting reports on the impact on operative morbidity and mortality of preoperative decompression for the management of obstructive jaundice (24–27). Initial uncontrolled, retrospective studies indicated that the frequency of postoperative complications was reduced if decompression was performed before surgical resection. The conclusion drawn from the initial studies was that reduction of the frequency of postoperative complications and improvement in the survival rate were due largely to restoration of physiologic bile flow and fluid and electrolyte balances and to improvement in nutritional status. A randomized study compared the complication and survival rates in patients in whom preoperative decompression was performed with the rates in patients in whom the procedure was not performed. No difference in complication or survival rate was found, and the authors concluded that preoperative decompression offered no advantage (28). It is necessary to reexamine the latter study and earlier reports to place them in proper perspective.

These reports analyzed the results obtained with the use of percutaneous techniques that incorporate external drainage, which eliminates the positive benefits of internal drainage, namely, restoration of fluid and electrolyte balances, enterohepatic circulation of bile salts and fluid volume of the bile. To date, no study has compared patients in whom internal drainage was provided by a percutaneous route with those in whom drainage was provided by a transpapillary endoscopic prosthesis. Cotton (personal communication) and his colleagues are currently studying this approach in a controlled manner. Cotton's group is undertaking a randomized trial to evaluate the relative benefits of decompression by use of percutaneous, endoscopic and surgical techniques in three respective patient groups. The results of this study should provide important findings relevant to the treatment of patients with biliary obstruction due to malignant processes.

Neff and associates (27), at Columbia Presbyterian Medical Center, were able to determine the prognostic implications of preoperative drainage by monitoring the decline in the serum level of bilirubin in three groups of patients. In the first group, the serum level of bilirubin had decreased to normal before surgical intervention, and the patients had an average postoperative survival of 198 days and a 30-day mortality of 10%. The second group of patients, in whom the bilirubin level had decreased by 50% before operation, survived 72 days and had a 30-day mortality of 33%. The third group of patients, in whom the bilirubin level had not decreased before operation, had a much shorter average survival, 12 days, and a much higher 30-day mortality, 88%. Regardless of the preoperative decline in the serum level of bilirubin, if hepatic metastases were present, the 30-day mortality was 47% for all groups. The latter data should serve as a criterion for selection of patients for surgical intervention.

Cooperman (29) has modified his indications for surgical intervention for the management of obstruction of malignant origin as a result of the report by Neff and associates (27) and subsequent experience. He attempts a definitive surgical procedure if the serum level of bilirubin returns to normal after preoperative drainage and if staging angiography indicates that resection is feasible. Only about 10% of patients with obstruction of malignant origin satisfy these criteria. Cooperman does not operate if the serum level of bilirubin does not decline when the drainage tube is patent. Instead, he continues long-term palliative drainage. This approach has avoided unwanted complications and has improved his overall operative success rate. However, surgical intervention is indicated when sepsis complicates biliary tract drainage or when obstruction of the gastric outlet occurs. This policy constitutes a logical approach for the management of biliary tract obstruction due to malignant processes.

ENDOSCOPIC TECHNIQUES

NASOBILIARY DRAINS

Shortly after the development of the percutaneous technique for biliary tract decompression, endoscopists in Europe and the United States submitted preliminary reports that described successful endoscopic decompression for the management of biliary tract obstruction (30–33). The initial reports described a technique in which nasobiliary catheters, or drains, are placed by use of an endoscope. The catheters are approximately 300 cm in length, a requirement for insertion through an endoscope and subsequent withdrawal of the endoscope over the catheter. The drains described in the initial reports were 5 French, leaving internal diameters of only 1.3 mm. Placement of the catheters provides not only drainage but also access to the biliary tree for repeat cholangiography, a distinct advantage for serial follow-up studies.

The nasobiliary drain is placed as follows: Once the endoscope is in place in the second portion of the duodenum, a cannula is selectively inserted through the papilla of Vater into the common bile duct. Contrast material is injected to define the level of osbstruction, the extent of obstruction and the degree of dilatation of the biliary tree proximal to the stricture. When the operator anticipates the need for placement of a prosthesis, he or she should prepare the accessory in advance. The tip of the cannula is dilated with an 18-gauge needle to accommodate the insertion of a guide wire. Standard, atraumatic guide wires are 0.035 inch in diameter. Dilatation of the tip allows immediate insertion of a guide wire when the diagnostic catheter is placed proximal to the site of obstruction and thus obviates exchange of catheters (i.e., removal of the diagnostic catheter and reinsertion of a larger one to accommodate the guide wire). In the author's experience, it is more difficult to negotiate a stricture a second and third time, and once a catheter has traversed a stricture, the operator should be prepared to place a more permanent drainage catheter.

With the guide wire inserted through the stricture and into the proximal portion of the biliary tree, the next step is to withdraw the diagnostic catheter over the wire as follows: The endoscopist carefully withdraws the catheter as the assistant continues to feed the guide wire. This maneuver is performed under fluoroscopic guidance to prevent dislodgement of the wire. After the diagnostic catheter has been removed, the nasobiliary catheter is placed onto the guide wire and advanced again under fluoroscopic guidance through the stricture and into the proximal portion of the biliary tree. At this point, the guide wire is carefully withdrawn to reform the pigtail but is withdrawn only into the endoscope, leaving the distal portion of the drain without the guide wire. Then, under fluoroscopic guidance, the nasobiliary tube is advanced through the endoscope channel while the endoscope is carefully withdrawn into the stomach, esophagus and oropharynx. With the guide wire still in place, the duodenal and gastric loops of the biliary drain can be adjusted. Once the position of the nasobiliary tube has been ascertained, the guide wire is removed.

Transferring the biliary tube from the oropharynx to the nose is performed in the following manner: A nasogastric tube or similar catheter is advanced through the nose and into the oropharynx, where it is visualized and grasped. This distal segment is pulled out of the mouth, leaving the proximal segment in place in the nose. The biliary tube is advanced through the distal portion of the catheter until it exits through the portion of the tube that remains in the nose. Once the nasobiliary drain has been passed through the larger tube, both it and the larger tube are grasped and withdrawn through the nose while the most distal portions of the tube in the bile duct, duodenum and stomach are carefully monitored. The tube in the oropharynx is held firmly by the endoscopist or assistant to maintain its position during withdrawal through the nose. This action prevents dislodgement of the drainage tube from the bile duct. The excess portion of the tube at the nose can be transected. After this maneuver has been done, a luer lock valve is attached, creating an adapter for an appropriate biliary tract drainage system.

Adequate decompression is provided even with the small catheter in the first 48 to 96 hours. However, after early decompression and subsequent reduction of back pressure, the flow rate begins to decline. A nasobiliary tube can remain in place indefinitely and provides continuous access to the biliary tree, obviating additional endoscopy. An estimation of the degree of decompression can

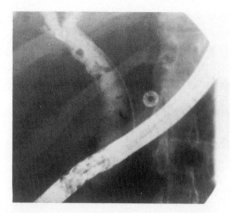 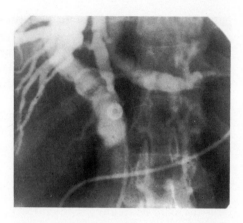

Fig. 1. A cholangiogram from a patient with cholangitis and obstructive jaundice shows a number of filling defects that represent calculi (*left*). A drainage catheter should be placed in this patient because stones remain in the duct after sphincterotomy and because the patient recently had cholangitis. A nasobiliary catheter is in place, and a subsequent cholangiogram obtained by injecting contrast material for follow-up study shows that the stones have passed spontaneously into the duodenum (*right*).

be ascertained in a serial manner by injecting contrast material and obtaining cholangiograms for comparison with previous studies (Fig. 1).

Nasobiliary drains provide initial decompression for the management of obstruction due to any cause, be it a stricture, a benign or malignant mass, or stones (30–33). Because access to the biliary tree is provided through this system, medication (monooctanoin or antibiotics), may be instilled to dissolve stones or to manage infection (Fig. 2) (32,34,35). If sphincterotomy has been performed and the stones have not passed, serial follow-up of stone dissolution or stone passage is effectively provided by this system.

The original configuration of the nasobiliary drain included a pigtail, or "C" form, at its distal end (Fig. 1). Subsequently, other configurations became available with the use of 5 or 7 French tubes. In another design, the pigtail has been eliminated; the anchor for this system conforms to the shape of the duodenal bulb (Fig. 3) (32). Therefore, the configuration of the catheter in the bile duct is straight and slightly tapered at the tip, and the catheter may be smooth or have side flaps to help anchor it. The loop-anchor conforms to the shape of the duodenal bulb to maintain its position. Larger tubing necessitates the use of an instrument having a larger channel, namely, a JF-1T (Olympus), a Duo XL (Fujinon) or an F32A (Pentax). This larger tubing not only provides an increased flow rate, which translates into an increased perfusion rate for therapy, but also helps prevent occlusion of the tubing by sludge and stone formation. Nasobiliary catheters are not difficult to place, provide drainage when needed and can prevent unnecessary complications (i.e., cholangitis) while providing continuous access to the biliary tree.

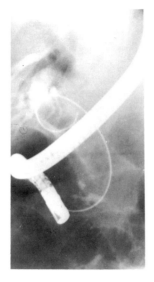 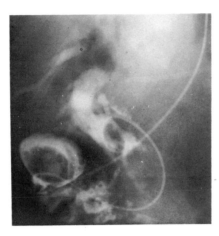

Fig. 2. A nasobiliary catheter is in place in an obstructed bile duct with the "C" loop catheter positioned above a large, radiolucent stone to provide drainage (*left*). A cholangiogram is readily obtained through a nasobiliary catheter to follow the course of perfusion therapy with monooctanoin (*right*). Frequently, radiographs of the common bile duct through such catheters are not of high enough quality to rule out small stones as opposed to air bubbles. Endoscopic retrograde cholangiopancreatography with balloon occlusion of the sphincterotomy may be necessary as a final procedure.

ENDOPROSTHESES

One of the most important advances in the field of endoscopic decompression has been the development and capability of placing biliary endoprostheses (32,33,36–38). The development of biliary endoprostheses and the subsequent availability of production model endoscopes with larger channels have enabled endoscopists to provide adequate preoperative drainage and long-term palliative decompression for the management of biliary tract obstruction. These endoprostheses have evolved from catheters with a single pigtail, used in initial applications, to catheters with a double pigtail and, finally, to the newest and most acceptable prosthesis, which is straight but which has side flaps that hold it permanently in the duct (Fig. 4, a and b). Recently, the latter configuration has been shown to decrease morbidity, maintain its position with infrequent dislodgement, provide maximal flow and decrease the risk for occlusion by sludge, stones or tumor (38).

The technique for insertion of an endoprosthesis is similar to that used for placement of a nasobiliary drain. An artist's diagram (Fig. 5) illustrates an obstructive lesion of the pancreas that is encroaching on the common bile duct. The initial endoscopic approach is to insert a diagnostic catheter selectively into the bile duct. It should be emphasized, again, that the operator must determine

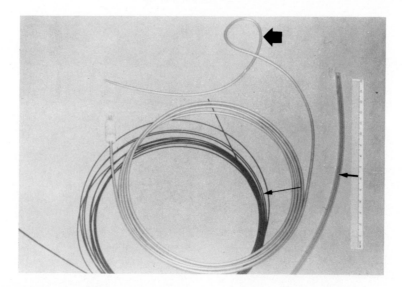

Fig. 3. This photograph shows a straight nasobiliary catheter (Wilson-Cook) with a duodenal loop configuration (large arrow). The catheter is continuous and has a luer lock adapter affixed to the proximal end to accommodate a syringe or perfusion system. The wire guide (long arrow) is included in the kit and a nasopharyngeal catheter (short arrow), is used to facilitate the transfer of the long catheter from the pharynx through the nose.

whether a guide wire can be easily passed through the distal tip of the dilated catheter; easy passage facilitates exchange of the catheter and wire, avoids delays and preserves the position of the instrument above a stricture. During the diagnostic portion of ERCP, contrast material is injected to define the level of obstruction and the degree of dilatation of the biliary tree proximal to the stricture. While the diagnostic catheter is being manipulated, an attempt is made to traverse the stricture with the catheter and, subsequently, with the guide wire. This maneuver facilitates exchange of the catheter and wire and the ultimate positioning and placement of the endoprosthesis. This technique usually is employed when small to medium-sized endoprostheses (5 to 8 French) are used. There is no evidence that sphincterotomy is a necessary prerequisite for placement of a small endoprosthesis. Certainly, however, sphincterotomy is helpful for insertion of large endoprostheses. There are three reasons for performing sphincterotomy before inserting large endoprostheses: to facilitate advancement of the accessory, to avoid occlusion of the pancreatic duct by the accessory and to provide access for two or more endoprostheses.

The difference between placement of an endoprosthesis and placement of a nasobiliary tube relates to differences in the configurations of the two devices. A nasobiliary tube is a continuous catheter, whereas an endoprosthesis is a prescribed length of tubing separate from the longer, pushing catheter. Because a nasobiliary tube is a continuous catheter, it can be pushed and withdrawn while it is being inserted through a stricture, wheras an endoprosthesis

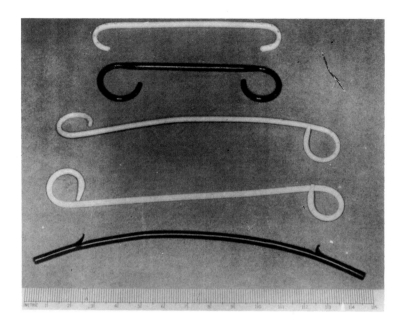

Fig. 4a. This photograph shows the configurations of different types of endoprostheses.

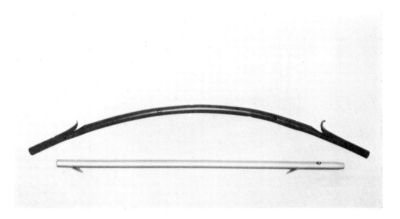

Fig. 4b. This photograph shows an Amsterdam Cotton-Leung 10 French prosthesis (*top*) and a Wilson-Cook 10 French prosthesis (*bottom*).

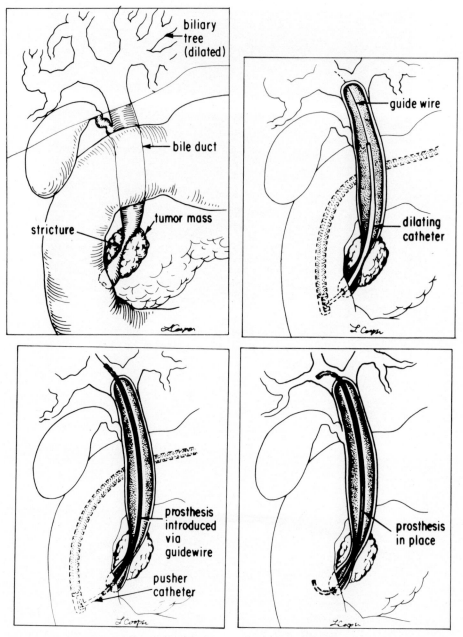

Fig. 5. The drawing at the upper left is an artist's conception of a pancreatic mass that is causing obstruction of the distal portion of the common bile duct and dilatation of the proximal portion of the biliary tree. In the upper right, an endoscopic guide wire and dilating catheter are shown being advanced through the stricture into the proximal portion of the biliary tree. The drawing at the lower left shows the prosthesis after it has been advanced through the stricture and placed above it. In the lower right, the prosthesis is shown placed correctly with its proximal portion beyond the stricture and its distal portion free in the duodenum. Reprinted from *Gastrointestinal Endoscopy* 30:21, 1984 (43), with permission.

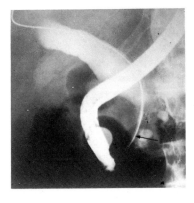 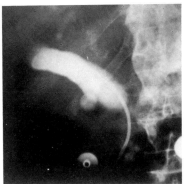

Fig. 6. The guide wire and dilating catheter (double line seen at the arrow in the distal portion of the common bile duct) have been passed through the stricture from the pancreatic mass (*left*). The prosthesis has been placed through the stricture to permit preoperative drainage (*right*).

is separate from the catheter and can only be pushed, not withdrawn. To make it possible to push an endoprosthesis through a stricture causing high-grade obstruction, the author has modified the technique of insertion in the following manner: Once the guide wire has been advanced into the proximal portion of the biliary tree and the diagnostic catheter has been withdrawn, dilating catheters are advanced in sequential order, from 5 to 10 French, over the guide wire (Fig. 6) (39). This maneuver enables the operator to prepare the stricture for insertion of an endoprosthesis and to calibrate the maximal diameter of an appropriate endoprosthesis. For example, in placing a 10 French endoprosthesis, a 10 French dilating catheter is used to calibrate and prepare the stricture before insertion.

Sphincterotomy is performed in the usual fashion after a diagnostic cholangiogram has been obtained to facilitate advancement of the endoprosthesis. No complication has resulted from this type of sphincterotomy because its length is limited to the length required for accommodation of the endoprosthesis. A special sphincterotome (American Endoscopy) is currently under investigation for use over a guide wire. As has been stated above, once the cannula and guide wire have traversed the stricture, the cannula can be removed and the sphincterotome can be advanced into position over the wire. After sphincterotomy has been performed, the sphincterotome is removed and the dilating catheter-endoprosthesis sequence can be performed without removing the wire.

After sphincterotomy has been performed, the guide wire, which is inside a smaller catheter, is inserted through the stricture into the proximal portion of the biliary tree, and dilating catheters of appropriate sizes are then advanced sequentially. Once the guide wire is in place and the smaller catheter has been removed, the endoprosthesis is advanced over it by use of a same-size pushing catheter, which is loaded next onto the wire. As the endoprosthesis is being advanced, resistance encountered by the wire is minimized by the assistant, who applies gentle traction on it. These maneuvers are all performed under fluoroscopic guidance to confirm the position of the wire and the endoprosthesis. Once the endoprosthesis has entered the papilla or sphincterotomy, it becomes even more essential that all subsequent manipulations be monitored to avoid displacement of the guide wire. The endoprosthesis and pushing catheter should be of different colors so that when the proximal end of the endoprosthesis is in the duodenum, the contrasting color of the pushing catheter can be recognized to assure accurate placement of the endoprosthesis. After the position of the endoprosthesis has been ascertained by endoscopic and fluoroscopic monitoring, the guide wire can be withdrawn. Separation of the endoprosthesis from the pushing catheter is visualized endoscopically. Although it is infrequently necessary to manipulate or adjust the endoprosthesis, fine-tuning adjustments can be accomplished while the endoscope is in place. By using a snare wire and advancing it through the endoscope into the duodenum, the endoprosthesis can be entrapped and advanced deeply into the bile duct or withdrawn to a more optimal level into the duodenum. The latter technique is used when an endoprosthesis is removed for the purpose of exchange.

In addition, sphincterotomy can be performed after a large endoprosthesis has been placed (Fig. 7, a to d). In this setting, sphincterotomy is performed by using a needle knife to cut down onto the accessory to prevent occlusion of the pancreas.

Since the introduction of endoscopes having large channels, large endoprostheses have become available, and these devices have provided more effective long-term decompression (38–44). Although many investigators agree that large endoprostheses are more effective than small ones, size as a measure of effectiveness continues to be a subject of controversy. Obviously, two or more endoprostheses having small diameters can be inserted to provide suitable drainage. In comparing large with small endoprostheses, one must refer to a principle of physics, Poiseuille's law, which states that the volume of fluid flowing through a tube is directly proportional to the drop in pressure along the length of the tube and to the fourth power of the radius of the tube. Therefore, under equal conditions, the rate of flow through a 10 French tube would be approximately 15 times the rate of flow through a 5 French tube. Certainly, in the author's experience, exchange of small catheters because of occlusion has been necessary more often than has exchange of large catheters, which rarely become occluded. In placing more than 200 large endoprostheses, the author has not had to replace any of them because of occlusion, and no fatal complications relating to the procedure have occurred (45).

An interesting study has been completed by Leung and colleagues (46) at the Middlesex Hospital in London. In a report to be published, these investigators measured the rates of flow of bile in tubes having different diameters and configurations. The flow of bile with gravity was measured in a 10 French straight catheter, which was used as the standard tube for the experiment. Subsequently, the experiment was repeated with 8 and 10 French catheters having the following configurations: single pigtail, double pigtail, straight, straight with slight distal tapering, straight with severe tapering and straight

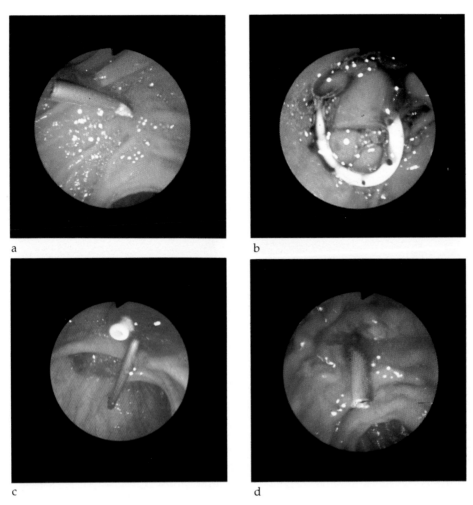

a

b

c

d

Fig. 7. (a) This endoscopic photograph shows a straight 10 French prosthesis protruding through an intact papilla into the duodenum. (b) A 10 French prosthesis is seen endoscopically with its pigtail in the duodenum. (c) A straight 10 French prosthesis is shown protruding through a short sphincterotomy (d). This endoscopic photograph shows two prostheses protruding through a sphincterotomy into the duodenum.

with formed configurations and side flaps. Leung and colleagues found that the rate of flow through straight catheters and straight catheters with slight tapering was nearly twice as fast as the rate of flow through catheters with pigtails. The formation of a pigtail requires tapering, and this conformity plus the angulation of a catheter having a pigtail reduced the rate of flow. For this reason, most investigators, including the author, use straight catheters when maximal long-term decompression is desired. On the basis of the above data and Poiseuille's law, effective long-term decompression will more likely be achieved when large, straight catheters are used.

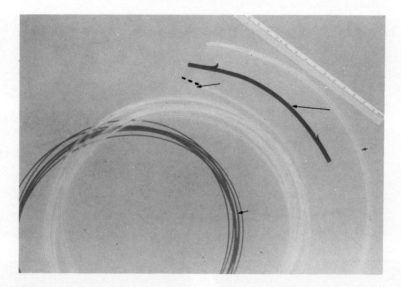

Fig. 8. This photograph shows an Amsterdam Cotton-Leung 10 French endoprosthesis kit (Wilson-Cook), including (a) an endoprosthesis (straight, dark catheter with flaps) and (b) a 6 French long, tapered catheter, which is placed over (c) the guide wire and into the proximal portion of the biliary tree. The endoprosthesis is advanced over the guide wire, and the 6 French catheter and is pushed into position with (d) the pushing catheter (clear, long catheter). Items a-d are identified by arrows of increasing length.

Large, straight catheters usually are easier to insert than are large, pigtail catheters and even small catheters. The reason for this greater ease of insertion will be evident as the procedure is described. Figure 8 is a photograph of a large endoprosthesis-catheter set. When such a large endoprosthesis is to be placed, sphincterotomy usually is performed. Once the guide wire has been inserted through the stricture and positioned in the proximal portion of the bile duct, a 6 French catheter is advanced over the wire. The Teflon-sheathed catheter serves to fill the empty space created in the large lumen of a 10 French catheter. When an attempt is made to advance a 10 French endoprosthesis over the wire, friction is created within the space, making it more difficult to advance the endoprosthesis. Filling the void with a 6 French catheter reduces the friction, facilitating advancement. If the wire should dislodge when the endoprosthesis is being advanced, the 6 French catheter is maintained in the proximal portion of the biliary tree to provide access for reintroduction of the wire. Once the prosthesis is in place, the wire and 6 French catheter are withdrawn and the pushing catheter is separated from the endoprosthesis.

Even though 10 French catheters are the largest catheters that can be advanced through an endoscope, endoscopists are not prohibited from inserting two endoprostheses of that diameter or smaller. Figure 9 illustrates placement of a 10 French catheter into the right hepatic system and subsequent placement of an 8 French endoprosthesis into the left hepatic system slightly proximal to

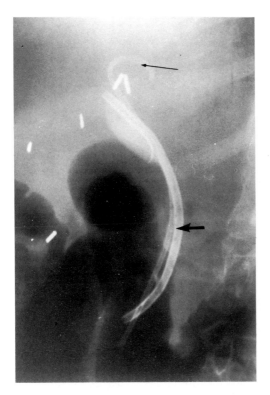

Fig. 9. A 10 French endoprosthesis is shown in the right hepatic system (short arrow), and an 8 French endoprosthesis is shown in the left hepatic system (long arrow). Both catheters have traversed a stricture of the common hepatic duct. The 8 French catheter was placed first because of persistent jaundice and sepsis.

the first catheter to permit drainage. In this instance, there was incomplete drainage of both hepatic systems due to an obstructing lesion at the bifurcation, which necessitated placement of a catheter in each system (Fig. 9).

The availability of endoscopes having large channels has permitted insertion of large endoprostheses, which have provided endoscopists with a potential for therapeutic success equivalent to that provided by percutaneous techniques and even surgical intervention (Fig. 10).

In the author's experience, the rate of successful drainage with adequately placed endoprostheses has exceeded 90% (success in 307 of 337 attempts). The 337 attempts have included 18 for benign disease, 76 for stone disease and 243 for obstruction of malignant origin.

Serial blood studies usually are performed after placement of large endoprostheses to follow up a patient's progress and to monitor the effectiveness of decompression. Although the serum level of bilirubin usually declines by a mean of 2 to 3 mg/dl per day, it is not unusual to observe a 50% drop in the bilirubin level in 24 hours (45). The bilirubin level continues to decline progressively until it is nearly normal; however, in some patients, the bilirubin

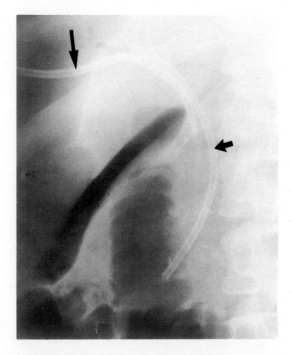

Fig. 10. A 10 French endoprosthesis has been placed through a stricture caused by a pancreatic carcinoma (short arrow). A percutaneous prosthesis (long arrow) had been in place for 2 months, but it caused persistent pain and recurrent episodes of cholangitis and was removed after the endoprosthesis had been placed.

plateaus at a higher level and does not decline further. This observation can be disconcerting to clinicians, but in patients with long-standing obstruction and liver disease or metastases, the bilirubin level never reaches normal.

The patency of an endoprosthesis can be assessed by means of radionuclide scans or "second-look" ERCP. It is less expensive to assess patency with radionuclide scans; if the radioisotope exits into the duodenum in a normal time frame, the hyperbilirubinemia is probably intrahepatic in origin. Therefore, no further manipulation is deemed necessary. However, if the radioisotope does not clear the bile duct normally, second-look ERCP is justified. At the second look, the large endoprosthesis is cannulated deeply with a standard or tapered cannula, and contrast material is injected. If part of the biliary tree is not opacified, a second endoprosthesis should be inserted because this finding indicates continued mechanical obstruction. The endoscopist should then attempt to cannulate the obstructed ductal system selectively by placing an endoprosthesis that is the appropriate size for traversing the one in place as well as the stricture. Here again, calibration is facilitated by using dilating catheters of the same size as the endoprosthesis that is being placed.

It must be kept in mind that regional and metastatic spread of a malignant lesion is responsible for continued cholestasis, and further prudent management is recommended in this setting. If the endoprostheses are patent and there is no other complicating condition, such as sepsis, further management is unnecessary. Too often, patients are subjected to needless additional procedures, such as attempts to decompress percutaneously or surgically. To reiterate, if the liver is infiltrated, further maneuvers are useless.

Other less reliable measures for following up such patients are the serum levels of alkaline phosphatase and gamma-glutamyl transpeptidase. In general, the serum levels of these enzymes decline at a slower rate than does the bilirubin level, which decreases by 30% to 70% on the average without reaching normal. Persistent cholestasis may be accounted for by long-standing obstruction, intrinsic liver disease, intrahepatic spread of tumor, a compromised nutritional status or, possibly, bone disease. Endoscopists should not intervene unless cholestasis is accompanied by hyperbilirubinemia and/or sepsis and unless the patency of the prosthesis(es) has been assessed by radionuclide scans.

Perhaps the most dramatic observation made in the follow-up of patients in this series was the mean survival of patients with obstruction of malignant origin. The mean survival of such patients was 108 days (range, 2 days to 2½ years). The relative success that these results reflect is manifest when the mean survival of such patients is compared with the mean survival of patients with carcinoma of the pancreas, which is only 2½ months; longer mean survivals have been reported for patients with ampullary lesions and cholangiocarcinoma who were poor surgical risks. Survival in the surgical series quoted by Cooperman (29) appears to be essentially the same. Considering the additional costs of hospitalization, ancillary care and postoperative convalescence, there is little doubt that nonsurgical techniques are cost effective.

ENDOSCOPIC-FLUOROSCOPIC TRANSPAPILLARY INSERTION OF A 15 FRENCH PROSTHESIS

The author has used a system from West Germany (MTW, Buderich) (47) that permits insertion of a 15 French endoprosthesis (Fig. 11) (42–45,48). The technique involves use of an endoscope with a 2.8-mm channel. After the endoscopist has obtained a cholangiogram that demonstrates a stricture (Fig. 12), he or she inserts a special guide wire that can be manipulated to angulate its distal tip; this wire provides an anchor for the system in the proximal portion of the biliary tree. Once this special guide wire is in the proximal portion of the biliary tree, the endoscope is carefully withdrawn over the wire under fluoroscopic guidance. The 15 French endoprosthesis is advanced over the guide wire, and the pushing catheter is then placed into position (Fig. 12). When the proximal end of the guide wire is free, a handle is attached and the internal wire is clamped onto it. The handle is tightened while the distal end of the guide wire is being monitored under fluoroscopic guidance. After the guide wire has been secured in the proximal portion of the biliary tree, it can be held firmly to

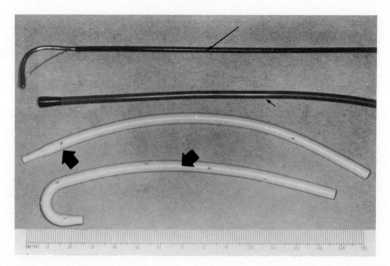

Fig. 11. These 15 French endoprostheses (large arrows; MTW, Buderich, West Germany) are inserted over a special guide wire (long arrow) and pushed with a catheter (short arrow) while tension is applied to the guide wire. For details of the technique of insertion, the reader is referred to the text. Reprinted from the *Am J Gastroenterol* 79:463, 1984 (48), with permission.

provide tension for advancement of the endoprosthesis. While the endoscopist maintains tension on the guide wire, he or she advances the endoprosthesis into position, releases the tension on the distal tip of the guide wire, firmly holds the pushing catheter in position, withdraws the internal guide wire to separate the endoprosthesis and then removes the pushing catheter.

A 15 French endoprosthesis is less likely to occlude, and use of such a large endoprosthesis has not been associated with the complications attendant with small ones. Neither bowel perforation nor catheter occlusion has occurred. Use of a 15 French endoprosthesis is suggested for long-term palliation in patients with obstruction of neoplastic origin (i.e., cholangiocarcinoma or ampullary carcinoma) and in those with obstruction due to benign processes that are not amenable to surgical intervention (stricture of the biliary tree and enterobiliary anastomosis). For decompression of obstruction due to carcinoma of the pancreas, the author prefers to use a 10 or 15 French drain. The 10 French drains have performed well in patients with cancer of the pancreas, and occlusion of these drains has not occurred during the short time that such patients survive. The author believes that one method for preventing occlusion of endoprostheses, large and small, is to administer chenodeoxycholic acid in therapeutic doses to prevent sludge and stone formation. A study is currently under way to evaluate the effectiveness of chenodeoxycholic acid, and longer functioning of the endoprostheses is an expected result of such therapy.

The development of catheters made of materials that help prevent adherence of bile is under consideration. These materials become slippery when set, which may prevent or retard adherence of bile and, therefore, occlusion. The author awaits the availability and use of such catheters.

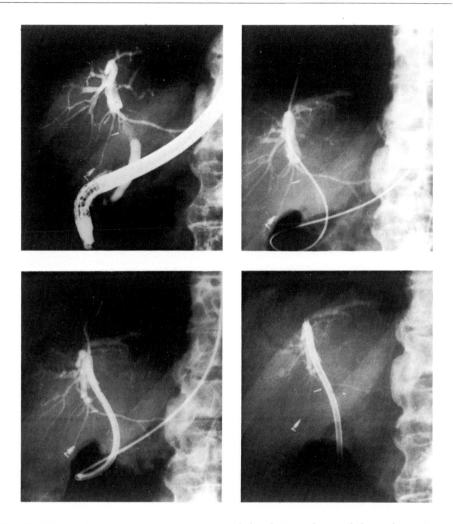

Fig. 12. The cholangiogram at the upper left shows a stricture in the common hepatic duct typical of cholangiocarcinoma. In the upper right, a special guide wire is shown after it has been advanced through a stricture and the endoscope removed. The endoprosthesis at the lower left is being advanced through a stricture over a guide wire by use of a pushing catheter. A 15 French endoprosthesis is shown in place at the lower right. This endoprosthesis was placed for long-term drainage in a patient with intense itching.

BALLOON DILATATION

Catheters similar to angioplastic balloon catheters have been modified for use in the biliary tree and pancreas (49–51). The balloons are made of durable polyethylene (Fig. 13) and are available in 4- and 6-mm diameters for use in endoscopes that have a 2.8-mm channel. A larger balloon, which inflates to 8

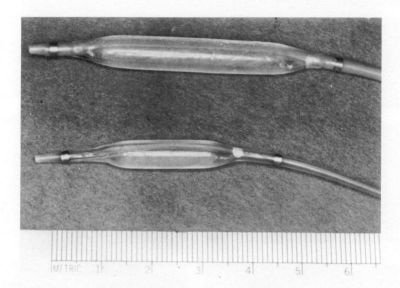

Fig. 13. These endoscopic balloons (upper, 3 cm in length, 8 mm in diameter) (lower, 2 cm in length, 6 mm in diameter) can be inflated under high pressure when they are placed across a stricture.

mm, can be used only with instruments having large channels, such as the Olympus JF-1T 3.7 mm channel. The indications for balloon dilatation include stricture of either ductal system or a hypertensive sphincter when it is the cause of recurrent symptoms. Examples of the versatility of balloon catheters have been reported, and the author has acquired extensive experience in this area treating a number of problems.

Posttraumatic and postoperative strictures of the bile duct can be alleviated by balloon dilatation. The technique is similar to that used for other manipulative procedures and is performed in the following manner: after the stricture has been demonstrated, a catheter and guide wire are advanced through the stricture into the proximal portion of the ductal system. The catheter is removed over the guide wire, and the balloon catheter is advanced into the stricture. The balloon is inflated to its maximal diameter with an equal mixture of 60% diatrizoate meglumine (Renografin) and saline so that the inflated balloon can be monitored under fluoroscopic guidance. The balloon is then deflated and removed. The fluoroscope monitor is viewed intermittently to observe drainage of the ductal system. Strictures of malignant origin can be dilated in this manner, as can strictures proximal to a sphincterotomy, preventing the removal or passage of retained stones (Fig. 14).

Recurrent cholangitis following choledochoduodenostomy may be a result of stenosis of the enterostomy. On several occasions, the author has had an opportunity to dilate an enterostomy and/or proximal or distal limbs involved

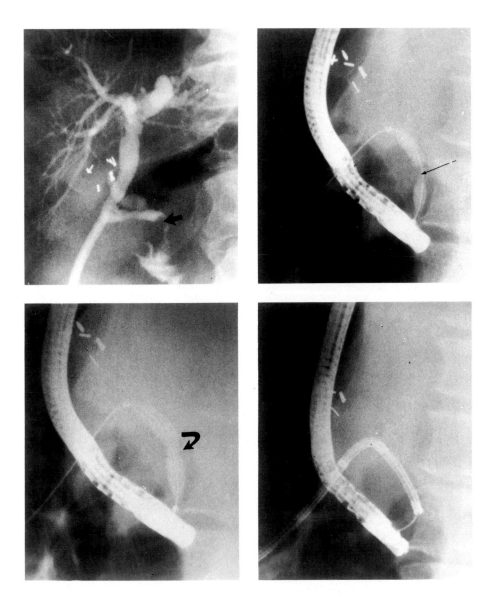

Fig. 14. The T-tube cholangiogram at the upper left shows a stricture of the distal portion of the common bile duct. The radiolucent area proximal to the stricture represents a stone (short arrow). At the upper right, ERCP and sphincterotomy have been performed. The T-tube has been removed, and a guide wire passed through the sphincterotomy; the stricture and the T-tube tract to the skin are seen (large arrow). A balloon catheter has been passed over the guide wire through the tract into the stricture (long arrow); inflation has been started. At the lower left, the balloon is shown nearly fully inflated, and narrowing at the stricture is decreased (arrow). At the lower right, the choledochoscope has been passed over the guide wire and through the T-tube tract to push the stone through the dilated distal portion of the common bile duct and into the duodenum. Extraction of the stone through the T-tube tract had been attempted previously, but that attempt had been unsuccessful, probably because of angulation to the common bile duct and the T-tube tract.

261

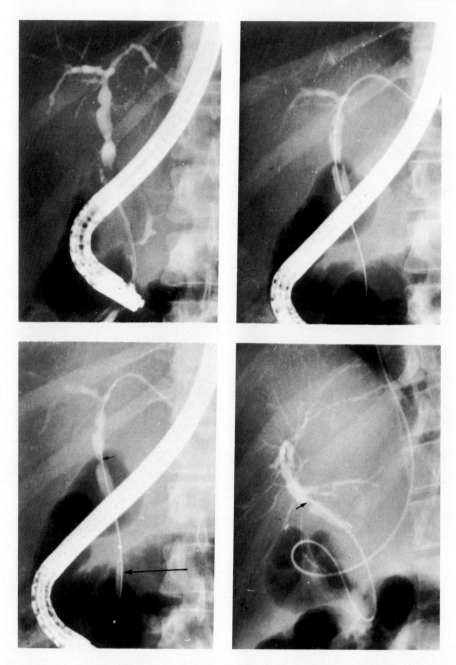

Fig. 15. The cholangiopancreatogram at the upper left shows slcerosing cholangitis involving the intrahepatic and extrahepatic systems. At the upper right, the guide wire and balloon are seen through a stricture in the common hepatic duct. The balloon is inflated. Because the balloon was small, it had a minimal effect on the stricture (arrow). At the lower left, the balloon is shown after it was pulled back to dilate the sphincter of Oddi (long arrow). At the lower right, a nasobiliary tube is shown after it was placed and a cholangiogram obtained. The stricture is essentially unchanged (arrow).

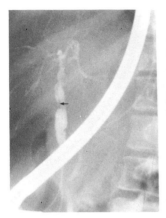 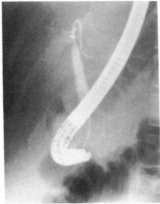 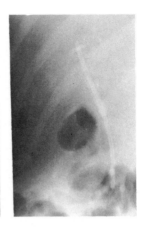

Fig. 16. This is the same patient as Figure 15. The nasobiliary tube is in place and ERCP is performed (*left*); a marked stricture (arrow) is again seen. A larger balloon was used to dilate the stricture of the common bile duct (*middle*). Because of continued uncertainty if the stricture was adequately dilated, an 8 French endo- prosthesis was placed in the proximal portion of the biliary tree (*right*). It is not known whether the primary difficulty with sclerosing cholangitis is stricturing of the large ducts or inflammatory disease of the small ducts. Further follow-up is needed to determine whether the dilated stricture will remain patent.

in the stenosing process. Use of balloon catheters in this clinical situation is safe and effective. The duration of the effect is not known.

Medical management of sclerosing cholangitis has been ineffective, and other forms of management are currently under investigation by the author. Guide wires can be advanced through tight strictures and balloon dilatation performed in an attempt to achieve mechanical palliation in patients with this disabling disorder. To date, balloon dilatation (Figs. 15 and 16) has been performed in eight patients, with encouraging results. In four patients, treatment has involved placement of nasobiliary tubes to provide access for continuous perfusion with medication (35). This protocol involves intermittent injection of antibiotics and saline for 8 to 12 weeks after continuous perfusion, which is initiated during hospitalization with an I-Med controller. Ultimately, the nasobiliary tube is removed and exchanged for a permanent 7 or 8 French endoprosthesis (Fig. 16). All patients have so far shown biochemical and clinical improvement with this regimen, and it is hoped that this improvement will continue throughout a long period of follow-up.

The author is currently managing strictures of the biliary tree of benign origin with catheter and balloon dilatation and insertion of endoprostheses (Figs. 17a and 17b). No complications have occurred, and the results have been encouraging. The catheters have remained patent, and cholangitis has not occurred. Endoprostheses have been placed in 76 patients with stone disease and in 18 patients with strictures due to benign processes. Chenodeoxycholic acid has been administered in three patients to prevent occlusion. All patients have been instructed to report signs or symptoms in an effort to prevent serious complications. To date, only one patient with benign disease, sclerosing cholangitis, has reported pain with cholestasis.

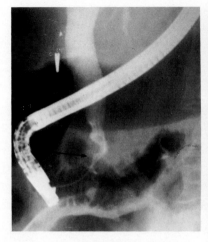 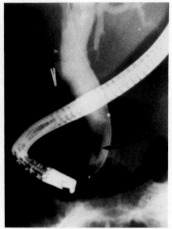

Fig. 17a. A cholangiopancreatogram (*left*) shows a stricture (long arrow) of the distal portion of the common bile duct with proximal dilatation after surgical sphincteroplasty. A large biliary balloon (*right*) was used to dilate the stricture (short arrow).

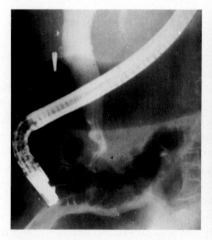 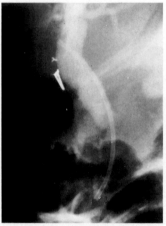

Fig. 17b. A cholangiogram (*left*) shows the stricture in Figure 17a. There is little, if any, increase in the narrowing (arrow). For this reason, a 10 French endoprosthesis was inserted (*right*). This elderly, high-risk patient has been maintained on endoprosthesis drainage for 1 year. A good-risk patient probably should undergo repeat dilatation or surgical therapy for strictures.

Endoprostheses have been used for the long-term management of retained stones (52). In situations where stones remain in the common bile duct after sphincterotomy, endoprostheses can be placed to prevent recurrent obstruction and cholangitis. In most cases, the endoprostheses have been placed permanently, remaining in place for 2 to 38 months, and the patients have been free of signs or symptoms. Three patients who were candidates for surgical intervention ultimately underwent common duct exploration and the stones were removed. At the time of this writing, 36 patients with endoprostheses are being followed. Although endoprostheses eventually occlude, cholestasis has not occurred because bile flows around them and through the patent sphincterotomies.

CONCLUSION

The impact of endoscopic transpapillary and percutaneous drainage techniques on the management of biliary tract obstruction is continuing to develop. As skilled endoscopists and radiologists become adept at performing these procedures, they will be done more successfully and frequently. They may reduce the costs of health care delivery. This point is well taken, considering that fewer than 10% of patients with carcinoma of the pancreas are considered candidates for surgical resection and that the 2-year survival rate is nearly zero. It has not been determined whether drainage of the biliary system improves either the length or quality of survival of patients with carcinoma of the pancreas. If studies of patient comfort and/or survival show improvement, our thrusts should continue in the present directions. Obviously, prevention, earlier detection and cure should be the highest priorities. The role of endoscopy in this setting and the future of endoscopy assure that interesting developments will take place.

REFERENCES

1. Oi I: Fiber duodenoscopy and endoscopic pancreaticocholangiography. *Gastrointest Endosc* 17:59–62, 1970.
2. Cotton PB: Cannulation of the papilla of Vater by endoscopic retrograde cholangiopancreatography (ERCP). *Gut* 13:1014–1025, 1972.
3. Dickinson PB, Belsito AA, Cramer GG: Diagnostic value of endoscopic cholangiopancreatography. *J Am Med Ass* 225:994–998, 1973.
4. Silvis SE, Rohrmann CA, Vennes JA: Diagnostic accuracy of endoscopic retrograde cholangiopancreatography in hepatic, biliary and pancreatic malignancy. *Ann Intern Med* 84:438–440, 1976.

5. Sivak MV, Sullivan BH: Endoscopic retrograde cholangiopancreatography. Analysis of the normal pancreatogram. *Am J Dig Dis* 21:263–269, 1976.

6. Cotton PB: Progress report, ERCP. *Gut* 18:316–341, 1977.

7. Stewart ET, Vennes JA, Geenen JE (eds): *Atlas of Endoscopic Retrograde Cholangiopancreatography*. St. Louis, Mosby, 1977.

8. Siegel JH: ERCP update: Diagnostic and therapeutic applications. *Gastrointest Radiol* 3:311–318, 1978.

9. Zimmon DS, Falkenstein DB, Kessler RE: Endoscopic papillotomy for choledocholithiasis. *N Engl J Med* 293:1181–1182, 1975.

10. Kawai K, Akasaka Y, Murakami K, et al: Endoscopic sphincterotomy of the ampulla of Vater. *Gastrointest Endosc* 20:148–151, 1974.

11. Classen M, Safrany L: Endoscopic papillotomy and removal of gallstones. *Br Med J* 4:371–374, 1975.

12. Safrany L: Duodenoscopic sphincterotomy and gallstone removal. *Gastroenterology* 72:338–343, 1977.

13. Geenen JE, Hogan J, Shaffer RD, et al: Endoscopic electrosurgical papillotomy and manometry in biliary tract disease. *J Am Med Ass* 237:2075–2078, 1977.

14. Siegel JH: Endoscopic management of choledocholithiasis and papillary stenosis. *Surg Gynecol Obstet* 148:747–752, 1979.

15. Siegel JH: Endoscopic papillotomy in the treatment of biliary tract disease: 258 procedures and results. *Dig Dis Sci* 26:1057–1064, 1981.

16. Classen M, Demling L: Endoscopic papillotomy now 10 years old, in *Proceedings of the Tenth Anniversary of Sphincterotomy Conference*, Erlangen, West Germany (To be published).

17. Okuda K, Tanikawa K, Emura T, et al: Nonsurgical percutaneous transhepatic cholangiography—Diagnostic significance in medical problems of the liver. *Am J Dig Dis* 19:21–36, 1974.

18. Nakayama T, Ikeda A, Okuda K: Percutaneous transhepatic drainage of the biliary tract: Technique and results in 104 cases. *Gastroenterology* 74:554–559, 1978.

19. Gold RP, Casavella WJ, Stern G, et al: Transhepatic cholangiography: The radiological method of choice in suspected obstructive jaundice. *Radiology* 133:39–44, 1979.

20. Kreek MJ, Balint JA: Skinny needle cholangiography. *Gastroenterology* 78:598–604, 1980.

21. Ring EJ, Oleaga JA, Feinman DB, et al: Therapeutic application of catheter cholangiography. *Radiology* 128:333–338, 1978.

22. Perieras RV Jr, Rheingold OJ, Hutson D, et al: Relief of malignant obstructive jaundice by percutaneous insertion of a permanent prosthesis in the biliary tree. *Ann Intern Med* 89:589–593, 1978.

23. Burchanth F: A new endoprosthesis for non-operative intubation of the biliary tract in malignant obstructive jaundice. *Surg Gynecol Obstet* 146:76–78, 1978.

24. Denning DA, Ellison EC, Carey LC: Preoperative percutaneous transhepatic decompression lowers operative morbidity in patients with obstructive jaundice. *Am J Surg* 141:61–65, 1981.

25. Wittenstein BH, Giacchino JL, Pickleman JR, et al: Obstructive jaundice: The necessity for improved management. *Am Surg* 47:116–120, 1981.

26. Pollock TW, Ring ER, Oleaga JA, et al: Percutaneous decompression of benign and malignant biliary obstruction. *Arch Surg (Chicago)* 114:148–151, 1979.

27. Neff RA, Fankuchen EI, Cooperman AM, et al: The radiological management of malignant biliary obstruction. *Clin Radiol* 34:143–146, 1982.

28. Hatfield ARW, Terblanche J, Fataar S, et al: Preoperative external biliary drainage in obstructive jaundice. *Lancet* 2:896–899, 1982.

29. Cooperman A: Periampullary cancer. *Semin Liver Dis* 3:181–192, 1983.

30. Cotton PB, Burney PG, Mason RR: Transnasal bile duct catheterization after endoscopic sphincterotomy: Method for biliary drainage, perfusion and sequential cholangiography. *Gut* 20:285–287, 1979.

31. Soehendra N, Reynders-Frederix V: Palliative bile duct drainage: A new endoscopic method of introducing a transpapillary drain. *Endoscopy* 12:8–11, 1980.

32. Wurbs D, Phillip J, Classen M: Experiences with long standing nasobiliary tube in biliary disease. *Endoscopy* 12:219–223, 1980.

33. Siegel JH, Harding GT, Chateau F: Endoscopic decompression and drainage of benign and malignant biliary obstruction. *Gastrointest Endosc* 28:79–82, 1982.

34. Witzel L, Wiederholt J, Wolbergs E: Dissolution of retained duct stones by perfusion with monooctanoin via a Teflon catheter introduced endoscopically. *Gastrointest Endosc* 27:63–65, 1981.

35. Siegel JH, Halpern G: A possible role for endoscopic therapy in the treatment of sclerosing cholangitis. (abstract) *Gastrointest Endosc* 30:161, 1984.

36. Zimmon DS, Clemett AR: Endoscopic stents and drains in the management of pancreatic and bile duct obstruction. *Surg Clin North Am* 62:837–844, 1982.

37. Laurence BH, Cotton PB: Decompression of malignant biliary obstruction by duodenoscopic intubation of bile ducts. *Br Med J* 280:522–523, 1980.

38. Huibregtse K, Tytgat GN: Palliative treatment of obstructive jaundice by transpapillary introduction of large bore bile duct endoprosthesis. *Gut* 23:371–375, 1982.

39. Siegel JH: Combined endoscopic dilatation and insertion of large diameter endoprostheses for bile duct obstruction. *Gastrointest Endosc* 30:91–92, 1984.

40. Siegel JH, Yatto RP: Approach to cholestasis: An update. *Arch Intern Med* 142:1877–1879, 1982.

41. Cotton PB, Safrany L, Schott B: Biliary prostheses using a 3.8 mm channel duodenoscope. (abstract) *Gastrointest Endosc* 28:129, 1982.

42. Siegel JH, Yatto RP: Transduodenal endoscopic decompression of obstructed bile ducts. *NY State J Med* 83:203–205, 1983.

43. Siegel JH: Improved biliary decompression using large caliber endoscopic prostheses. *Gastrointest Endosc* 30:21–23, 1984.

44. Siegel JH: Interventional endoscopy in diseases of the biliary tree and pancreas. *Mt Sinai J Med NY* (In press).

45. Siegel JH: Endoscopic placement of large caliber endoprostheses (ENP) in obstructive jaundice (abstract) *Am J Gastroenterol* 77:694, 1982.

46. Leung JWC, del Favero G, Cotton PB: Endoscopic biliary prostheses. A comparison of materials. *Gastrointest Endosc* (In press).

47. Kantz G: Tanspapillary bile duct drainage with a large caliber endoprosthesis. *Endoscopy* 15:312–315, 1983.

48. Siegel JH, Daniel SJ: Endoscopic and fluoroscopic transpapillary placement of a large caliber biliary endoprosthesis. *Am J Gastroenterol* 79:461–465, 1984.

49. Siegel JH, Guelrud M: Endoscopic cholangio-pancreatoplasty: Hydrostatic balloon dilatation in the bile duct and pancreas. *Gastrointest Endosc* 29:99–103, 1983.

50. Guelrud M, Siegel JH: Hypertensive pancreatic duct sphincter as cause of recurrent pancreatitis: Successful treatment with hydrostatic balloon dilatation. *Dig Dis Sci* 29:225–231, 1984.

51. Siegel JH, Yatto RP: Hydrostatic balloon catheters: A new dimension of therapeutic endoscopy. *Endoscopy* (In press).

52. Siegel JH, Yatto RP: Biliary endoprostheses for the management of retained common bile duct stones. *Am J Gastroenterol* 79:50–54, 1984.

12

Colonoscopic Polypectomy

Francis J. Tedesco

There is strong evidence that colonic polyps have a potential for malignant degeneration. This potential increases with the size of a polyp, certain histologic types and the degree of atypia, especially in polyps less than 1 to 2 cm in size (1,2). Before 1969, polyps detected by barium enema contrast examination or diagnostic colonoscopy had to be removed at the time of abdominal surgery. In the late 1960s, the technique of snare-cautery resection via a colonoscope was introduced (3). This chapter will review some basic features of the endoscopic applications of electrosurgery and the endoscopic approach to colonic polyps as well as the follow-up after colonoscopic polypectomy.

ENDOSCOPIC APPLICATIONS OF ELECTROSURGERY (4)

An understanding of the fundamental principles and knowledge of the hazards of electrosurgery are prerequisites for the safe use of colonoscopic polypectomy. Colonic tissue, like all other physical substances, offers resistance to the flow of electric current. As an electric current attempts to move through tissue, the electrons that constitute the electric current are constantly colliding with molecules of tissue. Through these collisions, energy is dissipated in the tissue, causing its temperature to rise. This effect can be described by the equation $P = I^2R$, where P is the electric power dissipated in the tissue (usually expressed in watts), I is the current (usually expressed in amperes) and R is the resistance of the tissue to the current (expressed in ohms). This equation reveals several features of passage of electric current through tissue: a) at a constant current, the power and, therefore, the temperature rise of tissue is directly proportional to the tissue's resistance. Tissue resistance depends on a tissue's vascularity, water content and other variables. Fat has a higher resistance to the passage of electric current than does muscle. In addi-

269

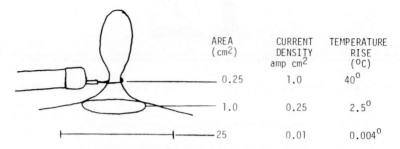

AREA (cm²)	CURRENT DENSITY amp cm²	TEMPERATURE RISE (°C)
0.25	1.0	40°
1.0	0.25	2.5°
25	0.01	0.004°

Fig. 1. Temperature rise compared to current density and cross-sectional area. Modified from: Barlow DE: Endoscopic applications of electrosurgery: a review of basic principles. *Gastrointestinal Endoscopy* 28:73, 1982, with permission.

tion, as tissue dries out, its resistance increases greatly, and the current passing through it falls off. b) Production of heat in the tissue is proportional to the square of the current passing through it. These principles can be demonstrated by using an ideal polyp, resting on a large return electrode (Fig. 1). Three areas should be noted: a thin section of the stalk, just below the snare, which has a cross-sectional area of 0.25 cm², the base of the polyp, which has a cross-sectional area of 1 cm², and the area of contact between the tissue and the plate electrode, which has an area of 25 cm². Assuming that the resistance to the passage of electric current is uniform throughout the tissue and that the current passing through each cross-sectional area is therefore uniform, when a current of 0.25 ampere is used, the current densities (dividing the current by the cross-sectional area) in these three areas are found to be 1.0, 0.25 and 0.01 ampere/cm², respectively. If the temperatures in the three cross-sectional areas were measured, the following temperatures might be observed. At the plate electrode, where the current density is extremely low, the temperature rise is barely noticeable, 0.004°C. At the base of the polyp, the cross-sectional area is 1/25 of the area of contact between the tissue and the plate electrode, and the current density is 25 times the density at the electrode. The temperature rise in this area is 625 (25 × 25) times the rise at the plate electrode, or 2.5°C; this rise does not result in tissue necrosis. In the area just below the snare, the current density is 100 times the density at the electrode. The temperature rise in this area is 10,000 (100 × 100) times the rise at the electrode, or 40°C; this temperature rise produces the desired desiccation of the stalk of the polyp. Tissue in contact with the snare wire will be rapidly heated to the point where cellular water instantly vaporizes, creating a cellular wall explosion that results in excision of the head of the polyp as the snare wire moves through the tissue.

An understanding of the above "ideal" example is important to practitioners of colonoscopic polypectomy, and many polypectomy techniques used by experts in the field have been developed on the basis of a thorough understanding of the effects of current density (5,6). For example, "tenting" of the wall during polypectomy tends to thin out and elongate the stalks of pedunculated polyps and reduces the cross-sectional areas of the stalks. Gently sliding a polyp back and forth along the wall of the colon spreads this heating effect over a larger area. When a large polyp is resected, caution should be exercised to ensure that the head of the polyp does not touch the opposite wall of the colon, an action that would create a point at which current becomes concentrated. If contact with the opposite wall is unavoidable, the polyp should be positioned so that this area of contact is as large as possible, thus reducing the heating that will take place at any given point.

Other important considerations are that coagulation of tissue also varies with the diameter of the snare wire, the thickness of the tissue and the traction placed on the snare wire. The greater the diameter of the snare wire, the slower it will cut through the tissue, and vice versa. If a very thin snare wire is used, the highly concentrated cutting effect quickly severs the tissue before the stalk has been sufficiently desiccated. The thicker the tissue, the greater its resistance and the more current that is necessary for coagulation. Strong traction on ensnared tissue allows for rapid transection, whereas weak traction allows for increased resistance of the tissue being coagulated and thus increases the cutting time.

Currents that have a "pure" cutting effect are never used in the performance of colonoscopic polypectomy. Some endoscopists use currents that have a "pure" coagulation effect, whereas others prefer currents that have a combined cutting and coagulation effect, which are known as blended currents. The electrocautery equipment, including the connections and ground plate, should be checked before each use. The amount of current used can be checked by sparking the active electrode to the ground plate. With the above as background, the general approach to colonoscopic polypectomy and the polypectomy technique can now be discussed.

EQUIPMENT: SNARE-CAUTERY APPARATUS

Although there are many types of commercial snares manufactured by various companies, there are only two basic types of snare-cautery devices. One is a strand of braided wire folded back on itself and then threaded through Teflon tubing. This homemade type of snare permits the use of a more sensitive method of applying tension to the wire loop created around a polyp. This type of snare can be more readily removed from the base of a polyp if the wire has become stuck in the polyp during cauterization but without complete transection of the tissue. In addition, this type of snare allows the size and shape of the loop to be adjusted precisely and individually for each polyp that one attempts to remove. Most snare-cautery devices used in the United States are commercial snares. The size and shape of the loop are predetermined, as is the diameter of the wire. These features necessitate that several types of snare-cautery devices be available to endoscopists who perform colonoscopic polypectomy. It is important to remember that the greater the diameter of a snare wire, the slower it will cut through tissue and, conversely, the thinner the wire, the faster it will cut through tissue. This feature may necessitate adjustments of the power settings on the electrosurgical unit. A number of electrosurgical units are available; examples are those made by Bovie, Cameron-Miller, Elmed and Valley Laboratories as well as the units made by endoscope manufacturers. The operator must be thoroughly familiar with the cauterization characteristics of the unit that he or she is using. For this purpose, it may be necessary to use, for example, a piece of raw steak and experiment with various snare wires and different power settings to determine the characteristics of the unit. Unfortunately, this method of testing a unit is less reliable than is testing the unit on a laboratory animal, but it is more readily available to a great number of endoscopists who perform colonoscopic polypectomy.

TECHNIQUE (7–12, 19–22, 31, 32,)

If colonoscopy to the cecum has not been previously performed, it should be carried out, when feasible, before colonoscopic polypectomy is done. This policy is an important consideration because approximately 40% of patients suspected of having one polyp are found to have additional polyps on complete examination. Usually, polypectomy is attempted on withdrawal of the colonoscope after a complete examination; however, if complete colonoscopy is not being performed, the colonoscope should be advanced approximately 20 to 25 cm beyond the polyp to remove fecal fluid to ensure that the bowel is clean and that fluid will not flow into the field during polypectomy. Once the polyp has been clearly visualized, the operator should assess its size and surface characteristics and determine whether or not it is pedunculated or sessile. It may at times be necessary to manipulate the polyp with the tip of the endoscope or with the tip of the snare-cautery device to determine these features. If the polyp cannot be adequately visualized, it may be necessary to alter the patient's position to determine whether better visualization of the polyp can be obtained. Once the polyp is thought to be in the proper position, the Teflon catheter with the snare inside is advanced out of the colonoscope, so that the tip is visible to the operator. The snare is advanced so that a wire loop is created, and the polyp is lassoed with the snare wire. The tip of the Teflon catheter is then advanced to the base of the polyp at the exact point where transection is desired, the loop is gently tightened and the polyp is tented slightly into the center of the lumen (Fig. 2). If excess colonic mucosa has been caught in the loop (Fig. 3), the snare can be gently opened, the excess mucosa can be released and the polyp can be resnared (Fig. 3). If normal colonic mucosa is included, there is much more resistance to transection than is encountered when only the polyp is being coagulated. Increased resistance and the need for prolonged coagulation should be warnings to stop application of

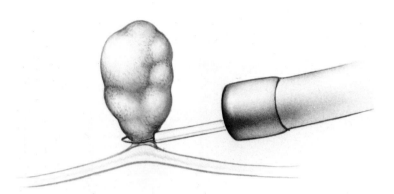

Fig. 2. Placement of a snare around the stalk of a polyp with tenting of the polyp into the lumen. Reprinted from Shinya H: Colonoscopy: Diagnosis and Treatment of Colonic Diseases. New York, Igaku-Shoin Medical Publishers, Inc., 1982, p 180, with permission.

current and reexamine the area being coagulated so that transmural burns and perforation do not occur. If the operator, after ensnaring the polyp, is able to tent the mucosa and move the polyp back and forth without moving the wall of the colon, he or she can feel more secure that only the polyp, and not adjacent, normal colonic mucosa, has been caught with the wire loop. Pedunculated polyps usually are transected within 2 to 4 seconds; mucosal blanching is noted adjacent to the snare wire during transection.

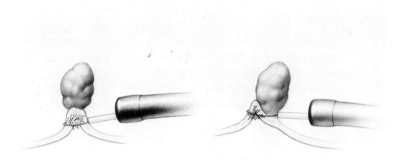

a   b

Fig. 3 (a and b). Placement of a snare with excess mucosa caught in the loop. Reprinted from Shinya H: Colonoscopy: Diagnosis and Treatment of Colonic Diseases. New York, Igaku-Shoin Medical Publishers, Inc., 1982, p 181, with permission.

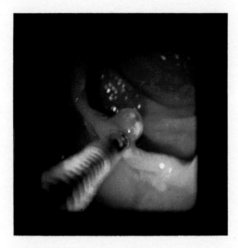

Fig. 4. Endoscopic view of a small, sessile polyp being approached with a hot biopsy forceps.

Because variability in types and sizes of polyps necessitates the use of different approaches, I will now describe the techniques employed to manage different types of polyp.

SMALL POLYPS

Polyps less than 0.5 cm in diameter (Fig. 4) can be removed by means of a hot biopsy forceps. The polyp is grasped at its head with the hot biopsy forceps and then is tented away from the wall of the colon. Current is applied, and mucosal blanching is noted at the base of the polyp. Because the polyp is tented away from the wall, its smallest diameter becomes the area between its head and the wall of the colon. With this technique, the polyp is destroyed, but tissue can still be obtained for histologic analysis.

SMALL, SESSILE POLYPS

Sessile polyps less than 1 cm in diameter (Fig. 5) can be removed in one piece by use of the snare-cautery technique if their bases are not wide and if a reasonable "pseudo-stalk" can be created at their bases. Such polyps are lassoed with the snare wire and, again, the tip of the Teflon catheter, which contains the snare wire, is advanced to the base of the polyp to the exact point where the operator desires to transect the polyp. The wire is gently tightened, forming a pseudo-stalk. The polyp is then gently tented toward the center of the lumen, and current is applied for transection. Even if a sessile polyp is transected too rapidly, the bleeding that occurs is usually negligible. Transmural burns and/or perforation from excessive coagulation is a more serious and more common complication with sessile polyps. The higher frequency of these complications may be related to capture by the snare of adjacent, normal colonic mucosa or to the fact that the bases of such polyps usually are very large, necessitating the application of greater current to overcome the increased resistance to permit transection.

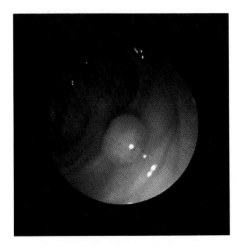

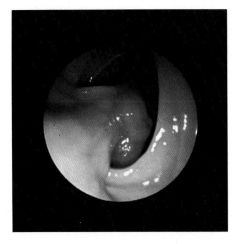

Fig. 5. Endoscopic view of a sessile polyp with a diameter of 1 cm.

Fig. 6. A pedunculated polyp with a broad stalk (pedicle) and a hyperemic, villous-appearing head.

PEDUNCULATED POLYPS

When a pedunculated polyp (Fig. 6) is being removed, the endoscopist should attempt to grasp the polyp toward its neck. If the polyp has a long stalk (Fig. 7), it is best to leave at least 1 cm of the stalk to avoid perforation and, if bleeding occurs after transection of the stalk, to permit the stalk to be resnared to achieve hemostasis. Polyps with short stalks are ensnared as close to their necks as is possible (Fig. 8, a and b). Placement of the snare for such polyps is

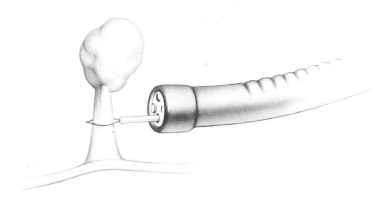

Fig. 7. Placement of a snare around the long stalk of a pedunculated polyp. Reprinted from Shinya H: Colonoscopy: Diagnosis and Treatment of Colonic Diseases. New York, Igaku-Shoin Medical Publishers, Inc., 1982, p 182, with permission.

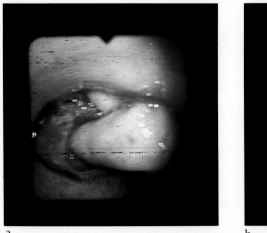
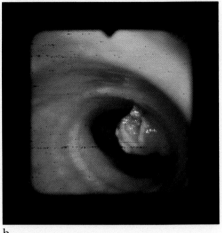

a   b

Fig. 8. (a) A polyp with a pedicle of moderate length. (b) View of the polypectomy site after the procedure. Approximately 1 to 1.5 cm of the pedicle adjacent to the wall was left.

similar to placement for other types of polyp. The polyp is encircled with the wire loop, which is then tightened loosely. Then, by positioning the tip of the Teflon catheter near the neck of a polyp with a short stalk, or approximately 1 to 1.5 cm from the wall if the polyp has a long stalk, before finally tightening the loop, one can easily obtain the desired area of transection. In the past, some experts have suggested that the stalks of pedunculated polyps be strangulated before electric current is applied. This approach seems unnecessary and is potentially dangerous because transection may be achieved prematurely, before electric current is applied, resulting in hemorrhage. In fact, once the snare has been tightened around the polyp or its stalk, it should not be released or loosened because if the tissue has been cut partially through with the wire, bleeding may occur and vision may be impaired. Therefore, once the snare has been applied and tightened around the polyp, that portion of the polyp should be transected by application of electric current. After this portion of the transection has been done, the snare can be repositioned in a more adequate place on the stalk and the polypectomy completed. In contrast to the situation with sessile polyps, the risk for serious bleeding is higher than the risk for perforation from excessive coagulation when pedunculated polyps are transected without adequate coagulation. This higher risk for serious bleeding is a major reason that some experts prefer to use currents that have a pure coagulation effect rather than blended currents, especially when they are removing pedunculated polyps.

PEDUNCULATED POLYPS WITH LARGE HEADS

Polyps with large heads may be a problem because visualization may not be satisfactory to ensure that their stalks and heads have not been lassoed to-

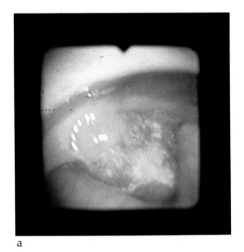
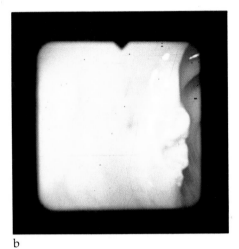

a   b

Fig. 9. (a) A large, sessile polyp that was
removed in a piecemeal fashion. (b) The
polypectomy site shows mucosal ulceration and adjacent edema.

gether requiring excessive coagulation. If such polyps are transected rapidly,
hemostasis may be inadequate as a result of incomplete coagulation of the
stalks. If a pedunculated polyp has a large or lobulated head, it may be necessary to ensnare part of the head, tighten the snare loop and then excise that
part of the head. After partial resection has been done, the wire snare can be
more easily and safely placed over the remaining portion of the head and
positioned around the neck for complete polypectomy. Homemade snares that
have a capability for creating large loops can be used to pass over a large head
and, at times, can be safely positioned around the neck if visualization is
adequate. Unfortunately, even with this type of snare, adequate visualization
of the stalk may not be possible, and segmental resection of the head may be
necessary before polypectomy can be completed.

BROAD-BASED PEDUNCULATED POLYPS

Because transection of broad-based, pedunculated polyps requires the application of strong electric currents that have a coagulation effect, thus increasing
the risk for perforation, they usually are managed by segmental, or piecemeal
resection, similar to the approach used for pedunculated polyps with large
heads.

LARGE, SESSILE POLYPS

Sessile polyps usually are more than 2 cm in diameter (Fig. 9, a and b). Before
an endoscopist removes large sessile polyps, he or she should consider the
patient's age and general physical condition, the morphologic characteristics of
the polyps and personal experience to decide whether the polyps should be

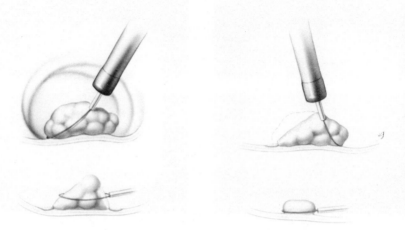

Fig. 10. Technique of polypectomy accomplished in a piecemeal fashion. At times, an entire polyp can be removed in one sitting. Sometimes, however, it may be appropriate to leave behind a portion of the base to provide time for the mucosal ulceration to heal and return later (after 4 to 8 weeks) to transect the remaining tissue completely. Reprinted from Shinya H: Colonoscopy: Diagnosis and Treatment of Colonic Diseases. New York, Igaku-Shoin Medical Publishers, Inc., 1982, p 187, with permission.

managed by abdominal or endoscopic resection. Once the endoscopist has decided to attempt endoscopic removal, he or she should remember that the risk for transmural burns and/or perforation is increased if a wide-based, sessile polyp that is 2 cm or larger is ensnared and coagulation attempted. This realization necessitates that such polyps be removed in a piecemeal, or segmental, fashion (Fig. 10). The technique is as follows: After the polyp has been well visualized, the wire snare is encircled on one end of its base, and the snare is tightened over the polyp in an oblique plane, usually encompassing one-quarter to one-third of the polyp. An important admonition is that it is better to encircle too little than too much of a polyp when piecemeal polypectomy is being performed. A small mucosal ulceration with minimal bleeding will be the result of this approach. The entire procedure is repeated with the wire snare encircling the opposite end of the base and, again, in an oblique plane and at a right angle to the first transection. With this approach, only the central portion of the polyp remains; this final portion can now be safely and, at times, completely ensnared and transected. However, the base of a polyp is not always transected during the initial polypectomy. The area of mucosal ulceration may be allowed to heal, resulting in some narrowing of the base. After 4 to 8 weeks, this area may be more safely transected endoscopically if the histologic characteristics of the polyp indicate that it is benign. All tissue removed by segmental resection should be examined histologically to determine the appropriate fol-

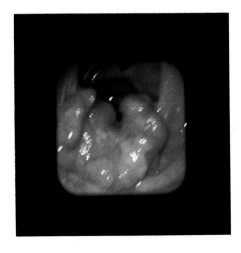

Fig. 11. This cancerous polypoid lesion was firm and friable and had a central depression with ulceration. Such lesions should be removed surgically.

low-up procedure (endoscopic or surgical) for the management of large, sessile polyps.

Although polyps larger than 3 cm can be removed by means of endoscopic polypectomy, this approach requires greater experience in evaluating the morphologic characteristics of polyps endoscopically as well as the use of endoscopic electrosurgical techniques. Sessile polyps, for example, those that are firm, granular, friable or ulcerated, should raise a high index of suspicion of malignant degeneration (Fig. 11). Such polyps should be managed with transabdominal resection, providing that a patient's age and general physical condition permit use of this approach.

After the endoscopist has performed colonoscopic polypectomy, it should be clear that only half of the job has been completed. The next important step involves retrieval of the polyp. A polyp can be retrieved by several methods. The tip of the colonoscope can be placed flush against the head of the polyp and suction applied. The polyp now impacted on the tip of the colonoscope can be retrieved by withdrawing the instrument. Another commonly used method is to lasso the cut polyp. Once the polyp has been ensnared, it can be withdrawn by use of the colonoscope. When the anal canal has been reached, the polyp is brought to the tip of the colonoscope, and the patient is asked to bear down, allowing the instrument and the polyp to be removed. This method is appealing, but endoscopists should be aware that when the wire snare encircles a polyp, it may cut through it or fragment it. The operator should attempt to ensnare the polyp at its stalk, which usually is firm, to decrease the risk for damaging the polyp.

Although the initial part of this chapter provides a reasonable approach to colonoscopic polypectomy, I think it is necessary to highlight again the following general principles of the procedure:

1. The operator should have familiarity with and check the electrosurgical unit. Settings on one type of electrosurgical unit may not provide the same current output as the same settings on other types of units.

2. Several types of snares may have to be used, and the characteristics of the wire snare may alter the power setting on a given electrosurgical unit.

3. The position of the tip of the Teflon catheter determines proper placement of the snare.

4. Before transection is started, the operator should attempt to move the polyp gently back and forth and to tent the mucosa so that an excess amount of adjacent, normal colonic mucosa is not caught in the loop.

5. With pedunculated polyps, the risk for bleeding from transection before adequate coagulation has been achieved is greater than the risk for transmural burns. By contrast, with sessile polyps, the risk for transmural burns and/or perforation from excessive coagulation is greater than the risk for bleeding. To prevent serious bleeding, many experts use currents that have a pure coagulation effect or blended currents that have mainly a coagulation effect. To prevent transmural burns and/or perforation, the operator should avoid ensnaring adjacent, normal mucosa and should perform resection in a segmental fashion instead of encircling too much of the polyp at one time.

6. With large, broad-based polyps or large, sessile polyps, it is better to ensnare too little than too much tissue. The endoscopist should plan to remove additional portions of such polyps at one sitting or at a later date.

7. Finally, the operator must be aware of his or her capabilities as well as the morphologic features of a polyp as seen endoscopically and, when necessary, should refer some patients for transabdominal resection rather than attempt endoscopic polypectomy.

Once a polyp has been retrieved, it must be sent for histologic evaluation. The results of the histologic evaluation guide the clinician in his or her approach and follow-up of the lesion (13,14). Colonic polyps can be divided into two major groups: neoplastic polyps, which include tubular adenoma (Fig. 12), tubulovillous adenoma (Fig. 13) and villous adenoma (Fig. 14), and carcinoma and nonneoplastic polyps, which include hyperplastic, inflammatory and hamartomatous varieties.

The most common type of polyp encountered in the distal portion of the colorectum is the hyperplastic or metaplastic polyp. Such polyps usually are sessile, the same color as or paler than adjacent, normal mucosa and small, although giant hyperplastic polyps have been reported. Recent work has demonstrated that tiny (less than 5 mm in size) colonic polyps are not always hyperplastic. Two studies (15,16) showed that 49% to 61% of polyps from 1 to 6 mm in size are neoplastic. In addition, islands of adenomatous tissue have been reported in as many as 13% of hyperplastic polyps. In view of this changing awareness of neoplastic tissue in tiny polyps, such polyps often are removed by use of a hot biopsy forceps during diagnostic or surveillance colonoscopy for neoplastic lesions. It has been suggested that the natural course of hyperplastic polyps is to remain small or, possibly, to regress. Hyperplastic polyps have an important clinical implication in that they may be associated with more serious lesions.

At the time of this writing, there is no evidence that routine follow-up exami-

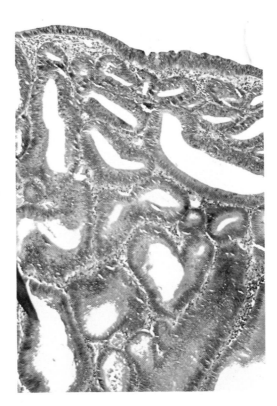

Fig. 12. This photomicrograph shows the branching tubules of tubular adenoma.

nation is necessary for patients with hyperplastic polyps. Likewise, there are no data concerning the need or timing for follow-up examinations in patients with tiny, mixed (hyperplastic-neoplastic) polyps that have been removed.

Inflammatory polyps usually are found in the regenerative and healing phases of any inflammatory colitis, including inflammatory bowel disease and infectious colitis. Such lesions have no intrinsic potential for neoplastic change.

Hamartomatous polyps include juvenile polyps and Peutz-Jeghers polyps. Juvenile polyps are characteristically round and have a smooth, bright red surface. Histologic examination reveals that such polyps consist of distended, mucus-filled glands, inflammatory cells and an edematous lamina propria. Juvenile polyps appear to have no potential for malignant degeneration. Peutz-Jeghers polyps are hamartomas that can reach a large size. They have a coarsely lobulated surface, and their characteristic histologic appearance is that of a treelike, branching core of smooth muscle surrounded by normal, mucin-secreting epithelium and lamina propria. Carcinoma of the colon and duodenum has been reported in patients with Peutz-Jeghers syndrome, but the incidence appears to be no more than 2% to 3%, and no specific follow-up surveillance has been defined for these polyps.

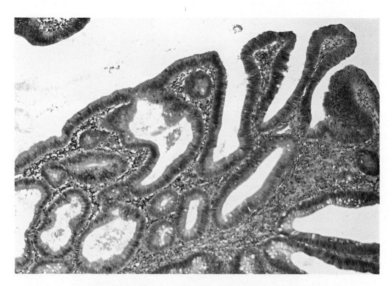

Fig. 13. This photomicrograph of a tubulovillous adenoma shows tubular epithelium on the left and villous fronds on the right.

The management and follow-up of neoplastic polyps will be discussed in the following section. It is now accepted that when neoplastic polyps have been excised completely, there is no need for further concern about dysplasia, carcinoma in situ or mucosal carcinoma if there has been no penetration through the muscularis mucosa. For example, if a pedunculated polyp has been completely excised endoscopically and shows evidence of dysplasia or carcinoma in situ, further resection is not required. In this situation, the patient should undergo follow-up colonoscopy in 1 year to look for additional polyps. If no new polyps are found, the patient should be placed on a program of colonoscopic surveillance at 3-year intervals. This approach may have to be modified as data from the ongoing National Polyp Study become available. If a completely or an incompletely excised neoplastic polyp was large and sessile, had a wide base and showed evidence of dysplasia or carcinoma in situ, segmental resection of the bowel might be advisable. However, in elderly patients, patients with other serious medical conditions and patients in whom surgical intervention is deemed inappropriate, repeat colonoscopy in 3 months and then at frequent intervals (3 to 6 months) to look for residual polypoid tissue or evidence of invasive carcinoma seems appropriate.

A subject of controversy is the approach that should be taken when a polyp with carcinoma in it has penetrated the muscularis mucosa. In general, it is important to make clear several distinctions. First, a malignant polyp, that is, a neoplastic polyp with a focus of invasive carcinoma, must be differentiated from polypoid cancer. Secondly, it is important to distinguish between malignant, pedunculated polyps and malignant, sessile polyps.

Many experts believe that even when a malignant focus penetrates through

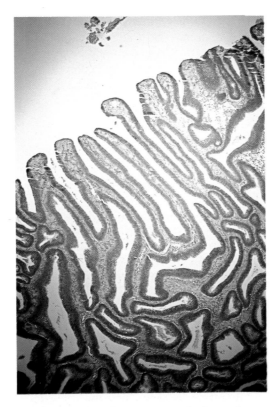

Fig. 14. This photomicrograph shows the finger-like projections of a villous adenoma.

the muscularis mucosa of a pedunculated polyp, colonoscopic polypectomy may be sufficient if there is an adequate margin between the plane of resection and the level of invasion (17). Although there are case reports of colonic wall involvement and/or distant lymphatic metastases in this situation, these findings appear to be unusual, being reported in only approximately 4% of cases. However, a recent report described 24 patients who had undergone colonoscopic polypectomy for the removal of pedunculated polyps that harbored invasive carcinoma but that had an intervening segment of uninvolved stalk (18). These 24 patients underwent colonic resection; in six patients (25%), one or two lymph nodes were noted to contain metastatic cancer. The authors suggested that all patients with polyps that harbor invasive cancer should undergo standard colonic resection, if feasible. The observations in this report, which differ from current wisdom, must be confirmed. It must be ascertained that the lesions described were truly pedunculated polyps that harbored invasive cancer rather than polypoid carcinomas initially. At best, it can be concluded that this issue remains a subject of debate.

Patients with sessile polyps that harbor invasive carcinoma and patients with pedunculated polyps with invasive carcinoma and have no clear margin of resection should undergo surgery, if feasible. For example, villous adenomas that harbor invasive carcinoma are associated with an incidence of nodal metastasis ranging from 16% to 39% and should be managed by surgical resection. However, the approach for patients with polyps in the lower portion of the rectum and for elderly patients and patients with other serious medical conditions may be individualized if the lesions harbor invasive carcinoma.

COMPLICATIONS

No chapter on colonoscopic polypectomy would be complete without a discussion of the potential complications of the procedure (23–34).

ADVERSE REACTIONS TO PREMEDICATIONS

Adverse reactions to such narcotics as meperidine are not uncommon and include hypotension, respiratory depression, bradycardia, nausea, vomiting and sweating. Respiratory depression can be reversed with naloxone. Bradycardia often responds to infusion of fluids and placement of the patient in Trendelenburg's position. With intravenous injection of diazepam, respiratory depression is a worrisome complication. The complication may be related to the rapidity of administration as well as to the total dose given. Diazepam should always be injected slowly while the effect on the patient is being monitored. Equipment for endotracheal intubation and artificial respiration should be readily available. Another potential danger with the use of diazepam is induction of burning and phlebitis at the injection site. To decrease the occurrence of this complication, the operator should avoid injecting diazepam into small veins. If injection into small veins cannot be avoided, it should be given slowly while the injection site is being flushed with a saline solution to dilute the concentration of the medication. Dilution is more adequately accomplished by using the side arm of a rapidly flowing intravenous solution.

VASOVAGAL ATTACK

This complication usually occurs when the colonoscope stretches the mesentery to such an extent that serious discomfort or pain ensues. Hypotension, bradycardia and cold, clammy skin are the clinical manifestations of vasovagal attack. The endoscopist should react to this complication by stopping the colonoscopy to allow it to pass, by giving saline intravenously and by placing the patient in Trendelenburg's position. At times, a small dose (0.4 mg) of atropine causes these clinical manifestations to abate. More often, however, and especially in elderly patients, giving a small dose (0.4 mg) of atropine before colonoscopy may help prevent vasovagal attack.

HEMORRHAGE

This serious complication is one of the most common occurences during colonoscopic polypectomy, being reported in 0.77% to 2.24% of cases in large surveys. Immediate bleeding during transection of the pedicle of a polyp results from inadequate coagulation. Coagulation is inadequate when a polyp is transected mechanically without application of adequate current. Also, when too much current is applied, a cutting effect results, but coagulation is inadequate, leading to hemorrhage. For this reason, when endoscopists are transecting pedunculated polyps, they should use currents that have a pure coagulation effect or blended currents that have mainly a coagulation effect. Although in most cases the bleeding that occurs after polypectomy ceases spontaneously as the vessels go into spasm and contract, the operator should be ready to react, especially if he or she observes serious bleeding or spurting from the transected stump of the pedicle. The snare should be reopened, and the loop should be passed over the stump of the pedicle and closed. The snare should be left in place for 10 to 15 minutes. This tamponade effect usually stops the bleeding. If the bleeding continues when the snare is opened, it should be closed again; if an adequate amount of pedicle remains, reapplication of current may be attempted. Current should be applied judiciously because overcoagulation may result in perforation. Other techniques for controlling hemorrhage, for example, injection of a vasoconstrictor solution (epinephrine, 1:10,000) through an endoscopic catheter, angiographic selective intraarterial perfusion and, at times, surgical intervention, may be used, if necessary.

Hemorrhage can occur from 24 hours to 21 days after polypectomy, although delayed hemorrhage usually occurs 5 to 9 days after the procedure. This late complication is related to sloughing of the coagulum at the site of resection. Late episodes of bleeding usually respond to conservative management with blood replacement as necessary, and surgical intervention is rarely necessary.

TRANSMURAL BURNS

The clinical picture of abdominal pain, leukocytosis and fever without evidence of free air or diffuse peritoneal signs suggest transmural burn injury. Conservative therapy is indicated in patients with transmural burns; surgical intervention should take place only if the clinical picture deteriorates with the development of diffuse peritoneal signs or other evidence of perforation.

PERFORATION

Although perforation is the most common serious complication of diagnostic colonoscopy, occurring in 0.14% to 0.26% of cases in large surveys, the incidence of perforation associated with colonoscopic polypectomy has ranged from 0.29% to 0.42% in several large surveys. Perforation can occur if a portion of the wall of the colon is ensnared, if too much current is applied for transection, especially with sessile polyps, or if there is substantial disruption of tissue by mechanical force during colonoscopy. The endoscopist can help avoid this complication by being sure that the ensnared polyp is freely movable over the underlying mucosa, by excising large polyps in a piecemeal fashion and by applying current judiciously.

Exploratory laparotomy and closure is the procedure of choice for the management of free perforation, and this procedure should be performed as soon as this complication has been recognized. There has been at least one report of a perforation that was managed conservatively, without surgical intervention, but such an approach seems warranted only in unusual situations and only if the patient remains free of symptoms and is showing clinical improvement.

EXPLOSION OF FLAMMABLE GASES

Combustible gases, such as hydrogen and methane, can be produced by bacterial fermentation in the colon. It has been clearly shown that standard preparations for colonoscopy, including fasting except for ingestion of clear liquids or bowel-cleansing substances, reduces the amount of flammable gases to undetectable levels. However, residual methane gas may be present, and it must be diluted by insufflation and aspiration of the air that is present during colonoscopy. Ideally, total colonoscopy allows the operator to confirm that the colon is clean and permits insufflation and aspiration of gas throughout the colon. Insufflation of carbon dioxide as a routine practice during polypectomy seems unnecessary in patients in whom adequate preparation has resulted in a clean colon. Great care must be exercised to ensure that all nonabsorbable carbohydrates (e.g., mannitol) are eliminated from the diet of patients undergoing colonoscopic polypectomy.

Even with an awareness of these potential risks, colonoscopic polypectomy is clearly preferable to transabdominal polypectomy.

CONCLUSION

Colonoscopic polypectomy can be accomplished safely and successfully only if the endoscopist has had thoughtful preparation for the various steps of the procedure and for the potential complications. The techniques of colonoscopy and colonoscopic polypectomy have revolutionized the diagnosis and management of colonic polyps.

REFERENCES

1. Morson BC: The polyp cancer sequence in the large bowel. *Proc R Soc Med* 67:451–457, 1974.

2. Day DW, Morson BC: *The Pathogenesis of Colorectal Cancer (volume 10 of Major Problems in Pathology)*. Philadelphia, Saunders, 1978, pp 58–71.

3. Wolff WI, Shinya H: Polypectomy via the fiberoptic colonoscope. *N Engl J Med* 288:329–332, 1973.

4. Barlow DE: Endoscopic applications of electrosurgery: A review of basic principles. *Gastrointest Endosc* 28:73–76, 1982.

5. Shinya H, Wolff WI: Colonoscopic polypectomy: Technique and safety. *Hosp Pract* 10:71–78, 1975.

6. Frühmorgen P: *Colonoscopy—Techniques, Clinical Practice and Colour Atlas*. London, Chapman and Hall; Chicago, Year Book Medical Publishers, 1981, pp 199–235.

7. Williams CB: Diathermy biopsy—A technique for the endoscopic management of small polyps. *Endoscopy* 5:215–218, 1973.

8. Cotton PB, Williams CB: *Colonoscopic Polypectomy—Practical Gastrointestinal Endoscopy* (2nd edition). Victoria, Australia, Blackwell Scientific Publications, 1982, pp 142–154.

9. Shinya H: *Colonoscopy—Diagnosis and Treatment of Colonic Diseases*. New York, Igaku-Shoin Medical Publishers, 1982, p 176.

10. Nivatvongs S, Goldberg SM: Results of 100 consecutive polypectomies with the fiberoptic colonoscope. *Am J Surg* 128:347–350, 1974.

11. Christie JP: Colonoscopic excision of large sessile polyps. *Am J Gastroenterol* 67:430–438, 1977.

12. Wolff WI, Shinya H: Modern endoscopy of the alimentary tract, in *Current Problems in Surgery*. Chicago, Year Book Medical Publishers, 1974, pp 1–62.

13. Shinya H, Wolff WI: Morphology, anatomic distribution and cancer potential of colonic polyps. *Ann Surg* 190:679–683, 1979.

14. Nivatvongs S, Goldberg SM: Management of patients who have polyps containing invasive carcinoma removed via colonoscope. *Dis Colon Rectum* 21:8–11, 1978.

15. Tedesco FJ, Hendrix JC, Pickens CA, et al: Diminutive polyps: Histopathology, spatial distribution, and clinical significance. *Gastrointest Endosc* 28:1–5, 1982.

16. Waye JD, Frankel A, Braunfeld SF: The histopathology of small colon polyps. (abstract) *Gastrointest Endosc* 26:80, 1980.

17. Shinya H, Cooperman A, Wolff WI: A rationale for endoscopic management of colonic polyps. *Surg Clin North Am* 62:861–867, 1982.

18. Colacchio TA, Forde KA, Scantlebury VP: Endoscopic polypectomy. *Ann Surg* 194:704–707, 1981.

19. Dagradi AE, Riff DS, Fort ET: Colonoscope polypectomy: Excision of a large villous adenoma. *Am J Gastroenterol* 66:464–466, 1976.

20. Hunt RH, Waye JD: *Colonoscopy—Techniques, Clinical Practice and Colour Atlas*. London, Chapman and Hall, 1981.

21. Nivatvongs S, Goldberg SM: Experience with colonoscopic polypectomy. Review of 700 polyps. *Minn Med* 62:197–199, 1979.

22. Williams CB, Hunt RH, Loose H: Colonoscopy in the management of colon polyps. *Br J Surg* 61:673–682, 1974.

23. Hall SC, Ovassapian A: Apnea after intravenous diazepam therapy. *J Am Med Ass* 238:1052, 1977.

24. Langdon DE, Harlan JR, Bailey RL: Thrombophlebitis with diazepam used intrave-nously. *J Am Med Ass* 223:184–185, 1973.

25. Langdon DE: Thrombophlebitis following diazepam. *J Am Med Ass* 225:1389, 1973.

26. Rogers BHG, Silvis SE, Nebel GT, et al: Complications of flexible fiberoptic colonos-copy and polypectomy. *Gastrointest Endosc* 22:73–77, 1975.

27. Smith LE: Fiberoptic colonoscopy: Complications of colonoscopy and polypectomy. *Dis Colon Rectum* 19:407–412, 1976.

28. Frühmorgen P, Demling L: Complications of diagnostic and therapeutic colonos-copy in the Federal Republic of Germany. *Endoscopy* 2:146–150, 1979.

29. Taylor R, Weakley FL, Sullivan BH Jr: Non-operative management of colonoscopic perforation with pneumoperitoneum. *Gastrointest Endosc* 24:124–125, 1978.

30. Williams CB, Tan G: Complications of colonoscopy and polypectomy. (abstract) *Gut* 20:903, 1979.

31. Norfleet RG: Colonoscopy experience in 100 examinations. *Wis Med J* 73:66–68, 1974.

32. Spencer RJ, Coates HL, Anderson MJ: Colonoscopic polypectomies. *Mayo Clin Proc* 49:40–43, 1974.

33. Geenen JE, Schmitt MG Jr, Wu WC, et al: Major complications of colonoscopy: Bleeding and perforation. *Am J Dig Dis* 20:231–235, 1975.

34. Carlyle DR, Goldstein HM: Angiographic management of bleeding following trans-colonoscopic polypectomy. *Am J Dig Dis* 20:1196–1201, 1975.

13

Laser Therapy for Esophageal and Gastrointestinal Neoplasms

John H. Bowers

Management of enteric cancer is a challenging problem. Although complete surgical resection of a localized lesion remains the best hope for a permanent cure, many patients' circumstances do not permit that approach. Nevertheless, obstruction and bleeding may necessitate treatment even when a tumor is not resectable. Not infrequently, patients' limited life expectancies make it difficult to recommend surgical intervention. Laser energy, delivered transendoscopically by means of a flexible waveguide, permits thermal destruction and coagulation of neoplastic tissue without incisional surgery.

The effects of laser energy on biologic tissues are thermal, occurring because absorbed light energy is converted to heat. The final result is determined by the magnitude of the temperature rise and ranges from simple coagulation necrosis through carbonization (charring) to vaporization of tissue. Depth of injury is predictable and largely dependent on the wavelength of the incident laser light (1,2). It is even possible to coagulate or vaporize discrete volumes of abnormal tissue selectively while sparing adjacent, normal tissue, thereby preserving bowel wall integrity. By contrast, the depth of tissue necrosis associated with the application of monopolar electrocautery is unpredictable (3), a fact that limits the usefulness of this technique in the management of enteric neoplasms. Taken together, these observations indicate that endoscopically directed laser energy has a potential role in the treatment of selected patients with benign or malignant gastrointestinal neoplasms.

Experimental animal studies performed with argon lasers have demonstrated the feasibility of rapid photocoagulation of large areas of the mucosal surface (Fig. 1a). Damage is restricted to the superficial layers, which are approximately 1 mm deep (Fig. 1b) (1). When argon laser energy is applied to normal tissue, the laser-induced ulcerations heal completely within a few days, leaving a normal-appearing mucosal surface (4).

Neodymium:YAG (Nd:YAG) laser energy penetrates more deeply than does argon laser energy and frequently causes full-thickness injury to normal colonic tissue in laboratory animals (Figs. 2a and 2b) (2,5,6). The risk for perfora-

289

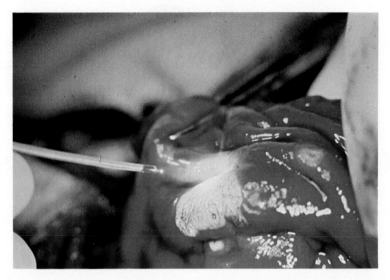

Fig. 1a. Argon laser photocoagulation of canine stomach. A large area of the mucosa has been coagulated. Figures 1a,b, 2a,b, 3a–c, 4a,b, 8a–d reprinted from Bowers JH: Laser therapy of colonic neoplasms. In Fleischer D, Jensen D and Bright-Asare P (eds): Therapeutic Laser Endoscopy in Gastrointestinal Disease. Boston, Martinus Nijhoff, 1983, pp 139–150, with permission.

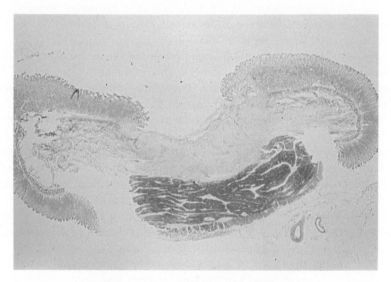

Fig. 1b. Argon laser photocoagulation of canine colon after 4 days. The mucosa is ulcerated, but damage is restricted to the submucosa.

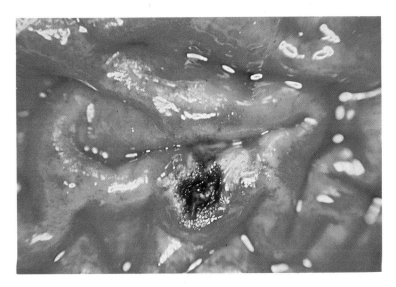

Fig. 2a. Nd:YAG laser photocoagulation of a canine gastric ulcer. Central excavation and carbonization are apparent.

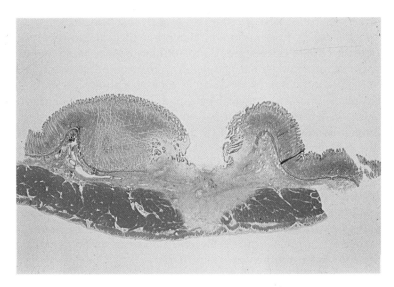

Fig. 2b. Nd:YAG laser photocoagulation of canine colon after 4 days. Damage extends to the serosa.

tion may be higher with Nd:YAG laser therapy than with argon laser therapy, especially in the colon, which has a thinner wall than that of the stomach. Bowel wall thickness is likely to be greater in areas of neoplastic involvement, perhaps enhancing the safety of Nd:YAG therapy in these areas. Greater penetration of Nd:YAG laser energy allows for more rapid photocoagulation of a given volume of tumor tissue. More rapid photocoagulation may be an advantage when bulky tumors are being treated. Unfortunately, the margin of tissue viability after application of the more deeply penetrating Nd:YAG laser energy is not immediately apparent and can be determined only by repeat endoscopic examination of the treated area after 48 to 72 hours. Several therapy sessions and careful follow-up often are necessary.

Carbon dioxide laser energy has a very shallow depth of penetration, approximately 0.1 mm in tissue. Carbon dioxide laser energy is, therefore, delivered to a smaller volume of tissue than is treated with argon or Nd:YAG laser energy. The greater magnitude of the temperature rise results in vaporization, rather than coagulation, of tissue. Carbon dioxide laser energy functions more as a scalpel than as a coagulator. Pulsed carbon dioxide laser energy might afford more rapid removal of relatively large volumes of tumor tissue, while maintaining the advantage of a discrete margin of necrosis. However, because a system for delivery of carbon dioxide laser energy by means of a flexible waveguide is not yet available, the usefulness of this technique in the gastrointestinal tract is limited. Perhaps the use of differing wavelengths, applied at different stages during tumor removal, will prove helpful. However, the choice of laser, best methods of treatment and ultimate role of laser therapy in the management of gastrointestinal neoplasms remain to be determined.

Some benign enteric polyps, because of their size and configuration, do not lend themselves easily to removal by standard endoscopic diathermy techniques. Also, malignant lesions of the bowel may be first manifested by local complications, such as obstruction or bleeding, that require treatment, even though the patient may already have disseminated or unresectable disease. Certain patients with benign or malignant bowel neoplasms may refuse surgical treatment or have an excessive risk for surgical intervention because of concomitant medical conditions. Alternative treatment modalities are needed for such patients. This chapter will present the results of the author's preliminary experience with argon and Nd:YAG laser therapy in the management of bowel neoplasms, a review of the literature and comments regarding future expectations for laser photocoagulation therapy.

BENIGN POLYPS AND VILLOUS ADENOMA

Because adenomatous polyps of the bowel are true neoplasms, they have a potential for malignant degeneration; prompt removal of such polyps is therefore advisable (7). Villous adenomas are especially worrisome. More than 50%

of large (greater than 2 cm in diameter) villous adenomas are found to harbor cancer at the time of removal (8). Whereas most polyps can be easily removed with electrosurgical snare and biopsy devices, removal by this technique is not always possible. Large, broad-based (sessile) polyps present special problems. Attempts at removal with a snare can lead to perforation if the serosal surface is entrapped. Fulguration with a ballpoint electrode can also cause full-thickness injury to the bowel wall, leading to perforation. Broad-based, polypoid lesions often are excised surgically, but it would be desirable to have an effective and safe endoscopic technique for removal. Laser photocoagulation therapy offers an alternative form of management because of the precise nature of the interaction between laser energy and tissue.

TECHNIQUE

Adenomatous polyps chosen for removal by means of laser photocoagulation should be sessile, at least 5 mm in transverse diameter and judged difficult to remove by standard endoscopic techniques. Specimens for histologic examination must be obtained before laser coagulation therapy is begun. Treatments usually are performed on an outpatient basis unless hospital admission is required for other reasons. Access to the treatment site usually is obtained by means of a flexible, fiberoptic therapeutic endoscope. Occasionally, a rigid proctoscope affords the best access to low-lying rectal lesions.

The choice of laser depends on the location, size and configuration of the polyp to be treated. In most cases, argon laser therapy is chosen as the first treatment modality for colonic lesions because its limited depth of penetration affords greater safety. However, large, protruding polyps may be managed with Nd:YAG laser therapy; the choice of laser depends on the operator's judgment. Rectosigmoid and gastroduodenal neoplasms can be managed more aggressively than can lesions of the upper part of the colon because the wall is thicker.

Argon laser energy is applied at a power setting of 5 to 10 watts, in the continuous-wave mode, at a distance of 0.5 to 2.0 cm from the area being treated (9,10), whereas Nd:YAG laser energy is applied at a power setting of 40 to 70 watts in pulses of up to 2 seconds in duration, at a distance of 1.0 to 2.0 cm (9–11). Photocoagulation is begun centrally and continued until the entire surface of the polyp has blanched. Small colonic polyps usually require only a few seconds of argon laser photocoagulation. Large adenomas subjected to Nd:YAG laser photocoagulation typically require 500 to 3000 joules (12,13). For large polyps, several courses of therapy usually are necessary (10–13), a problem that may be partially overcome if diathermic resection of polypoid projections is performed before laser therapy (10). Subsequent courses of therapy are scheduled at intervals of 2 to 10 days until the tumor has been obliterated. Follow-up endoscopy is then performed at intervals of 3 to 6 months, with additional laser therapy given as needed (9,10). Biopsy specimens obtained at the time of follow-up examinations may help establish whether there is persistence of neoplastic tissue (10).

RESULTS AND DISCUSSION

Small, benign gastric polyps and adenomas usually can be removed in one or two sessions (11,12,14). Absence of tumor in specimens that have been resected surgically after Nd:YAG laser therapy has been demonstrated (14). However, long-term follow-up data are lacking.

Argon laser therapy is effective for the removal of small, benign colonic polyps (9). No recurrence was noted after 14 months. However, one large (20 mm) tubular adenoma recurred 1 year after laser photocoagulation. Additional Nd:YAG laser therapy was required; the lesion did not recur during the next 12 months of observation (Figs. 3a to 3c) (9).

Impressive clinical results have been obtained with Nd:YAG laser therapy for the management of villous adenomas (10,15,16). Lambert and Sabben (15) reported cures for 35 of 39 villous adenomas; 12 of these tumors contained foci of malignant change. Brunetaud and colleagues (10) treated 21 patients. Ten patients showed complete healing after 3 to 9 months of observation. Six patients were still undergoing laser therapy. Two patients underwent surgical removal of villous tumors because carcinoma in situ was found in biopsy specimens. However, histologic examination of the surgically excised specimens showed that complete removal of cancer had been achieved with Nd;YAG laser therapy. Kiefhaber and Kiefhaber (16) reported cures in 14 patients. There were three recurrences, but complete removal was accomplished in all three cases with additional laser therapy.

Major complications are rare, although there have been reports noting hemorrhage (15), perforation (15) and rectal stenosis (10,15). Rectal stenosis is most likely to occur in patients who initially have circumferential tumors (10).

Experience with and length of observation in such patients are limited. However, these initial studies indicate that laser photocoagulation therapy has a potential role in the management of benign enteric tumors in selected patients.

POLYPOSIS SYNDROMES

Persons with Gardner's syndrome or familial polyposis have myriads of adenomatous polyps scattered throughout the bowel (17). These colorectal tumors have a strong potential for malignant change, a circumstance that dictates early removal of the colon (17). However, the rectum often is retained by the surgeon to avoid creation of an ostomy. When this approach is taken, the patient must have polyps periodically removed transrectally to prevent development of rectal cancer. Argon (4,10) and Nd:YAG (18) laser therapy has been used successfully for the management of this problem.

TECHNIQUE

Patients with Gardner's syndrome or familial polyposis who have had subtotal colectomies with ileorectal anastomoses are candidates for this form of treat-

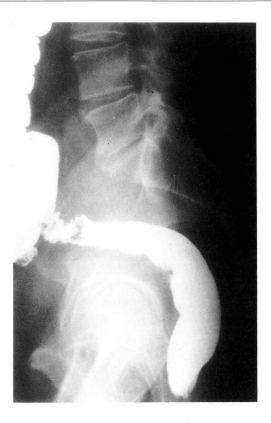

Fig. 3a. Sessile adenoma on the anterior
wall of the rectum.

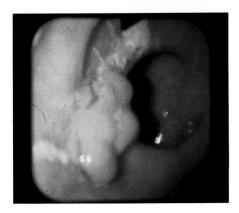

Fig. 3b. Appearance of the lesion shown
in Figure 3a before laser photocoagulation.

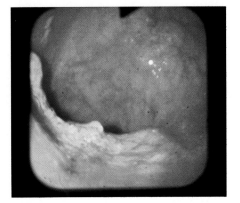

Fig. 3c. The lesion shown in Figures 3a
and 3b immediately after argon laser
photocoagulation.

ment. Laser therapy is administered on an outpatient basis after cleansing enemas. A flexible, fiberoptic sigmoidoscope is used for access to most polyps. Insufflation of gas at constant pressure, as described later in the section on gastrointestinal cancer, is helpful. Polyps in the lower portion of the rectum are sometimes most easily treated with a hand-held laser fiber through a short (10 to 15 cm) proctoscope.

Argon laser therapy (4,10) is administered at a power setting of 3 to 10 watts in the continuous-wave mode. The optimal treatment distance is 0.5 to 2.0 cm. A typical small polyp requires only a few seconds of treatment. With Nd:YAG laser therapy (18), 50 to 70 watts and pulses of 0.5 second in duration are used. Each polyp requires about 300 joules for photocoagulation. Treatment is considered complete when the entire surface of the polyp has blanched. Repeat treatments, usually at intervals of 2 to 4 weeks, must be administered until all polyps have been obliterated. Subsequent examinations and treatment sessions are scheduled at intervals of 3 to 6 months.

RESULTS AND DISCUSSION

A large kindred of patients with Gardner's syndrome has been followed up at the University of Utah for the past several years. At intervals, the patients have returned for reevaluation and removal of new polyps from their rectal remnants. Twelve of the patients agreed to undergo argon laser therapy for the management of rectal polyps. Short-term and long-term studies were carried out (4).

One patient with Gardner's syndrome was scheduled for surgical removal of the rectum because of inability to control polyp regrowth with monopolar electrofulguration. Four days before the surgical procedure was scheduled, 15 rectal polyps were photocoagulated with argon laser energy. The surgical specimen was studied histologically and found to show ablation of polyps with thrombosis of submucosal vessels. Tissue injury was limited to the submucosa (Figs. 4a and 4b).

In the other 11 patients, 211 rectal polyps were photocoagulated with argon laser energy. Follow-up endoscopy was performed at 4 and 12 days to assess the effects of treatment. At 4 days, the polyps were gone, having been replaced by small, superficial ulcerations. After 12 days, the mucosal surface had healed completely and no polyps were encountered. The same 11 patients have continued to return at intervals of 3 to 6 months for laser photocoagulation of new polyps; at the time of this writing, more than 500 polyps have been removed in this manner. These treatments have been given on an outpatient basis and have been well tolerated; no serious complication has occurred. Subsequent endoscopic examinations have shown that the number of polyps has been reduced. It seems likely that it will be possible to obliterate all polyps and stay ahead of new polyp growth. After the polyps have been removed with argon laser therapy, the mucosal surface heals completely, leaving a normal appearance, without scar (10). Spinelli and coworkers (18) have used Nd:YAG laser therapy to remove polyps in three patients with familial polyposis. One patient

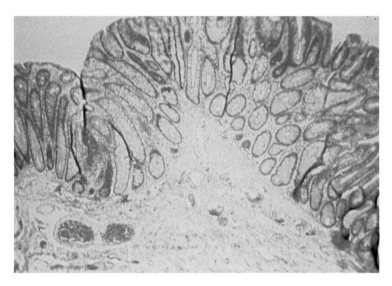

Fig. 4a. Typical adenomatous polyp from a patient with Gardner's syndrome.

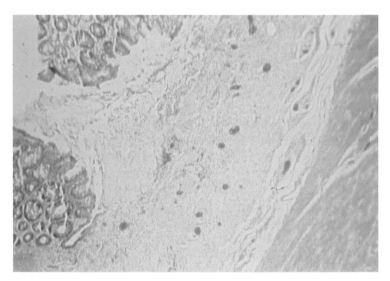

Fig. 4b. Surgical specimen from the patient with Gardner's syndrome 4 days after removal of a small polyp by argon laser photocoagulation. The mucosa is ulcerated and the submucosal vessels are thrombosed, but damage is limited to the submucosa.

was completely free of polyps after such therapy. However, the follow-up period was short. No complication occurred with either type of laser therapy. It remains to be seen whether Nd:YAG laser photocoagulation will have a tendency to promote rectal scarring and stenosis in these patients, as has been observed in patients with villous adenomas (10,15).

The technique of laser removal of new polyps in patients with familial polyposis seems promising. All patients have had subtotal colectomies. The remaining surface area of the colon is small and can easily be subjected to fiberoptic sigmoidoscopy at regular intervals. Periodic removal of new polyps will, hopefully, allow such patients to maintain normal defecatory function for prolonged periods without development of cancer.

GASTROINTESTINAL CANCER: GENERAL CONSIDERATIONS

Local complications of enteric cancer, such as obstruction and hemorrhage, may necessitate treatment even when the tumor is not amenable to curative therapy. Surgical therapy cannot be used in all cases and is invariably attended by some degree of morbidity. Ionizing radiation and chemotherapy are effective in some patients but have the following limitations: relief of local symptoms, if it occurs, may be delayed; systemic effects may be disabling; and the total amount of treatment that can be administered is limited.

A histologic diagnosis of cancer must be established for each patient. Because laser therapy is only palliative, patients in whom the cancer is potentially curable should not ordinarily be considered for such therapy. However, concomitant medical conditions may preclude an attempt at curative surgery in some patients. All available modes of palliative treatment, in addition to laser therapy, should be considered in order that the best possible course of action be offered the patient.

Preliminary radiographic studies are mandatory for delineating the anatomic structure of the tumor and for determining its anatomic relationships to surrounding structures. Computerized tomography often is helpful in this regard. Patients usually are hospitalized for their initial treatments in order to maintain hydration, provide nutritional support and observe for possible complications of treatment. However, choice of inpatient or outpatient status is based on the patient's clinical circumstances. After the initial phase of laser therapy has been completed, subsequent treatments often can be perfomed on an outpatient basis, once local symptoms have been controlled.

Access to such tumors usually is gained via a flexible, fiberoptic endoscope. Patients are sedated for laser endoscopy with intravenous meperidine and diazepam. Allowance must be made for evacuation of gas during laser therapy because the bowel may rupture spontaneously with high gas pressure (19). Overdistention of the bowel causes discomfort and increases the risk for laser-induced perforation. A two-channel, therapeutic endoscope is used to facilitate removal of gas. The second channel is connected to a constant-pressure gas-recirculation system built into the laser system. Not all laser systems have this capability, but a water manometer system can be assembled and incorporated to provide this capability. Pressure in the system should not exceed 65 cm of water (50 mm of mercury) (20). Instead of a two-channel, fiberoptic endoscope, two alternatives can be used. A single-channel therapeutic instrument can be used, provided that the channel is sufficiently large to allow for effective suction through the space around the laser fiber. Some authors favor placing a small gas-evacuation tube alongside, or attaching it to, the endoscope. This tube, if desired, can also be routed through a constant-pressure apparatus.

Choice of a laser is determined by the location, size and configuration of the tumor, the specific medical problems and the tumor's anatomic relationships to surrounding structures. Therapy with argon laser energy, because of its limited depth of tissue injury, might be chosen for initial management of a malignant, sessile polyp located in the intraabdominal portion of the colon. However, elsewhere in the gastrointestinal tract (esophagus, stomach, rectum), Nd:YAG laser energy can be applied safely, because the wall is thicker. Sometimes, the two types of laser are used in combination. The more deeply penetrating Nd:YAG laser energy might be applied for initial management, whereas argon or carbon dioxide laser energy could be used to photocoagulate residual tumor. The use of carbon dioxide laser therapy is limited to the rectum because flexible delivery systems are not yet available. Exact power settings, pulse durations and other technical aspects will be discussed in greater detail in the sections to follow.

Methods of delivering laser energy to a tumor bed are a point of controversy. Usually, surface photocoagulation of the tumor is employed; this approach results in thermal vaporization or coagulation necrosis. Only a limited volume of tumor is removed from the surface. A major disadvantage is that several treatments often are necessary to achieve complete removal. One approach to this problem has been termed "interstitial" treatment of tumors (20). A bare laser fiber is embedded into the bulk of a tumor at several sites to more effectively coagulate deeper layers of the neoplasm. Because lower power settings must be used to avoid carbonization and laser fiber damage, longer pulse durations must be used to achieve the desired total energy application.

Standard methods of laser photocoagulation are nonselective. Normal and abnormal tissues are destroyed concurrently by heat. Another potentially useful approach is photoactivation of neoplastic tissue by use of chemical compounds, such as hematoporphyrin derivative, that are selectively taken up by neoplastic tissue (21,22). After sensitization, laser energy is applied at a very low power setting for a long duration. Normal tissues are preserved. Photoactivation of hematoporphyrin derivative after uptake by cancer cells causes selective, delayed necrosis of tumor cells. This is not a thermal effect. For the gastrointestinal tract, the technical aspects of optimal laser wavelength, dosimetry and laser delivery remain to be clarified.

Possible complications (10,15,23) of laser therapy for enteric cancer include perforation, bleeding and submucosal fiberosis leading to luminal stenosis. Perforation can be avoided by careful selection of patients, proper choice of laser and conservative application of laser energy to the treatment area. Bleeding rarely occurs and usually can be controlled with additional photocoagulation. If a major vessel is disrupted, angiographic or direct surgical intervention might be required. Great care must be taken not to aggressively treat tumors that are adjacent to large vascular structures. Submucosal fibrosis commonly occurs after Nd:YAG laser therapy. Luminal stenosis has been reported but often is asymptomatic. However, this complication could ultimately necessitate dilatation or other surgical intervention.

Damage to a flexible, fiberoptic endoscope may occur if laser energy is absorbed by the tip of the endoscope. The mechanism of damage is believed to be reflection of laser light from the target surface to the tip of the endoscope. This type of damage is more likely to occur when the tip of the endoscope is constructed of black plastic, which has a relatively low melting point. Moreover, the sheath of such endoscopes is highly flammable. In either case, damage to the instrument or the patient could occur. Damage to the tip of the endoscope is not likely to occur if the following three precautions are observed: endoscopes used exclusively for laser therapy are manufactured with stainless-steel or white porcelain, reflective tips; endoscopists make certain that the laser fiber is well outside the endoscope channel, clearly visualized in the field of view, before activating their lasers; and endoscopists do not work too closely to the target surface during extensive coagulation.

Fires have been reported in the bronchopulmonary tree during laser endoscopy (24). A high concentration of oxygen seems to be a prerequisite for the occurence of this event. Although fires and explosions caused by laser endoscopy have not been reported in the gut, care should be taken to eliminate flammable gases, especially from the colon. A thoroughly prepared colon and low-oxygen environment are desirable. To produce this result, patients should be prepared, when possible, with a saline or polyethylene glycol purge.

The specific goals of treatment must be carefully defined for each patient. Laser therapy is not presently considered a curative treatment modality. When obstruction is already present or imminent, the intent should be to remove enough tumor tissue to relieve or prevent that problem. Additional laser therapy may be administered as necessary. When bleeding is a problem, the objectives are to reduce the surface area of the tumor and to coagulate tumor vessels to reduce the severity of hemorrhage to a tolerable level. Selected patients may be considered for an attempt at cure with laser therapy if they are not candidates for complete surgical resection. In this circumstance, small, circumscribed neoplasms are treated; the operator begins treatment at the center of a tumor and works toward its margins. Care should be taken not to disrupt normal tissue. Even so, selective destruction of all tumor tissue should be attempted, if possible. Careful follow-up examinations at regular intervals are necessary. Reduction of tumor mass might also be helpful, especially if laser therapy is to be used in conjunction with other treatment modalities, such as chemotherapy or radiation therapy.

ESOPHAGEAL CANCER

Patients with cancer of the esophagus commonly have progressive dysphagia, malnutrition and weight loss (25). Their long-term survival rate is dismal (26). Because such patients are unable to eat, their quality of life is poor. Even surgical gastrostomy, which reestablishes access to the gut, is unsatisfactory because such patients remain unable to eat and even unable to swallow their own saliva. In many cases, radiation therapy and chemotherapy are not helpful.

The major objective of laser therapy is to reestablish luminal patency to allow such patients to eat normally. Neoplastic tissue is vaporized and coagulated by the thermal effect of Nd:YAG laser energy. Only the portion of a tumor that obstructs the lumen is removed. This technique is considered palliative, not curative. However, there is no limit to the number of times that laser therapy can be employed, and it can be used in conjunction with other treatment modalities.

TECHNIQUE

Patients are hospitalized for their initial treatments so that health care personnel can maintain hydration, provide nutritional support and observe for possible complications of treatment. Sedation in preparation for laser endoscopy is accomplished with intravenous meperidine and diazepam. Careful attention should be directed to maintenance of airway patency. However, endotracheal intubation and/or general anesthesia usually is not required. For the management of obstructing esophageal carcinoma, Nd:YAG laser energy is used, because its greater depth of penetration allows a greater volume of tumor to be removed with each application of laser energy. The variables of laser therapy are adjusted as indicated in Table 1.

Laser treatments (23,27) are begun where the center of the esophageal lumen would normally be. A circular area, up to 12 to 13 mm in diameter, is coagu-

**TABLE 1. Nd:YAG Laser Photocoagulation Therapy
for Esophageal Cancer**

Power	50–70 watts
Maximal pulse duration	2.0 seconds
Treatment distance	0.5–3.0 cm
Gas flow, basal	20–30 ml/second
Gas flow, maximal	40–60 ml/second
Number of treatment sessions	2–13
Total energy per treatment	1200–6500 joules
Total energy per lesion	2500–70,000 joules

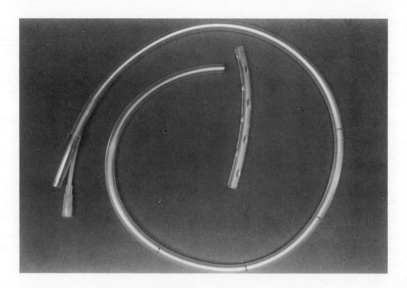

Fig. 5. A 34 French double-lumen, polyvinyl gastric lavage tube that has been modified for debridement of necrotic tissue after Nd:YAG laser therapy for obstructing esophageal carcinoma. The reader is referred to the text for details.

lated and, to some degree, vaporized. The total energy delivered usually is 4000 to 6000 joules (range, 2000 to 7000) at each treatment session. The actual duration of laser activation is normally less than 15 minutes. Subsequent treatments are carried out at intervals of 48 to 72 hours. This period is sufficient to allow edema to resolve and some necrotic tissue to slough. A line of demarcation between divitalized and living tissue becomes apparent after only 24 to 48 hours. Patients should be warned that dysphagia (due to tissue edema) may actually worsen for 24 hours after treatment.

Before subsequent treatments are given, necrotic debris must be removed to afford access to the underlying neoplasm. For this purpose, a modified 34 French polyvinyl gastric lavage tube with a second channel for irrigation is prepared (Fig. 5). The tube is transected with scissors just above the most proximal side hole. Sharp edges are softened with heat, and the tube is well lubricated. This device is then passed perorally into the tumor region and gently wedged into place. Vigorous suction is applied, and the tube is retracted. Irrigation through the second channel helps loosen debris. Large fragments of necrotic material often are removed in this manner.

Subsequent treatments are carried out in the same manner as the first treatment. Each treatment session allows removal of approximately 1 to 2 cm of additional tissue along the axis of the esophagus. Relief of obstruction is achieved only after several treatments. At least two, and often as many as six, treatment sessions are necessary. Dysphagia is not relieved until the entire length of the neoplasm has been treated. The duration of treatment can be discouraging. Patients must be informed of this problem before laser therapy is begun; even so, enthusiastic encouragement between treatment sessions often is necessary. Patients must be prepared to continue with treatment until the goals of laser therapy have been achieved.

In another approach, guided dilatation is applied to the tumor before laser therapy is initiated. This approach permits endoscopic access to the lower margin of the tumor. Laser photocoagulation is applied in a radial manner, beginning at the lower margin and working upward. With this method, fewer treatment sessions may be required for relief of obstruction.

RESULTS AND DISCUSSION

Fleischer and colleagues (23,27) found that the average length of esophageal tumors was 8.2 cm (range, 5 to 11) and that a mean of 5.3 treatments (range, two to 13) was required for restoring luminal patency. The mean energy delivered per treatment session was 4615 joules. The total energy delivered throughout the course of therapy ranged from 2592 to 70,217 joules.

Completion of the initial phase of treatment restores sufficient luminal patency to afford adequate deglutition and food intake in most patients (Figs. 6a to 6e) (23,27–29). Almost all patients can expect substantial relief of dysphagia and odynophagia, even though their swallowing after treatment may not be entirely normal (23,27). Survival of patients with advanced cancer is short, usually 2 to 4 months (23). However, the quality of life is greatly improved; many patients are able to eat solid foods until they die of other complications of cancer.

Minor complications, such as fever, leukocytosis, transient chest pain and temporary worsening of dysphagia, occur in some patients (23,27). These complications apparently accompany the edema and inflammation associated with laser therapy and usually resolve in 1 or 2 days. Perforation of the esophagus was reported by Fleischer and colleagues (23,27) in two of 14 patients (14.3%). In one patient, an esophagopleural fistula was successfully managed with chest tube drainage. An esophagotracheal fistula developed in the other patient; it was managed by placement of an esophageal stent. Perforation might be related to the concomitant use of forceful dilatation (23,27). Nonetheless, dilatation often is necessary for debridement and luminal enlargement. Perforation and fistula formation may occur spontaneously in patients with esophageal carcinoma and as a complication of radiation therapy or dilatation in patients who have not previously had laser therapy (23,25–27).

In any case, Nd:YAG laser therapy offers an opportunity for relief of dysphagia in patients with advanced cancer of the esophagus or esophagogastric junction. Several treatment sessions usually are necessary, and patients should be forewarned of this possibility. Treatment can be administered without general anesthesia or incisional surgery. The most important complication, perforation, occurs in 10% to 15% of patients but usually can be managed successfully. The quality of life is improved, but survival remains short for patients with advanced cancer.

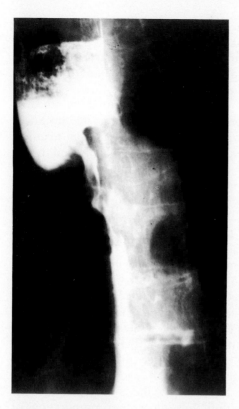

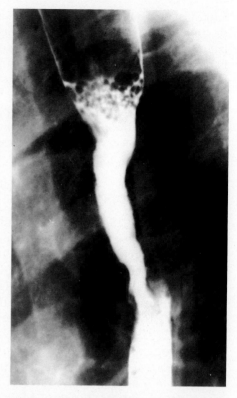

Fig. 6a. Radiographic appearance of an obstructing squamous cell carcinoma of the esophagus before Nd:YAG laser photocoagulation.

Fig. 6b. The lesion shown in Figure 6a after Nd:YAG laser photocoagulation. Luminal patency has been restored, and the patient is able to eat.

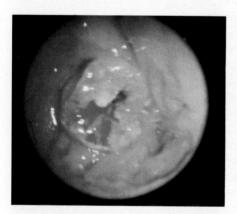

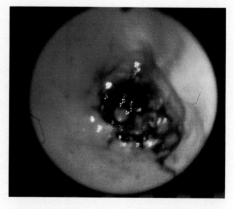

Fig. 6c. Endoscopic appearance of the tumor shown in Figures 6a and 6b before Nd:YAG laser photocoagulation.

Fig. 6d. The lesion shown in Figures 6a to 6c immediately after Nd:YAG laser photocoagulation.

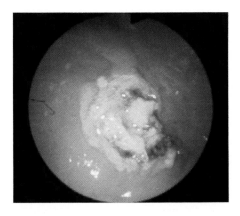

Fig. 6e. The lesion shown in Figures 6a to 6d 2 days after Nd:YAG laser photocoagulation. Necrotic tissue must be removed before the next laser treatment.

GASTRIC CANCER

Patients with gastric cancer present with a variety of symptoms (30), including weight loss, abdominal pain, anorexia, vomiting and chronic upper gastrointestinal tract bleeding. Some cancers cause obstruction, particularly when they recur locally after resection. The long-term cure rate is low; the 5-year survival rate is less than 10% (30). Laser therapy may be offered to patients who are not candidates for curative surgical intervention. Indications include gastric outlet obstruction, chronic bleeding and the need to reduce tumor bulk. Other palliative treatment modalities, such as surgical intervention, radiation therapy and chemotherapy, should also be considered in all patients. The goals of treatment and the method of approach must be individualized; consideration must be given to the extent and location of the tumor and the possible roles of other treatment modalities. In selected Japanese patients with early gastric cancer, laser therapy has resulted in probable cures (11,14,31–33). However, this patient population is not analogous to the patients with advanced gastric carcinoma who are seen in North America and Europe (30).

TECHNIQUE

Nd:YAG lasers are preterred over argon lasers by most authors (10,11,13,16,23,33–35) for the management of gastric cancer. The number of treatments, total energy delivered and method of approach are dictated by individual circumstances. However, representative laser therapy variables are given in Table 2. Argon laser therapy has rarely been used for the management of gastric cancer (23,36,37). In most cases, the size and depth of the tumor have necessitated the application of the more deeply penetrating Nd:YAG laser energy (Table 2).

In patients with advanced gastric cancer, palliative laser therapy is instituted to relieve or prevent obstruction, control hemorrhage and, possibly, reduce tumor bulk. For relief of obstruction, treatments are directed along the ex-

TABLE 2. Nd:YAG Laser Photocoagulation Therapy for Gastric Cancer

Power	40–90 watts
Maximal pulse duration	2.0 seconds
Treatment distance	0.5–3.0 cm
Gas flow, basal	20–30 ml/second
Gas flow, maximal	40–60 ml/second
Number of treatment sessions	1–10
Total energy per treatment	1000–12,000 joules
Total energy per lesion	1500–30,000 joules

pected luminal axis; treatment is begun in the center of the tumor and is continued toward the periphery until a circular area 13 to 15 mm in diameter has been coagulated, which usually requires 3000 to 6000 joules per treatment session. A waiting period of at least 48 to 72 hours ensues, during which time the margin of necrosis becomes evident and some necrotic tissue sloughs. At all subsequent treatment sessions, devitalized tissue is mechanically removed with forceps or brush to expose underlying tumor. Laser treatments are repeated until the lumen has been reestablished. Directed dilatation, accomplished with the tip of the endoscope, often is helpful. Ordinarily, a lumen sufficiently large for passage of a therapeutic instrument that is 13 mm or greater in diameter is adequate to allow passage of liquids and soft, solid foods.

In patients with chronic bleeding from gastric cancer, the problem usually is diffuse oozing from the friable surface of the neoplasm. Nd:YAG laser energy is systematically directed across the bleeding surface at a power setting of 70 to 90 watts until the entire surface of the neoplasm has been photocoagulated. One or two treatments usually are sufficient. Additional laser treatments may be necessary if bleeding recurs.

For reduction of tumor bulk, Nd:YAG laser energy at a power setting of 40 to 70 watts is used. The surface of the neoplasm is systematically photocoagulated, first centrally and then peripherally. Subsequent treatments are performed at intervals of 48 to 72 hours, or longer if desired. Patients who are able to take liquids by mouth can be treated on an outpatient basis. Reduction of tumor bulk is not necessarily beneficial. However, it might be helpful when obstruction is imminent or when it is anticipated that the effectiveness of radiation therapy or chemotherapy will be enhanced.

Laser therapy for early gastric cancer with the intent to cure can be undertaken in selected patients. This approach should be reserved for patients who cannot tolerate surgical excision of their tumors. The technique is applicable to polypoid, sessile, localized lesions. Large portions often can be removed first with a snare. This approach greatly reduces the number of laser treatments that are necessary. Residual tumor is photocoagulated with Nd:YAG laser energy at a power setting of 40 to 70 watts until the entire surface of the tumor has been photocoagulated. Subsequent treatments should be continued at intervals of 2 to 10 days until the entire lesion has been destroyed. Careful endoscopic follow-up examinations (with biopsies) should be done at intervals of 1 to 3 months.

RESULTS AND DISCUSSION

In patients with advanced gastric carcinoma, relief of stenosis can be expected in 60% to 80% of cases (13,16,23,33). As many as eight laser treatments may be required, depending on the length of the obstructed segment. Treatments should be continued until the obstruction has been relieved.

In patients with chronic bleeding, laser therapy often controls the hemorrhage (10,29). However, this effect often is only temporary (29) unless the entire tumor can be removed. In some cases, laser-induced fibrosis might reduce blood flow to the surface of a tumor even though the entire neoplasm has not been removed. When other treatment modalities are available, they may be used concurrently.

Tumor volume is reduced after laser photocoagulation (12,13,29,33). Anaplastic and undifferentiated cancers do not respond as well as do the better differentiated ones (35), probably because growth of anaplastic and undifferentiated tumors is more rapid. There is no published information regarding the survival of patients with such cancers. A beneficial role for laser therapy, when applied for the purpose of reducing tumor mass, is not yet clearly evident in patients with advanced gastric cancer.

In patients with early gastric carcinoma, complete removal can be achieved in 80% to 100% of cases (11,14,31–33). The reported follow-up periods are short, but tumor-free survival of up to 4 years has been noted (11). Treatment failures also have been reported (13,35). American and European experience with early gastric cancer is scant (16). The results noted above may apply only to Japanese patients because early gastric cancer observed in this patient population may have a distinct clinical course. Nonetheless, it seems reasonable to conclude that early gastric cancer in non-Japanese populations might also be effectively managed with laser photocoagulation therapy. At this time, laser therapy for early gastric carcinoma should be undertaken only in patients who are not considered candidates for curative surgical intervention.

COLORECTAL CANCER

Persons with symptomatic colorectal carcinoma commonly have rectal bleeding, anemia, alteration in bowel habits, abdominal or perineal pain and bowel obstruction (38). The most desirable treatment is complete surgical excision to produce a cure. Unfortunately, this goal cannot be achieved in many cases because the cancer has disseminated or extended locally and because some patients would not be expected to survive an attempt at curative surgery due to concomitant medical conditions. Surgical removal, particulary of tumors in the lower portion of the rectum, can be technically difficult; abdominoperineal resection and placement of a colostomy sometimes are necessary. Some patients simply refuse to undergo surgical procedures if their risks for surgical intervention are high or if placement of a colostomy is anticipated. Nonetheless, local complications, such as bleeding and obstruction, may necessitate some form of treatment in patients who are unable to tolerate surgical intervention. Laser therapy can be used in such patients to relieve established or imminent obstruction, control bleeding, and reduce tumor bulk; such therapy also can be used in an attempt to cure early cancer in nonsurgical cases. The use of laser photocoagulation for cancer of the colon should generally be regarded as a palliative, or noncurative, measure.

TECHNIQUE

Patients who do not require intravenous fluids or special nursing care can be treated on an outpatient basis. Preparation of the colon, when possible, is achieved with an oral saline or polyethylene glycol purge that affords good visualization and removes flammable gases. Patients who undergo a series of treatments need not take saline purges before every treatment, provided that they are continued only on clear liquids between treatments. Broad-spectrum antibiotic prophylaxis should be employed in patients with valvular heart disease and in patients who are at high risk for infection.

Normally, argon laser energy should be applied first to carcinomas located within the intraabdominal portion of the colon because the lesser depth of tissue penetration as compared to the depth of penetration of Nd:YAG laser energy affords greater protection against perforation (1,2,4–6). Nd:YAG laser energy may be applied in the lower portion of the rectum and to bulky tumors, provided that great care is taken to avoid damaging adjacent, normal bowel. The wall of the sigmoid colon usually is thicker than that of the transverse or right colon, a factor that might afford some degree of safety should it be necessary to use Nd:YAG laser therapy in that area. Often, lobulated or polypoid carcinomas can be partially removed with an electrocautery snare before laser treatments are begun, an approach that greatly reduces the amount of laser photocoagulation that is required. Electrosurgical fulguration may be considered in some patients, but its use should be restricted to patients with low-lying, noncircumferential tumors located on the posterior wall of the rectum (39,40). Typical laser variables used in the management of carcinoma of the colorectum are given in Table 3.

For relief or prevention of obstruction, treatments are begun centrally in the region where the bowel lumen would normally be. A circular area, up to 1.5 cm in diameter, is photocoagulated. Even when obstruction is not complete, portions of tumor that project into the lumen can be photocoagulated as a preventive measure. Several treatments often are necessary, particularly if the strictured area is long. Treatments are scheduled at intervals of 48 hours or longer. The interval between treatments should not be so long that appreciable tumor regrowth occurs. Treatments are continued until luminal patency has been restored.

TABLE 3. Laser Photocoagulation Therapy for Colorectal Cancer

	Argon Laser	Nd:YAG Laser
Power	5–10 watts	30–70 watts
Maximal pulse duration	Continuous	1.0–2.0 seconds
Treatment distance	0.5–2.0 cm	0.5–3.0 cm
Gas flow, basal	10–30 ml/second	20–30 ml/second
Gas flow, maximal	(continuous)	40–60 ml/second
Number of treatment sessions	1–5	1–5
Total energy per treatment	N.A.	1000–5000 joules
Total energy per lesion	N.A.	1000–20,000 joules

Patients with bleeding from neoplasms with friable surfaces can be treated to achieve control of hemorrhage. The surface of such a tumor is sytematically photocoagulated until the entire area of involvement has been treated. One or two treatment sessions usually are adequate for short-term control.

For reduction of tumor bulk, lobulated projections of the tumor are first excised with a monopolar electrosurgical snare. Residual tumor is then photocoagulated, first centrally and then outward toward the periphery. For early cancers, this approach may afford complete removal, resulting in a cure. As has been indicated previously, attempts at curative removal with laser therapy should be reserved for patients who are unable to tolerate surgical intervention.

Carbon dioxide laser energy has been applied through rigid endoscopes to vaporize or excise anorectal lesions (41,42), but this form of laser energy cannot be delivered through a flexible waveguide. The shallow depth of penetration of carbon dioxide laser energy affords great safety, but treatment of large tumors would be expected to take a long time.

RESULTS AND DISCUSSION

In patients with advanced colorectal carcinoma, relief of stenosis has been reported (16,29). One of the author's patients, an 87-year-old man with a sigmoid adenocarcinoma causing partial obstruction, was maintained in an asymptomatic state with argon and Nd:YAG laser therapy given alternately at regular intervals for a period of 15 months until his death from cardiovascular disease. Hemorrhage may be controlled for short periods (10,29), but bleeding may recur unless the entire tumor can be removed (29). Follow-up treatments may be necessary in that case. Tumor bulk can be reduced in patients with advanced colorectal cancer, but such patients usually survive only 2 to 5 months (29).

The potential for cure with laser therapy in some patients with early colorectal cancer seems promising (Figs. 7a and 7b). Short-term cures, as evidenced by the observation of complete healing on endoscopic examination, have been achieved in 12 of 13 patients with small (less than 4 cm in diameter) adenocar-

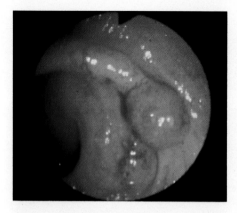

Fig. 7a. Endoscopic appearance of early adenocarcinoma of the rectum before laser photocoagulation.

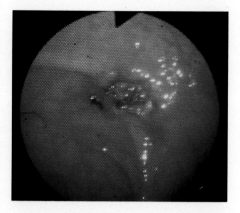

Fig. 7b. The lesion shown in Figure 7a immediately after Nd:YAG laser photocoagulation.

cinomas and in four of 32 patients with large (greater than 4 cm) adenocarcinomas of the colon (15). These investigators have reported cures for 35 of 39 villous adenomas after Nd:YAG laser therapy; 12 of the 35 tumors were malignant (15). At the University of Utah, three patients with early rectal adenocarcinoma have been treated, and the tumors appear to have been completely obliterated. Two of these patients died of unrelated causes 2 and 4 months after laser therapy had been completed. The third patient, a 90-year-old man, has survived without evidence of cancer for 18 months after the Nd:YAG treatments were completed (Figs. 8a to 8d). Harada and associates (43) have re-

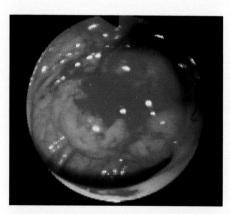

Fig. 8a. Endoscopic appearance of a multilobulated, polypoid adenocarcinoma of the rectum in a 90-year-old man before treatment.

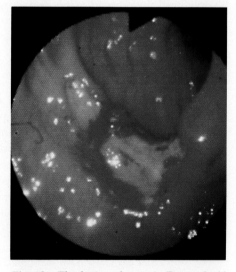

Fig. 8b. The lesion shown in Figure 8a 11 days after partial removal with an electrocautery snare.

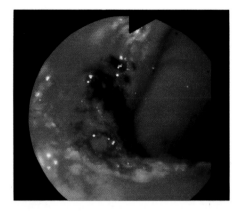

Fig. 8c. The lesion shown in Figures 8a and 8b immediately after Nd:YAG laser photocoagulation.

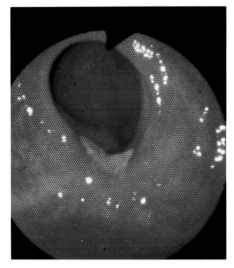

Fig. 8d. The lesion shown in Figures 8a to 8c 1 month after Nd:YAG laser photocoagulation. The treatment site has nearly healed, and mild rectal stenosis is evident. During the ensuing 18 months, the patient has remained free of tumor, and complete healing has occurred.

ported cures in two patients with early rectal carcinomas after Nd:YAG laser therapy; the results of these investigators, however, are preliminary.

Serious complications are uncommon, occurring in less than 5% of patients. Although perforation can be dangerous, it has been managed conservatively, with good results (15). Nonetheless, it seems likely that in some patients, this complication might necessitate surgical exclusion of the affected bowel segment. Rectal stenosis, due to submucosal fibrosis, has occurred after extensive treatment of circumferential tumors (10). Surgical relief from laser-induced stenosis is not necessary unless symptomatic obstruction occurs. Minor complications, such as fever, proctalgia and minor bleeding, occur but usually are of no clinical consequence.

SUMMARY

Laser photocoagulation therapy for enteric neoplasms is an embryonic field. The exact circumstances in which laser therapy might be preferred to surgical intervention remain to be clarified. However, promising short-term results have been obtained in the management of early gastric and colonic cancers. Complete removal of many rectal villous adenomas can be achieved. Nonetheless, laser therapy is now best regarded as a palliative, or noncurative, measure because removal of regional lymph node metastases is not possible by endoscopic means alone. Patients with advanced gastrointestinal cancer may benefit from palliative laser therapy when local complications occur. Obstruction and, to a lesser extent, bleeding are the major indications for palliative laser therapy. The depth of tissue damage is precise, a factor that allows safe transluminal treatment of local complications. The recovery period after successful laser therapy is short as compared to the recovery period after surgical intervention. This is an important advantage for persons with limited life expectancies. New technical advances in phototherapy are forthcoming. The most notable is photosensitization of tumors with such compounds as hematoporphyrin derivative. This approach may allow selective removal of cancer cells without damage to adjacent normal tissue. Although laser therapy may not replace surgical intervention for the management of gastrointestinal neoplasms, it may well be the treatment of choice in selected patients.

REFERENCES

1. Kelly DF, Bown SG, Salmon PR, et al: The nature and extent of biological changes induced by argon laser photocoagulation in canine gastric mucosa. *Gut* 21:1047–1055, 1980.

2. Bown SG, Salmon PR, Storey DW, et al: Nd:YAG laser photocoagulation in the dog stomach. *Gut* 21:818–825, 1980.

3. Piercey JRA, Auth DC, Silverstein FE, et al: Electrosurgical treatment of experimental bleeding canine gastric ulcers: Development and testing of a computer control and a better electrode. *Gastroenterology* 74:527–534, 1978.

4. Dixon JA, Burt RW, Rotering RH, et al: Endoscopic argon laser photocoagulation of sessile colonic polyps. *Gastrointest Endosc* 28:162–165, 1982.

5. Protell RL, Silverstein FE, Auth DC, et al: The Nd:YAG is dangerous for photocoagulation of experimental bleeding gastric ulcers when compared to argon laser. (abstract) *Gastroenterology* 74:1080, 1978.

6. Dixon JA, Berenson MM, McCloskey DW: Neodymium-YAG laser treatment of experimental canine gastric bleeding. Acute and chronic studies of photocoagulation, penetration and perforation. *Gastroenterology* 77:647–651, 1979.

7. Welch CE: Polyps and cancer of the colon. *Am J Surg* 138:625–626, 1979.

8. Day DW, Morson BC: The adenoma-carcinoma sequence, in Bennington JL (ed): *The Pathogenesis of Colorectal Cancer.* Philadelphia, Saunders, 1978, pp 58–71.

9. Bowers JH: Laser therapy of colonic neoplasms, in Fleischer D, Jensen D, Bright-Asare P (eds): *Therapeutic Laser Endoscopy in Gastrointestinal Disease.* Boston, Martinus Nijhoff, 1983, pp 139–150.

10. Brunetaud JM, Mosquet L, Bourez J, et al: Laser applications in nonhemorrhagic digestive lesions, In Atsumi K (ed): *New Frontiers in Laser Medicine and Surgery.* Amsterdam, Excerpta Medica, 1983, pp 455–461.

11. Mizushima K, Namiki M, Harada K, et al: Endoscopic laser therapy of gastric cancer

and polyps, in Atsumi K (ed): *New Frontiers in Laser Medicine and Surgery.* Amsterdam, Excerpta Medica, 1983, pp 470–478.

12. Sasako M, Iwasaki M, Konishi T, et al: Clinical application of the Nd:YAG laser endoscopy. *Lasers Surg Med* 2:137–147, 1982.

13. Iwasaki M, Sasako M, Konishi T, et al: Clinical application of the Nd:YAG laser endoscopy, in Atsumi K, Nimsakul M (eds): *Laser-Tokyo '81.* Tokyo, Japan Society for Laser Medicine, 1981, pp 5–14 to 5–17.

14. Tsujimura D, Masui H, Yamamoto H, et al: Safety and efficacy of Nd:YAG laser photocoagulation: Experimental and clinical studies, in Atsumi K, Nimsakul M (eds): *Laser-Tokyo '81.* Tokyo, Japan Society for Laser Medicine, 1981, pp 20–13 to 20–16.

15. Lambert R, Sabben G: Laser therapy in colorectal tumors: Early results. (abstract) *Gastroenterology* 84:1223, 1983.

16. Kiefhaber P, Kiefhaber K: Present endoscopic laser therapy in the gastrointestinal tract, in Atsumi K (ed): *New Frontiers in Laser Medicine and Surgery.* Amsterdam, Excerpta Medica, 1983, pp 439–446.

17. Bussey HJR: Polyposis syndromes, in Bennington JL (ed): *The Pathogenesis of Colorectal Cancer.* Philadelphia, Saunders, 1978, pp 81–94.

18. Spinelli P, Pizetti P, Mirabile V, et al: Neodymium-YAG laser treatment of the rectal remnant after colectomy for familial polyposis, in Atsumi K, Nimsakul M (eds): *Laser-Tokyo '81.* Tokyo, Japan Society for Laser Medicine, 1981, pp 23–49 to 23–50.

19. Kozarek RA, Earnest DL, Silverstein ME, et al: Air-pressure-induced colon injury during diagnostic colonoscopy. *Gastroenterology* 78:7–14, 1980.

20. Bown SG, Coleridge-Smith PD, Mills TN, et al: Interstitial treatment of tumours with the Nd:YAG laser. (abstract) *Lasers Surg Med* 3:137–138, 1983.

21. Dougherty TJ, Boyle DG, Weishaupt KR, et al: Photoradiation therapy of malignant tumors, in Atsumi K (ed): *New Frontiers in Laser Medicine and Surgery.* Amsterdam, Excerpta Medica, 1983, pp 161–165.

22. Wile AG, Dahlman A, Burns RG, et al: Laser photoradiation therapy of cancer following hematoporphyrin sensitization. *Lasers Surg Med* 2:163–168, 1982.

23. Fleischer D, Bown SG: Endoscopic laser therapy of upper gastrointestinal carcinomas, in Fleischer D, Jensen D, Bright-Asare P (eds): *Therapeutic Laser Endoscopy in Gastrointestinal Disease.* Boston, Martinus Nijhoff, 1983, pp 117–137.

24. Casey KR, Fairfax WR, Smith SJ, et al: Intratracheal fire ignited by the Nd:YAG laser during treatment of tracheal stenosis. *Chest* 84:295–296, 1983.

25. Pope CE II: Tumors (of the esophagus), in Sleisenger MH, Fordtran JS (eds): *Gastrointestinal Disease.* Philadelphia, Saunders, 1983, pp 479–490.

26. Lowe WC: Survival with carcinoma of the esophagus. *Ann Intern Med* 77:915–918, 1972.

27. Fleischer D, Kessler F: Endoscopic Nd:YAG laser therapy for carcinoma of the esophagus: A new form of palliative treatment. *Gastroenterology* 85:600–606, 1983.

28. Kiefhaber P, Kiefhaber K, Huber F, et al: Tumour irradiation by Nd:YAG laser of stenosing carcinomas and neoplastic polyps in the upper and lower gastrointestinal tract. (abstract) *Lasers Surg Med* 3:137, 1983.

29. Bowers JH, Dixon JA: Laser palliation of gastrointestinal cancers. (abstract) *Lasers Surg Med* 3:138, 1983.

30. Davis GR: Neoplasms of the stomach, in Sleisenger MH, Fordtran JS (eds): *Gastrointestinal Disease*. Philadelphia, Saunders, 1983, pp 578–601.

31. Takemoto T, Oshita Y, Ariyama S, et al: Laser endoscopy, treatment for G-I bleeding and early gastric carcinoma, in Atsumi K (ed): *New Frontiers in Laser Medicine and Surgery*. Amsterdam, Excerpta Medica, 1983, pp 462–469.

32. Ito Y, Sigiura H, Kano T, et al: Endoscopic laser treatment of borderline lesions and early gastric carcinomas, in Atsumi K, Nimsakul M (eds): *Laser-Tokyo '81*. Tokyo, Japan Society for Laser Medicine, 1981, pp 20–10 to 20–12.

33. Imaoka W, Okuda J, Ida K, et al: Treatment of digestive tract tumor with laser endoscopy—Experimental and clinical studies, in Atsumi K, Nimsakul M (eds): *Laser-Tokyo '81*. Tokyo, Japan Society for Laser Medicine, 1981, pp 5–7 to 5–10.

34. Sakita T, Koyama S, Ishii M, et al: Early cancer of the stomach treated successfully with an endoscopic Neodymium-YAG laser. *Am J Gastroenterol* 76:441–445, 1981.

35. Ichikawa T, Nakasawa S, Ema Y: Effects of Nd:YAG laser irradiation on gastric cancers, including histology, in Atsumi K, Nimsakul M (eds): *Laser-Tokyo '81*. Tokyo, Japan Society for Laser Medicine, 1981, pp 5–18 to 5–21.

36. Rösch W, Frühmorgen P: Endoscopic treatment of precancers and early gastric carcinoma. *Endoscopy* 12:109–113, 1980.

37. Fukutomi H, Kawakita I, Nakahara A, et al: Endoscopic diagnosis and treatment of gastric cancer by laser beam, in Atsumi K, Nimsakul M (eds): *Laser-Tokyo '81*. Tokyo, Japan Society for Laser Medicine, 1981, pp 20–16 to 20–28.

38. Winawer SJ, Sherlock P: Malignant neoplasms of the small and large intestine, in Sleisenger MH, Fordtran JS (eds): *Gastrointestinal Disease*. Philadelphia, Saunders, 1983, pp 1220–1249.

39. Crile G, Turnbull RB: The role of electrocoagulation in the treatment of carcinoma of the rectum. *Surg Gynecol Obstet* 135:391–396, 1972.

40. Eisenstat TE, Deak ST, Rubin RJ, et al: Five year survival in patients with carcinoma of the rectum treated by electrocoagulation. *Am J Surg* 143:127–132, 1982.

41. Ishii W, Kawai K, Matai K, et al: CO_2 laser surgery applied for anorectal diseases and its clinical assessment. Use of newly developed optic fiber waveguide, in Atsumi K, Nimsakul M (eds): *Laser-Tokyo '81*. Tokyo, Japan Society for Laser Medicine, 1981, pp 23–47 to 23–48.

42. Giler S, Ben Bassat M, Taube E, et al: The use of the CO_2 laser in palliative surgery for cancer, in Atsumi K, Nimsakul M (eds): *Laser-Tokyo '81*. Tokyo, Japan Society for Laser Medicine, 1981, pp 23–12 to 23–15.

43. Harada K, Mizushima K, Namiki M, et al: Endoscopic YAG laser treatment of lesions in the distal colon with experimental studies. (abstract) in Atsumi K, Nimsakul M (eds): *Laser-Tokyo '81*. Tokyo, Japan Society for Laser Medicine, 1981, p 20–32.

Index

Chandresh Saraiya
- 312-430-7224.

- K. C. JHAH.
  ↳ 818-445-7333
  ↳ Arcadia.